PRINCIPLES OF PHARMACOLOGY:
A tropical approach

Principles of Pharmacology:
A tropical approach

D. T. OKPAKO
Department of Pharmacology & Therapeutics, College of Medicine, University of Ibadan, Nigeria

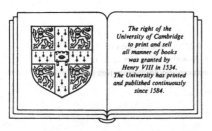

. *The right of the University of Cambridge to print and sell all manner of books was granted by Henry VIII in 1534. The University has printed and published continuously since 1584.*

CAMBRIDGE UNIVERSITY PRESS
Cambridge

New York   Port Chester

Melbourne   Sydney

CAMBRIDGE UNIVERSITY PRESS
Cambridge, New York, Melbourne, Madrid, Cape Town, Singapore,
São Paulo, Delhi, Dubai, Tokyo

Cambridge University Press
The Edinburgh Building, Cambridge CB2 8RU, UK

Published in the United States of America by Cambridge University Press, New York

www.cambridge.org
Information on this title: www.cambridge.org/9780521121569

First published 1991
This digitally printed version 2009

A catalogue record for this publication is available from the British Library

Library of Congress Cataloguing in Publication data
Okpako, D.T.
Principles of pharmacology: a tropical approach/D.T. Okpako.
  p. cm
Includes bibliographies and index.
ISBN 0-521-34095-0
1. Pharmacology. I. Title
(DNLM: 1. Drug Therapy. 2. Pharmacology. 3. Tropical Medicine.
WB 330 (O41p)
RM300.036 1989
615'.1'0913—dc20 89-9866 CIP

ISBN 978-0-521-34095-3 Hardback
ISBN 978-0-521-12156-9 Paperback

To four lovely people:
Obien, Gweneth, Branwen and Edore.

Contents

and toxicology) in which pharmacology is a major subject, Part VI consisting of 10 chapters is devoted to systematic pharmacology. These cover the principles of drug action in major organs and systems in the body.

Some of the subjects dealt with in the early chapters have been put together as a student text for the first time. I hope that the availability of the material in this form should help to give the pharmacology curriculum in the tropics a better orientation. I have written this book with people in the tropics in mind, but I hope that 'Western' readers will also find my approach interesting.

D.T. Okpako

ACKNOWLEDGEMENTS

I wish to acknowledge with thanks the various authors and publishers who have kindly permitted reproduction of data from published work. These are:

The C. V. Mosby Company, the Publisher of *Journal of Paediatrics*. The Physiological Society, Elsevier Science Publishers B.V. (Biomedical Division) Amsterdam, Raven Press Publishers/New York; British Medical Bulletin; Macmillan Press Ltd.; Professor L. A. Salako, Professor A. W. Cuthbert, Professor John Barrett, Professor Lucio Luzzatto.

In writing this book, I have received help and encouragement from a large number of people. I wish to express my gratitude to all of them and in particular the following:

Students and colleagues in the Department of Pharmacology and Therapeutics, University of Ibadan for allowing me a Sabbatical to write this book, and for helping to refine some of the views expressed therein; The Master and Fellows of Corpus Christi College Cambridge for electing me Senior Research Scholar in the 1983/84 session and for providing wonderful hospitality and a research grant, which enabled me to read for this book; Professor A. W. Cuthbert, FRS, Fellow of Jesus College, Cambridge and his staff at the Department of Pharmacology, University of Cambridge, for putting at my disposal the excellent facilities of the Department during the 1983/84 session when I was accepted there as Visiting Scientist; The British Council for the award of a Senior Fellowship. I wish to express my sincere thanks to the following for critical review of initial drafts of several chapters: Dr B. A. Callingham, Professor Dinah M. James, Professor Lucio Luzzatto; Dr S. O. Fagbemi, Department of Pharmacology & Therapeutics, and Dr E. U. Nduka, Postgraduate Institute for Medical Research and

Training, University of Ibadan for assistance with the preparation of Chapters 21 and 23 respectively. I thank Dr Joyce Lowe, for assistance with the botanical names of the plants mentioned in the text and for reading the entire book in proof. All persisting errors of omission and commission are however entirely mine. I am grateful to the following for typing various drafts of the manuscript: Helen Gibson, Rufus Owoyokun, Agnes Adesuyi, Titus Shipe, and most of all, Johnson Akinlade.

Without the hard work and encouragement of the editors, Fay Bendall and Peter Silver this book would never have seen the light of day.

PART I

General Background to Drug Usage in the Tropics

1

Traditional medicine

1.1 INTRODUCTION

Modern medicine is based on scientific principles. Its practice therefore demands a degree of rationalisation on the part of both physician and patient. The physician makes a diagnosis after a systematic analysis of symptoms, and for the treatment to be optimally effective, the patient must understand the reasons for the prescription and cooperate with the physician by complying with the latter's instructions. In Africa and many third world countries, this form of medicine exists alongside traditional forms whose practice is based on what are described as 'irrational animistic beliefs'. Many patients come to the modern doctor after being treated by the traditional healer and many return there if they are not satisfied with the scientific method. We therefore have a situation in which modern medicine is being practised by people who hold strong traditional beliefs about disease, its cause and its treatment. Some of these beliefs conflict with the principles upon which the practice of modern medicine is based.

The purpose of this chapter therefore is to consider the impact of traditional medical beliefs on the outcome of modern drug therapy. Traditional African Medicine (TAM) will be used as the basis of the discussion and the following points will be raised:

    (i) What are the theories of causation of disease in African traditional medical systems?

    (ii) Are there elements in traditional beliefs which may adversely affect the individual's attitude to modern drug treatment?

    (iii) What is the theoretical basis for the use of plant parts in traditional African medicine and are we justified in expecting that herbal remedies used by traditional healers will yield 'drugs' on scientific analysis?

3

Such a discussion forms an appropriate background against which drug action and drug use in the tropics can be discussed.

There are other reasons for including a chapter on traditional medicine in this book. Firstly, although modern medicine has made and continues to make great advances, man's desire to have an effective cure for every conceivable ill is far from being satisfied. Therefore, everywhere, attention is being drawn to the possibility of finding cures in alternative medical systems. The importance of testing alternative approaches is underlined by the fact, for example, that acupuncture, a traditional form of treatment in ancient China, has proved to be of value and is being increasingly incorporated into modern medical practice; useful drugs have been developed from plants originally employed by traditional healers. Facts such as these lead scientists to expect that other spectacular discoveries can be made through a critical evaluation of traditional medicine. Secondly, many African countries find the idea of research into traditional medicine attractive. For it embodies the hope that traditional medicine can supplement or even replace the orthodox form of health care which these countries are unable to provide adequately. It is also a basis for the preservation of a heritage which was scorned by European colonialists and is now in danger of being obliterated by modern medicine.

Attempts are presently being made to introduce the subject of traditional medicine into medical and pharmacy syllabuses in some African Universities. Continuous critical analysis of different aspects of traditional medicine is necessary for it to become a serious subject of academic study. This chapter is meant to represent one approach. In conformity with the rest of the book an attempt is made to evaluate the theoretical basis of traditional African medical practice. Detailed clinical procedures are not described. Such information may be found in recent books some of which are listed at the end of the chapter. In discussing this vast subject, I have deliberately been dogmatic with some statements in order to provide a firm basis for discussion. Thus here and there it may appear that I have overlooked crucial examples which represent an opposing point of view.

The discussion is based on traditional African medicine (TAM), but readers from other third world countries should find that the problem of a potential or real conflict between traditional and orthodox medicine is of general interest. The reader ought to be aware too that other well known alternative systems of medicine exist which are not discussed in this chapter. Examples are Homeopathy, Christian Science, Osteophathy, Chiropractic. The principles upon which all these systems are based often conflict with those of scientific medicine. That these alternative systems continue to flourish in spite of being 'irrational', is evidence that faith and suggestion play significant roles in healing.

There is one more apology to make. The term *herbal remedies* as used in this chapter, refers to preparations prescribed by qualified traditional physicians in the treatment of serious illness. There are several popular folk remedies used extensively in Nigeria for the treatment of fevers or other minor ailments, as it were, without the doctor's prescription or divination. Such popular remedies e.g. dongo yaro (*Azadirachta indica*) or mango bark (*Mangifera indica*) are used entirely for their physical effects and are not usually major components of the traditional healers' armamentarium.

1.2.   TRADITIONAL AFRICAN MEDICINE
Definitions

Traditional medicine is defined by the World Health Organisation (WHO, 1976) as the sum total of all knowledge and practices whether explicable or not, used in diagnosis, prevention and elimination of physical, mental or social imbalance and relying exclusively on practical experience and observations handed down from generation to generation whether verbally or in writing.

The following elements embodied in the above general definition apply to traditional African medicine:

(a) *Unwritten knowledge.* The body of knowledge pertaining to traditional African medicine is largely unwritten. Until recently, most of its practitioners were illiterate and the ideas upon which its practice is based have never been subjected to systematic critical evaluation. The only available records have been derived largely from observations made on contemporary practitioners of the art by outsiders. In contrast, the traditional medical systems of India (Ayurveda, Siddha and Unani) and of China have literatures going back for several centuries.

(b) *Empiricism.* The system is not based on any recognised scientific framework, but rather on the accumulated experience of what has proved effective. Empirical knowledge thus derived has been handed down from generation to generation through apprenticeship or family lineage.

(c) *The role of supernatural forces.* The practice of traditional African medicine assumes the existence and participation of supernatural forces – gods, spirits etc. – in the causation of disease or other human misfortune. The system has therefore been described as *non-scientific* in the sense in which epistemologists such as Karl Popper would use the word. According to this usage, a body of knowledge is scientific only if its composite parts (hypothesis/propositions) are capable of being verified. The proposition must contain assertions which if disproved experimentally should lead to a rejection or modification of the proposition. The idea that supernatural forces are involved in the causation of disease cannot be experimentally verified. Therefore aspects of traditional medicine which assume participation of such forces are regarded as non-scientific.

Theories of the causation of disease in TAM
In African thought all living things, including man, are united with one another and with the gods and ancestral spirits, through vital forces which each generates. A state of health exists when there is perfect harmony between man and his total environment. On the other hand, ill-health and other misfortunes can result from a disturbance in harmony in the relationship between man and his social and spiritual environment, or from forces directed at him by witches, evil spirits or offended ancestral spirits. This is the reason why divination, ritualistic sacrifices, incantations, and potions made from animal and or plant parts are essential components of traditional medical treatment. These are meant to re-establish the patient's harmony with his environment and/or counteract the influence of evil spirits. This may be compared with the Homeopathic concept of pathology, namely that the body is controlled by vital forces and

> any disturbance of this vital energy or forces results in a disfigured or disturbed development of the whole human economy . . . That brings us to the point of looking upon disease as a dynamic expression of the disturbance of the harmony and rhythm of the vital energy. (A.H. Roberts cited by Burn, 1948).

Similarities in the concept of disease causation in different African societies
The belief that supernatural forces and disturbances of harmonious relationships can be the cause of disease is widespread in most traditional African societies. This is despite differences in language and other aspects of culture. This universal acceptance of supernatural forces as a cause of illness constitutes justification for the use of the expression *traditional African medicine*. Observations made in

different parts of the African continent show this. Lambo (1969) who has studied the traditional medical systems of the Yorubas extensively observes that to the African

> 'reality consists in the relation not of man with things but of man with man and of all with the spirits'.

Among the Ndembu people of Zambia, the Tivs of Northern Nigeria and the Urhobos of Southern Nigeria, it is believed that a seriously ill patient will not recover until all tensions and aggressions in the community's inter-relations have been brought to light and exposed to ritual treatment. In serious illness, one of the first things the traditional healer does is to extract confessions of wrong doings from the patient. In the case of a child, the mother in particular must seriously examine her previous moral conduct since it is believed that offended ancestral spirits can visit the sins of the mother on her child. It is the responsibility of the traditional physician to determine appropriate ritual sacrifice and to which god or spirits it should be made. Confessions are believed to be both healing and prophylactic. From Angola, Burkina Faso, Ghana and Nigeria to Zaire and Zambia, divination in some form is employed in diagnosis of illness, death or other misfortune. Even the essential features of divination (throwing a number of objects e.g. cowries, cola nuts, and interpreting events from their pattern of fall) are similar.

Primary and secondary elements in disease causation

From the foregoing, it can be said that in TAM serious illness results from a primary supernatural cause. The symptoms are secondary. The traditional practitioner can accept a diagnosis that the symptoms of an illness are due to malaria or salmonella infection, cancer, or high blood pressure. But he would ask 'who put the disease in the victim? or why should the particular victim suffer from the disease rather than someone else? People do not just suffer serious illness by chance'. The presence of the disease is believed to be due to the operation of supernatural forces – the primary cause.

Treatment often concentrates on the primary cause by the application of suitable rituals, but treatment may also be directed at the symptoms (see Fig. 1.1). The well known Nigerian herbalist Apata (1979) implies a dual conception of disease when he states that herbal remedies are used for:

(a) Real treatment and
(b) Psychological treatment.

Real treatment is for those who require no incantations or other ceremonies. Psychological treatment is for those who do require incantations and other ceremonies such as sacrifices before the medicine can act. Both are inextricably tied, since we require the services of the two together to cure the two aspects of sickness.

In modern medicine, disease is caused by a malfunction which can be identified by diagnosis. The disease is treated by correcting the malfunction, for instance, by drug therapy. The drug used is chosen for its known, clearly defined physicochemical and pharmacological properties. The modern approach is said to be *materialistic* whereas the traditional approach is *spiritual* and *holistic*. The spiritual emphasis in TAM can be rationalised in scientific terms by saying that stress, caused by a breakdown in relationships with neighbours, sins against the gods and lore of the community, and feelings of guilt can cause diseases by damaging the cardiovascular system or by lowering the body's defences. Modern medicine increasingly recognises the contribution

Fig. 1.1. *Factors affecting the health of the traditional African.* In traditional medical belief systems, the primary cause of disease is attributed to supernatural agencies such as witchcraft and ancestral spirit anger. Treatment is directed at the primary cause as well as the disease itself (arrows with black shaft). In modern medicine, treatment is directed at the disease (arrow with unshaded shaft).

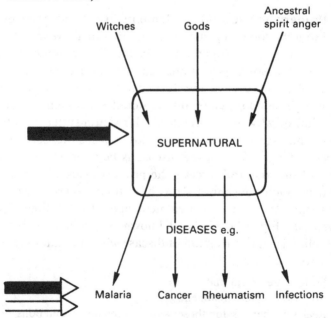

of psychosomatic factors to ill-health.The well known placebo effects of inert substances in bringing relief in certain disease conditions is evidence that faith and suggestion can play a part in healing even in modern medicine. A recent study showed that the placebo effect is as high as 60% in peptic ulcer in some countries. Possibly, this aspect does not receive enough attention in modern medicine, and it could be that it is in this respect that modern medicine may benefit from the accumulated wisdom of traditional African medicine.

The role of herbs in TAM

Traditional healers use herbal preparations as part of their regimen to prevent or cure disease. These preparations consist mainly of parts of plants – roots, leaves, bark etc. – although some concoctions may also contain animal tissues. This is the part of TAM that is most amenable to rational scientific analysis; research into traditional medicine usually refers to analysis of herbal remedies.

However, the scientists' assumption that herbs in TAM serve the same purpose as drugs do in modern medicine is an over-simplification. For there is ample evidence that traditional physicians use herbal remedies not necessarily for the pharmacological action of their chemical constituents, but for their power to restore health by operating as agents of supernatural forces.

Some observations support this view:

(1) The vital force in plants

The use of plants in the treatment of disease derives from the basic idea that all living things generate vital forces which can be harnessed to advantage by those who know how. The traditional physician is almost always both diviner and herbalist. He knows not only how to prepare mixtures, he must also be able to administer them with the appropriate incantation without which the medicine would be ineffective. The incantation and other rituals (these may also accompany the collection of the plant to be used in the preparation of the remedy) are meant to release the vital energy contained in the plant for the benefit of the patient. These ideas are not fundamentally different from those of ancient European physicians (e.g. Galen and Dioscorides) who believed that

> there were four constituent elements in the body – the hot, the cold, the wet and the dry and that in a healthy body all were in balance . . . the function of a medicinal plant (in the treatment of disease) was simply to restore this balance . . . (Shellard, 1979).

(2) Absence of a system of dosage

None of the studies of traditional practice carried out in different parts of Africa has revealed an indegenous system of dosage. Osuntokun (1975) observed that one characteristic feature of the Yoruba pharmacopoeia is the absence of dosage. Dosage is not just a matter of how much of the concoction the patient must take. Dosage determination begins with knowing the *weight* of plant material and *volume* of liquid used in making the mixutre. Now, there are no indigenous systems of weights and measures or precise time consciousness in most African traditional cultures. It is therefore not surprising that precise dosage is not a feature of traditional African medicine nor indeed is it of other activities such as cookery in which fairly precise measurements may be indicated. Accurate dosage is critically important in modern drug therapy because we know that a drug is worthless if too little is taken, effective at the right dosage and harmful if too much is taken. Therefore, not only must the optimum dosage be determined for individual drugs, it is also crucially important for the patient to adhere strictly to the dosage schedule. In TAM, the efficacy of the herbal remedy is not perceived in physical terms and toxicity resulting from traditional medicine appears not to be a complication as it is known in modern medicine.

(3) Methods of application

In modern medicine the drug is applied topically, rectally, parenterally, orally, sublingually or by inhalation. The choice is governed by considerations such as the property of the drug, the site of the ailment etc. (see Chapter 3). In traditional African medicine, the oral and topical routes are also commonly used, so is inhalation; sometimes the physician makes scarifications on the skin in an appropriate area and rubs in the medication. However, frequently, the herbal remedy prepared to cure or prevent an internal ailment is neither taken internally nor even applied topically. The ingredients can be mixed, encapsulated and worn as amulet, necklace or around the waist or ankle. For instance, to make child delivery easy, the remedy prescribed by a traditional healer highly respected for his successes in an Urhobo community consists of a band which the pregnant woman must wear round the waist. In some cases, the preparation may not even come into contact with the patient at all. It is believed that the remedy can be just as effective if placed across the lintel above the door, or under the pillow or sleeping mat.

It is thus clear that in traditional usage the herb is perceived to have powers beyond those which are due to its chemical constituents.

(4) The choice of plants to be used as remedy in TAM

It is often stated that the traditional pharmacopeia of remedies in TAM has been arrived at by trial and error. It is not easy to argue against this. On the other hand there is not much evidence that the selection of herbal remedies was preceded by any form of therapeutic trials. Rather, there is evidence that remedies might have been selected on the principle that the plant or animal part bore some resemblance to the condition to be treated. Thus *Rauvolfia serpentina*, a climbing plant with a strong resemblance to a snake was used by Indian traditional healers to treat snake-bite; preparations made from rhinoceros horn have a reputation for strengthening male erection and are employed as male aphrodisiacs. Similar principles which govern the choice of particular plants in the preparation of medicines among the Ndembu have been enumerated by Turner (1981) as follows:

> trees from which bark rope or bark string can be made are never used in ritual to make women fertile, as these would tie up their (the women's) fertility. Many of the trees used . . . had many fruits . . . the doctors trusted that the patient would have many children. Other trees had honey-filled flowers attractive to bees. By using them, the doctors hoped to attract many children to the patient . . .

The general theory seems to be that the plant with healing powers is revealed to man by the supernatural through certain physical attributes of the plant. Some of these attributes (or signatures) may be quite subtle so that only experts (traditional healers) with appropriate knowledge can recognise them. This principle is similar to the Homeopathic 'principle of signatures', or *similia similibus curentur*, that is, similars should be cured by similars. The principle of signatures has no scientific basis but it is widespread in traditional medical systems. The Yoruba proverb which says 'it is a curse that we use in order to cure a curse' is an apt expression of the principle. It explains why red-coated ferrous gluconate tablets are more acceptable as 'blood tonic' than green-coated ferrous sulphate tablets.

Summary

So far we have attempted to articulate the characteristic features of traditional African medicine and have shown that the basis of the practice is both spiritual and physical. There is reason to believe that the role of herbs in TAM is esoteric and different from the role of drugs in modern medicine. In TAM herbs may exert beneficial effects by mechanisms other than those due to their content of pharmacologically active constituents. It may be concluded that the major beneficial effects of herbal remedies are placebo effects. This means that the whole treatment of which herbal remedies are only a part allows nature to heal. Such a conclusion is inevitable given the traditional theory of disease causation, the basic principles governing the selection of remedies and the methods of use of the remedies. However, this conclusion can be challenged by pointing out that some traditional remedies have turned out to contain chemical substances with pharmacological activities appropriate to their use in the traditional pharmacopoeia. An example is *Rauvolfia vomitoria* which Yoruba healers used for centuries in the treatment of psychosis and which turned out on scientific analysis to contain, *inter alia*, the alkaloid reserpine. Examples of this sort are so rare, however, that one suspects that the correlation between traditional medical usage and the occurrence of appropriate pharmacological activity might be insignificant. This issue is discussed in more detail later in this chapter.

The effects of traditional beliefs on the outcome of modern therapy

The patient who comes to the modern practitioner from a background of traditional African medical practice must be bewildered and confused by the strange environment in which the modern physician works and the whole approach to treatment which he encounters. Moreover, deep-rooted beliefs in the traditional method can adversely affect the way he responds to treatment. What the patient expects on the basis of his experience with traditional physicians, is not what he finds in the modern clinic. For example:

(1) Patients' expectation from the doctor

In TAM, the patient is accustomed to the physician knowing what has brought him to the clinic. Being in touch with the spirits of the ancestors and the gods, it is the physician who, through divination, tells the patient what his problem is. Osuntokun (1975), points out that when the peasant Yoruba patient approaches the modern doctor with the same expectations, he (the patient) is surprised that the doctor is *asking* him questions instead of *telling* him why he has come to the clinic. In such circumstances, the patient's confidence in the doctor, initially at least, is less than 100%.

(2) Patients' expectation from drugs

We have seen from the previous section that in TAM the primary cause of disease is attributed to the operation of supernatural forces, and that herbal remedies act in esoteric ways. Treatment is frequently aimed at the primary supernatural cause and since this can manifest in different disease forms, one remedy can be used to treat many different kinds of diseases. In fact the number of diseases which certain traditional herbal remedies are reputed to be able to cure is quite staggering. An interesting case in point is the plant *Zizyphus mauritania* which is reputed to cure such antithetic diseases as constipation, dysentery and diarrhoea. In contrast, the modern doctor may use many drugs to treat one ailment. He might treat pneumonia with penicillin or other antibiotic to which the causative organism is sensitive. He might also use an antipyretic drug to lower the body temperature and prescribe vitamins or iron. Sometimes the doctor's prescription may contain a drug whose purpose is to prevent the adverse effects of another drug in the prescription etc. All this is confusing to one brought up in the practice of traditional medicine and who is likely to regard each drug in a multiple prescription as equally important in serving one purpose, namely, to eliminate the disease.

The confusion which a misunderstanding by the patient can give rise to is illustrated by a personal experience with an elderly relation. On being discharged from Eku Baptist Hospital, Mr. O.A. was given five different types of drugs (tablets and capsules) in separate brown envelopes marked with instructions for use. When I arrived at the hospital to take the old man home, I found to my dismay that he had instructed his wife to discharge the contents of the envelopes into one large screw-capped plastic container – to protect the medicines from the rain. How would he take the medicines now that he had destroyed the doctor's instructions? I asked. He said he would take *some from time to time* when he did not feel well and it did not matter which he took and when, since he would eventually take them all. In any case, medicine is medicine and they are all going into the same place – his stomach.

Much can be learnt from this experience. The doctor had good reasons to prescribe five different drugs for the patient *after* he was well enough to be discharged. To his traditional patient, the reasons were not obvious. Even more confusing for the patient, was why he could not take the five medicines in the same way – one was to be taken 'one, three times a day', another 'one, four times a day', and another 'two at night' etc.

The lesson here is that (a) drugs for the traditional ambient patient should be as few as possible, and (b) instructions for their use must be as clear and as simple as possible, otherwise, not understanding or not remembering what he has been told, the patient is likely to take matters into his own hands in the light of his more extensive experience with traditional remedies.

This idea that *medicine is medicine* adversely affects the use of drugs in another way in a traditional community. The modern doctor usually prescribes, for example, a course of sixteen doses of an antibiotic in the treatment of a bacterial infection. It is quite common for the patient to stop taking the drug after the first few doses when he feels better. It is also common for him to dispense the remnants of his medicine to neighbours who are ill, no matter what from, with the result that pathogenic micro-organisms are repeatedly exposed to sublethal doses of antimicrobial agents with consequent development of resistance.

It is therefore clear that fundamental attitudes acquired in traditional medical practice can lead to the misuse of drugs, unless the physician and the pharmacist make the effort to educate the patient very carefully on how to use modern drugs.

(3) The patient expects the medicine to do good only

The idea that a drug can cure disease at a certain dose level and can be harmful at higher doses which is a crucially important principle in modern therapeutics is not widespread in TAM. Indeed, drug-induced toxicity would be inconceivable, in relation to some of the ways herbal remedies are used (p. 10). Generally, the medicine prescribed for the treatment of disease by the doctor is *good medicine*, as distinct from *bad medicine* which can be used to do harm. The attitude is that if the expected good does not materialise quickly, more of the medicine should be taken. Many patients in fact do the same with modern drugs. Since people are brought up to believe that remedies used to treat disease can only do good, violent toxic reactions to drugs such as diarrhoea and vomiting, or general malaise are sometimes viewed positively as signs that *the medicine is working* especially if the patient gets over the illness. Therefore the patient must be educated in the idea that the drug which can cure disease can also cause disease and possibly kill if taken incorrectly.

(4) The patient expects a quick response

In traditional practice, once the cause of illness has been identified and the appropriate rituals have been applied visible improvement usually follows medication in a matter of days. The course of recovery in modern medicine is less dramatic. A patient may have to take medication for long periods in, for instance, cases of leprosy, stroke, tuberculosis or for life in hypertension, diabetes. This is probably why many relatives switch the patient from hospital to traditional healer or why many patients abandon their prescriptions.

In summary, there are certain expectations among traditional patients accustomed to TAM which conflict with the scientific basis of modern medicine. Such conflict can adversely affect the individual's ability to benefit optimally from modern drug therapy. Unless these conflicts are recognised and catered for, they can lead to misuse and wastage of drugs. Some of the major differences between traditional African medicine and modern medicine, and the different expectations of the patient in both systems are summarised in Table 1.1.

On herbal remedies as sources of drugs

Many African governments and peoples and international funding agencies (e.g. Organisation of African Unity, World Health Organisation etc.) are convinced that research into traditional African medicine is worthwhile. The focus is on medicinal plants, the spiritual aspect being considered too esoteric for scientific study. Odelola (1979) the then Executive Secretary of the Scientific, Technical and Research Commission of the O.A.U., stated, in an address to a Pan African Conference on medicinal plants held in 1974 at Ife, that his organisation supported research in this field to ensure:

(a) the scientific exploration of African fauna and flora for the benefit of the peoples of Africa;
(b) *a diversification in the sources of our medicaments and a reduction in our dependence on importation of drugs* (my italics)
(c) the codification of oral tradition in Africa which at present is confused with our culture and religious rites.

Why has there been such high expectation that research into plants used in traditional medicine should yield drugs in sufficient quantity to reduce our dependence on drug importation?

The high expectation is based on the following reasoning:

The plants have been effective in traditional medicine. Therefore it should be a simple matter for pharmacologists, pharmacognosists and chemists to obtain information from traditional healers about their remedies and to extract the active principles for development into drugs.

One fact on which this reasoning rests is that some of the most potent drugs in use today were extracted from plants and several synthetic drugs are made from starting molecules extracted from plants. Up to 25% of all prescriptions in Europe and America, it is said, contain

Table 1.1   *Characteristic features of traditional and modern
medicine*

Characteristic features	Medical systems	
	Traditional	Modern
Primary cause of disease	supernatural	physical
Psychosomatic components of disease	important	relatively unimportant
Diagnosis of disease	by divination	by physical examination
Role of ritual incantations and sacrifice in cure	important	unimportant
Role of pharmacologically active ingredients in medication	relatively unimportant	important
Dosage of remedy	relatively unimportant	strictly regulated
Time interval between doses	not regulated	strictly regulated
Duration of treatment	normally relatively short	variable but can be for life
Side effects due to medication	unknown	important

plant products or were originally derived from them (Jaroszewski, 1984).

Two approaches are recommended for the exploitation of medicinal plants for drugs. One is to extract the active ingredients from the remedy, identify it chemically, establish its detailed pharmacology and make it into a drug for clinical trial and distribution. The other is to evaluate the herbal remedy as it is used by the traditional healer without purification. If it is found to be efficacious, then after further scientific studies on toxicity, dosage standardisation and clinical trials, the preparation can be included in the modern pharmacopoeia.

Why research into medicinal plants may not lead to the discovery of drugs

The idea of obtaining drugs from medicinal plants is so powerful and plants are so plentiful in the tropical rain forests that even very intelligent people in these countries believe that a handful of scientists should be able to make a tropical country self-sufficient in drugs.

The fact of the matter is that after several decades of research into medicinal plants, there is very little to show in the form of drugs. Failure can be explained by saying that the research efforts have not been sufficiently concerted and multidisciplinary and funding has not been adequate. But there is a more fundamental reason and that is that the high expectation is misplaced, being based on the assumption that the effectiveness of the traditional remedy is due to pharmacologically active ingredients in these plants. Modern scientists are entitled to assume that a plant remedy can be therapeutically effective only if it contains pharmacologically active ingredients. But we have to remember that the traditional physician makes no such assumptions in using plants and to expect drugs from his remedies would be to commit what some sociologists refer to as a fallacy of retrospective determinism, that is, the assigning of current values and patterns to past systems of thought. Traditional healers use herbs as part of a complex treatment schedule. The major component are the ritual sacrifices designed to harmonise the sick person with his total environment. The point being made here is that the use of a herb in traditional healing should not *ipso facto* suggest that the plant contains drugs and the acceptance of TAM should not be predicated on whether its herbal remedies possess appropriate pharmacological activities or not. After all, many people accept homeopathic medicine even though it cannot be proved *in the laboratory* that the potency of a drug increases with dilution. The scientist who approaches the problem of research into herbal remedies with narrow and overoptimistic expectations is likely to find (as many have found) that the traditional healers' remedy does not contain what he is looking for.

Inconsistency in plant use

To begin with, those who advocate that the traditional remedy is a potential source of drugs assume a certain degree of consistency in the use of a plant for the treatment of a given disease. This is not so in general. A traditional healer may be consistent in the use of a certain plant for a given disease condition and a number of herbalists in a community may recognise the same plant for certain qualities, but there is also evidence that even practitioners in the same district or village may use the same plant for completely unrelated purposes. A good example to illustrate this point is the medicinal use of the plant *Crotalaria retusa*, known in Yoruba as Koropo. Maclean (1971), in a survey of 100 herbalists practising in a district of the city of Ibadan asked what the plant was used for.

> Some seemed to prescribe it primarily as an analgesic for rubbing on swollen joints, or any painful area; there were numerous advocates

for its use for eye trouble, for dysentery and for applying to the swollen
breasts of pregnant women, . . . it was regarded by some as aid to conception, being said to retain sperm in the vagina, . . . it was reputed to
bring on labour when this was overdue.

Other herbalists were more esoteric and thought that *Koropo*

would persuade an *abiku** child to stay; . . . induce a divorced wife to
return to her husand; guard a house and its occupants against dangerous medicines; or . . . assist in the arrest of evil doers and lunatics.

One herbalist considered it a

. . . valuable aid to school children's memory when taken along with
fish.

Poisonous plants

There are a number of other reasons why one should not
expect herbal remedies to contain potent chemicals, which drugs are.
Unless they are used within certain well controlled dosage limits, drugs
are poisons. In the evolution of the traditional pharmacopoeia, and in
the absence of accurate dosage systems, plants containing potent
chemicals and therefore giving rise to toxic effects would have been
eliminated. Many *Strophanthus* species containing cardiac glycosides
grow in West Africa. Traditional healers tend to avoid them because
they know these plants to be toxic. In fact, Bambara Sorcerers of Mali
use *Strophanthus* seeds in the preparation of poisonous potions (See
Imperato, 1977). It is also the case that many plants, fruits and seeds
used in the treatment of disease are edible – foods and spices. It is not
surprising that herbalists might go for fairly innocuous plants knowing
that the efficacy of their treatment comes at least partly from supernatural intervention.

There is one more point to make on this issue. The fact that many
drugs were originally extracted from plants is used to urge research
into medicinal plants. But many such drugs were obtained from plants
which were known to be poisonous – fish poisons, arrow poisons,
ordeal poisons, poisonous mushrooms etc., and were avoided by traditional healers (see Table 1.2). Possibly, a majority of the plants from
which useful drugs have been obtained were never used as traditional
therapeutic remedies at all. Indeed our search for drugs among plants
might be more successful, if, instead of traditional herbal remedies, we
focused on plants deliberately avoided by traditional healers. The
point being made is that if we select a plant for scientific investigation

*Abiku: a 'spirit' child believed to be fated to a cycle of early death and rebirth to the
same woman.

because it is claimed to be an effective traditional remedy, we should still approach the work with the same care, seriousness and even skepticism as we would if we selected the plant on a different basis and our expectations should be no less realistic.

How to choose plants for investigation

The plant kingdom is a rich source of potential drugs. But with over 250,000 species of higher plants to choose from, it is important to determine some rational basis for the selection of plants for investigation. Four selection procedures can be roughly identified, namely:

Selection based on traditional medical usage

We have seen that the fact of a plant being part of a traditional treatment regimen is not sufficient ground to expect it to contain potential drugs. Nevertheless, usage over many generations in TAM should be one criterion for selecting a plant for investigation. There are a number of reasons for this:

(a) There is the probability that the plant contains active principles with biological activity appropriate to its use in TAM. There is no contradiction between this statement and what went on before; one is simply saying that everything considered, the probability of discovering useful drugs through this approach is not necessarily better than other approaches. But the possibility is there and is underlined by discoveries of quinine from *cinchona*, reserpine from *Rauvolfia* and quinghaosu from *Quinghao*, etc.

(b) If a given plant has been taken as medicine for generations, it is reasonable to assume that its constituents are not toxic, at least in the form in which the preparation is used in TAM. Therefore if a drug is derived from such a plant, it is likely to be safe. This reasoning can break down when pure constituents are isolated from the plant as the example *Oldenlandia affinis* has shown. In Zaire, aqueous extracts of this Rubiaceous plant are drunk by women just prior to child birth to bring about easy delivery. Danish scientists attempted to isolate active principles which might explain the beneficial effect of this plant in women. In doing so they isolated a number of oxytocic polypeptides, one of them being extremely potent. *In vivo* however, this polypeptide was found to be cardiotoxic at a dosage several times lower than that at which it was oxytocic; so clinical trials were abandoned.

(c) The plant may contain active principles which are useful for the treatment of diseases other than the one for which it was used by traditional healers. A well known example of this is the Rose Periwinkle, *Vinca rosa (Catharanthus roseus)* which was used by Jamaican traditional healers for the treatment of diabetes, yet does not appear to have any useful effect on blood sugar levels. However detailed phytochemical investigations of the plant led to the discovery of a number of alkaloids some of which are now in use in the treatment of cancer (see Table 1.2). As a result of this unexpected discovery, all species of *Vinca* have been examined further and other useful alkaloids have been isolated. One of these is *vincamine* which acts as a hypotensive exclusively on cerebral vessels.

Another example is *Fagara zanthoxyloides* lam (orin-ata in Yoruba). The roots of this tree are used in Nigeria as chewing sticks (chewed to a brush and used to clean the teeth) as well as a remedy for fevers. In view of the observation that the teeth of fagara users appeared to be generally free of dental caries, Nigerian scientists considered that the roots of fagara might contain active ingredients with antimicrobial activity. Crude aqueous extracts were indeed found to possess antimicrobial activity. But even more striking was the observation that the extract prevented red cells in the investigators' blood agar from haemolysing. This led the research in an entirely different direction. The crude extract was tested for, and found to prevent and reverse, sickling of Hb-S erythrocytes *in vitro* (Isaacs-Sodeye et al., 1975). Fagara and the interesting compound, dimethylbenzopyran butyric acid (DBA) derived from it, have not found clinical application in the treatment of sickle cell disease, but have undergone extensive preclinical investigations which have stimulated great excitement in this area (see p. 325 for a detailed discussion). What these examples show is that when a plant is chosen for investigation on the basis of its use as a traditional remedy, it should nevertheless be screened for as many different types of pharmacological activity as possible in order not to miss an unexpected property.

Random selection

Some laboratories select plants for investigation in search of a particular pharmacological activity. The most ambitious programme of this sort is that of the National Cancer Institute in the U.S.A. which selects plants on a random basis and evaluates the extracts against one or more *in vitro* tumor systems, and also for *in vitro* cytotoxicity. Many would consider this approach too expensive for a commercial pharmaceutical organisation but it is recommended by some investigators. Fansworth and his group have used the approach to search for anti-inflammatory activity with encouraging results.

Selection of plants on the basis of their chemical constituents

For this approach plants are screened for the presence of a particular type of chemical compound e.g. alkaloid. Any plant showing the presence of alkaloids is then extracted and the extract subjected to a variety of pharmacological screenings. Other types of chemical compounds e.g. glycosides, terpenes etc. may be extracted for investigation depending on the general interest of the research group. Some multinational pharmaceutical companies base their search for natural products on this approach.

Selection based on a combination of criteria

Selection can also be based on traditional medical usage on the knowledge that the plant contained, e.g. alkaloids. The approach is to take a number of plants reputed to be effective in traditional or folkloric medicine and to extract those known to contain a type of chemical constituent and subject the extract to a wide variety of pharmacological screening e.g. antitumor, behavioural, antimicrobial, antiviral, antiinflammantory, insecticide etc. It is possible nowadays to predict from computer data the most likely chemical constituents of different plant species.

This is the approach used by Eli Lilly Scientists in the U.S.A. which yielded from *Catharanthus roseus (Vinca rosea)* the antitumor alkaloids vincaleukoblastine (Vinblastine) and leurocristine (Vincristine) used clinically in the treatment of Hodgkin's disease, choriocarcinoma and other human neoplasms. Other alkaloids from this programme having antitumour activities are still undergoing preclinical and clinical studies. The programme spanned twenty years (1956–76).

In conclusion, plants to be investigated for medicinal properties can be selected on at least four different criteria. The cost-benefit ratio of each approach depends on several factors which a research group must evaluate. Traditional medicinal usage can be an important basis for selection in the African environment; but the chances of finding new drugs may be optimised if traditional usage is combined with other criteria.

Some examples of drugs derived from natural products

It is useful to describe some drugs of natural origin because they have interesting histories and also illustrate the point that poisonous plants have been important sources of drugs in the past (see also Table 1.2).

Digitalis (Digitalis purpurea Linn. also known as Witch's Glove. Foxglove, Blood Fingers, Dead Man's Thimbles)

Foxglove grows wild and cultivated throughout most of Europe where it has been known for its poisonous and medicinal properties for centuries. According to European mythology, the mottled marks on the flowers of the foxglove were put there by the gods to warn man of the dangerous nature of the juices secreted by the plant. The foxglove was employed by ancient European herbalists for various treatments which are mostly unrelated to the valuable properties for which it is used in modern medicine today. According to old manuscripts, Welsh traditional physicians of the thirteenth century frequently used foxglove to treat fresh wounds, sores and ulcers, bruises and boils as an external preparation. Foxglove was introduced into the London Pharmacopoeia in 1650 but it took over 100 years before William Withering, in 1785, drew attention to its beneficial effects in dropsy (oedema associated with a failing heart). Digitalis leaf is still an official drug in the British Pharmacopoeia. Its therapeutic effects are due to glycosides such as digoxin present in the leaf. It is instructive to note that digitalis was used in the treatment of one form of ailment or another for over 500 years before the cardiac properties for which it is used in modern medicine were discovered.

Physostigma venenosum Balfour (Etu Esere Nut, Calabar Bean)

Calabar bean was used as an 'ordeal poison' in trials of witchcraft by the Ibibios in the Cross River State of Nigeria. The bean was taken to England in 1840 by a British medical officer stationed in Calabar. Investigations of the crude extract were undertaken by Fraser in 1863. In his very detailed paper on the pharmacological properties and therapeutic uses of the ordeal bean of Calabar, Fraser proved to be a keen observer of the political, social and religious organisation of the Ibibio people. He wrote:

> The government is oligarchical. Several chiefs rule the towns, each of which separately forms an independent government, joining with

others in times of danger for the common cause and possessing with them a common council. This is presided over by one of their number who on this account, receives the title, king . . . Next in power are the medicine men – 'mbia-idiong' and 'mbia-ibok'. In their condition of ignorance, superstitution reigns supreme. Everything unexplainable – sorrow, disease and death are ascribed to the mysterious agency of witchcraft. And it is for the discovery of the operations of this evil genius that the discriminating power of the ordeal bean is required.

The charge of witchcraft was made before one of the chiefs who then summoned a council of the neighbouring chiefs to hear the charge and the defence of the accused person, who usually opted for trial by the esere nut. The ordeal was administered in public watched by large crowds of onlookers. The bean, or its infusion, was administered in increasing amounts until the victim either vomited (proof of inno-cence) or died (proof of guilt).

Fig. 1.2. Digitalis glycosides. Aglycones of digitoxin and digoxin. The corresponding glycosides consist of the aglycone joined to hexose sugars at the -OH groups marked 3.

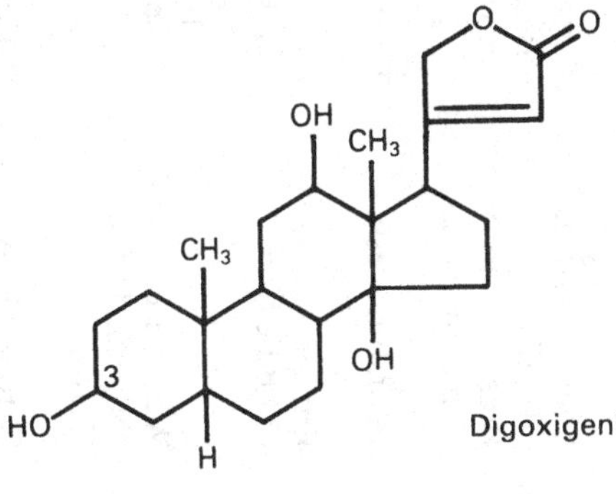

Digoxigenin

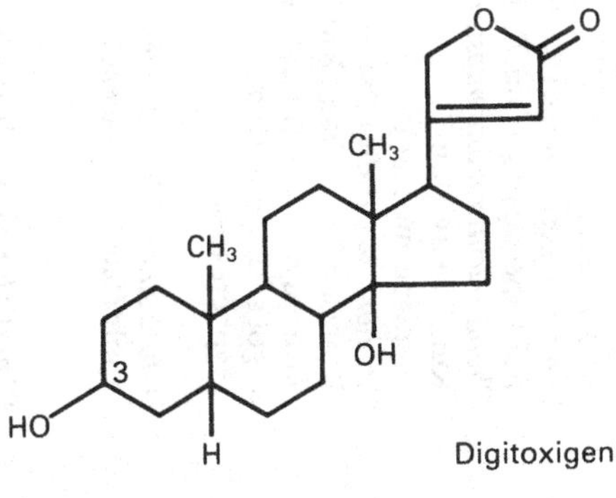

Digitoxigenin

Table 1.2 *Some biological sources of drugs*

Plant	Geographical sources	Traditional use	Active ingredient	Modern use
Anamirta cocculus Wight & Arn. – (*Cocculus indicus*), fish berries (fam. Menispermaceae)	Malabar, S. East Asia	Fish poison	picrotoxin	Formerly used as barbiturate antidote, experimental in CNS studies
Atropa belladonna L., deadly nightshade leaves (fam. Solanaceae)	India, Europe	Poison, beauty cosmetic	dl-hyoscyamine (atropine), scopolamine (hyoscine)	Various in ophthalmology, anaesthesia, peptic ulcer
Cephaelis ipecacuanha (Stokes) Baill, ipecac root (fam. Rubiaceae)	South America, Brazil	Various medicinal uses, diarrhoeas	Alkaloids: emetine, cephacine	Amoebiasis
Chondrodendron tomentosum Ruiz. & Pav. (fam. Menispermaceae)	Brazil (Orinoco and Amazon Rivers)	Arrow poison	d-tubocurarine	Muscle relaxant
Cinchona succirubra Pav. ex Klotzsch (bark) (fam. Rubiaceae)	Peru, Indonesia	Treatment of fevers	Quinine Quinidine	Antimalarial Anti-arrhythmic
Claviceps purpurea (Fries) Tul – ergot sclerotium (fam. Hypocreaceae)	Europe, Russia, Middle East	Poison (caused St Anthony's fire – gangrenous outbreak of 1676)	Ergot alkaloids: ergotamine ergometrine	Migraine, post-partum haemorrhage
Datura stramonium L., Devil's apple (fam. Solanaceae)	West Africa, Nigeria, India, Europe	Poison	Atropine	Various uses in ophthalmology anaesthesia, peptic ulcer
Digitalis lanata Ehrh. (fam. Scrophulariaceae)	Europe, U.S.A.	Various unrelated medicinal uses	Digitoxin, gitoxin Digoxin lanatocides	Congestive heart failure

Plant	Distribution	Traditional use	Active compound	Clinical use
Digitalis purpurea L. (fam. Scrophulariaceae)	Europe, U.S.A.	Various unrelated medicinal uses, e.g. epilepsy, skin ulcers, fresh wound, dropsy	digitoxin, gitoxin, gitalin	Congestive heart failure
Erythrina senegalensis DC. *E. excelsa* Bak. (fam. Leguminosae)	West Africa, Nigeria	Arrow poison	β-erythroidine	Muscle relaxant
Erythroxylum coca Lam. – coca leaf (fam. Erythroxylaceae)	South America, Peru	Suppression of hunger and fatigue	Cocaine	Local anaesthetic, frequently abused
Rauvolfia serpentina Benth. *Rauvolfia vomitoria* Afzel. (fam. Apocynaceae)	Nigeria, India	Snake bites, mental illness	Reserpine, deserpidine, rescinanine	Antipsychotic, anti-hypertensive, experimental
Strophanthus gratus (Hook.) Franch. (seed) (fam. Apocynaceae)	East and Central Africa	Arrow poison	Ouabain	Congestive heart failure
Strophanthus kombe Oliv. (seed) (fam. Apocynaceae)	East and Central Africa	Arrow poison	K-strophanthin-B, K-strophanthoside, cymarin	Congestive heart failure
Strophanthus sarmentosus DC. (fam. Apocynaceae)	West Africa	Usually recognised as poisonous – sometimes used to induce emesis or diuresis	Cardioactive glycosides	None
Strychnos nux-vomica L. (seed) (fam. Loganiaceae)	India, Calabar, Cameroons	Pesticide (rat poison)	Strychnine	Experimental in CNS studies, rat poison
Strychnos toxifera Schomb. ex Benth. (fam. Loganiaceae)	South America	Arrow poison	Toxiferine	Muscle relaxant
Catharanthus roseus (L.) G. Don. syn. *Vinca rosea* L. (fam. Apocynaceae)	Jamaica	Treatment of diabetes	Vincaleukoblastine (vinblastine), leurocristine (vincristine)	In various malignancies e.g. Hodgkin's disease, choriocarcinoma, leukaemias

> The confidence of the natives in the power of the bean is remarkable. They do not believe that any peculiar virtue resides in it, or even that it possesses any disagreeable or dangerous properties, but consider it an instrument, indifferent in itself but employed by the gods to show who is and who is not guilty. (Fraser, 1863).

The people believed

> that the esere or Calabar bean possesses the power to reveal and destroy witchcraft. (Holmstedt, 1972).

The people were aware that accidental ingestion of the esere nut was fatal, but if the bean was administered under circumstances other than as specified by the traditional practitioners, and death occurred, the perpetrator was guilty of murder and punished. However, the victim's death was not attributed to an inherent property of the bean, but to the anger of the gods *at the victim for taking the bean without sanction.* As a result of Fraser's extensive studies, the use of the crude extract of the bean in the treatment of glaucoma followed in 1877. A pure alkaloid, named physostigmine or eserine was isolated in 1865 but it was not until 1923 that its structure was elucidated. Synthesis was achieved in 1925.

Physostigmine is a powerful inhibitor of the enzyme acetylcholinesterase. Loewi and Navratil were the first to show that eserine owes its powerful pharmacological action to its anticholinesterase effect; i.e. it causes the transient, synaptic effect of acetylcholine, released from nerve endings to become excessively prolonged and intensified. The effects of the ordeal bean on its victims as described by Fraser are consistent with generalised anticholinesterase poisoning. Physostigmine (see Fig. 1.3) remains the classical inhibitor of cholinesterase enzymes, but its main clinical use now is in the treatment of glaucoma. The quaternary-nitrogen containing neostigmine lacks the central nervous system side effects of physostigmine since it crosses the blood–brain barrier with difficulty. Neostigmine is therefore safer than physostigmine for systemic use, e.g. in the treatment of myaesthenia gravis, and for reversing the effects of tubocurarine overdose.

Physostigmine's ability to preserve acetylcholine enabled investigators since the early 1930s to establish that acetylcholine is the neurotransmitter substance at:

(a) all postganglionic parasympathetic nerve fibres;
(b) some postganglionic sympathetic fibres, e.g. sweat glands;
(c) preganglionic fibres of the sympathetic (Feldberg and Gaddum, 1934);

(d) motor nerves of skeletal muscle (Dale, Feldberg and Vogt, 1936);

(e) certain neurones in the central nervous system; thereby making physostigmine one of the most important drugs ever to be discovered in a plant.

Atropa belladonna (Deadly nightshade leaves)

Belladonna was known as a potent poison in many parts of the world. It was known to the ancient Hindus of India. During the Roman Empire and in the middle ages the deadly nightshade was a common ingredient in the potions of professional poisoners. It produced a prolonged and obscure poisoning which led to certain death. This prompted Linne to name the plant *Atropa* after Atropas (meaning inflexible) – the name of the Greek Fate who cuts the thread of life. 'Belladonna' means beautiful lady and refers to the practice of Roman ladies who instilled a decoction of the leaves into their eyes to dilate the pupils. This was fashionable and considered becoming at the time. Throughout Europe and North America belladonna was a notorious source of poisoning to children who accidentally ingested it.

The most important alkaloid from the deadly nightshade is atropine (dλ-hyoscyamine) first isolated in 1831. But it took another 35 years before its fundamental mode of action was elucidated in 1867 by Bezold. Atropine has been studied extensively and used clinically for over 100 years and today there are few drugs about which there is more secure knowledge than atropine. It was one of the first materials used

Fig. 1.3. Structural formulae of physostigmine, neostigmine and pyridostigmine.

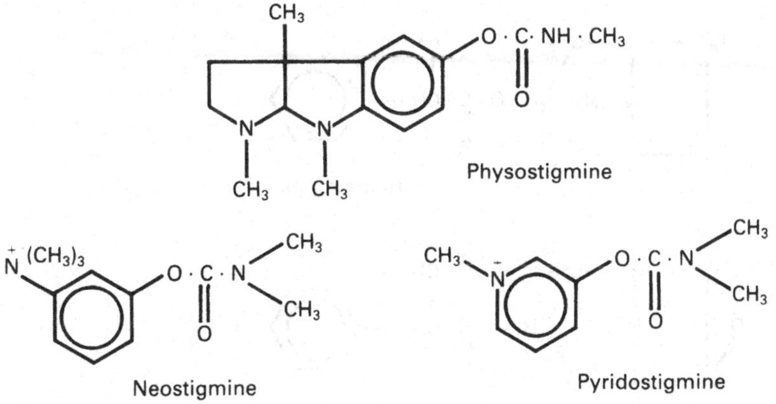

Physostigmine

Neostigmine

Pyridostigmine

to demonstrate that a drug can inhibit neurotransmission, not by preventing the release of the transmitter, but by blocking its receptor. Its action as a muscarinic receptor antagonist is so consistent and specific that the muscarinic effects of acetylcholine are defined as those actions of the neurotransmitter that are blocked by a low concentration of atropine. (See Fig. 1.4).

Atropine is also found in several *Datura stramonium* species some of which are found in West Africa. It is noteworthy that *strammonium* rarely features in traditional herbal remedies, but it has been used as an ordeal poison.

Scopolamine (Hyoscine) occurs in *Hyoscyamus niger* (Henbane). Homatropine, a shorter-acting analogue of atropine is synthetic.

Curare

The term curare was originally used to describe various South American arrow poisons. The term is now generally used to refer to compounds with skeletal muscle paralysing properties. Indians living in the Amazon and Orinoco river basins used curares to kill wild animals for food. Basically the leaves or bark of the tree were extracted in

Fig. 1.4. Structural formulae of atropine, homatropine and scopolamine.

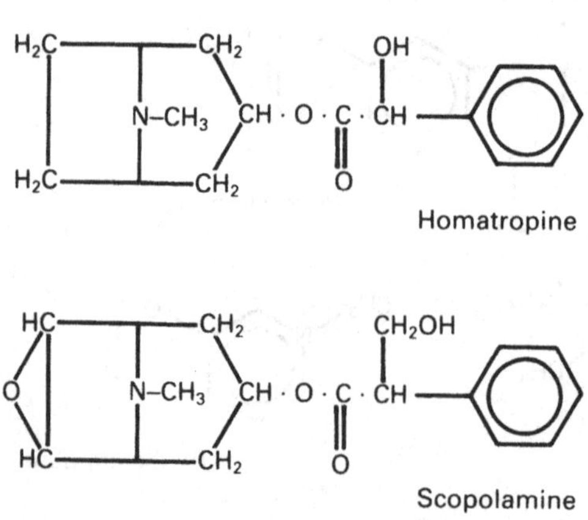

Atropine

Homatropine

Scopolamine

water and the extract concentrated by boiling or drying in the sun. The dark brown gummy mass was used to smear the hunters' arrows. After the animal had been shot, the hunter would track the wounded animal until the latter collapsed from muscle paralysis. Sir Walter Raleigh and other explorers brought curare to Europe in the early sixteenth century.

The history of curare, one of the most romantic and mysterious in medicine, has been told in numerous monographs and reviews. The following is typical.

> The technique of preparation of curare by the South American Indians was long shrouded in mystery and was entrusted only to tribal witch doctors. It varied with the tribe, the season, the whim of the maker and the ingredients available. Much secret ritual and magic accompanied the actual preparation and often many extraneous plant and animal materials were incorporated in the mixtures ... For many years the samples of curare which reached civilisation were classified on the basis of the containers in which they were stored and transported. Thus, three 'types' of curare were identified: tube curare (tubocurare) in bamboo tubes, pot curare in earthenware jars, and calabash curare in gourds.

Curare was made from different species of plants which were subsequently found to contain skeletal muscle paralysing alkaloids. Native South Americans made their curares from various species of *Strychnos* e.g. *Strychnos toxifera* which contain toxiferines, the most potent of all curare alkaloids. Note that the Asian and African species of *Strychnos* e.g. *Strychnos nux-vomica* contain tertiary nitrogen alkaloids such as strychnine with no skeletal muscle paralysing properties. Certain species of *Chondrodendron* were also used by native South Americans e.g. *C. tomentosum* which yields the clinically familiar d-tubocurarine.

Another source of curare alkaloids are the bean-like seeds of the trees and shrubs of the genus *Erythrina*. These grow in the tropical and subtropical areas of the American continent, Asia, all over Africa and Australia. Of the over one hundred species of Erythrina, several have been tested and found to contain curare alkaloids. The most potent of these alkaloids, β-erythroidine isolated from *E. americana* has been tested extensively as a muscle relaxant. It has the unusual characteristic of being a tertiary amine alkaloid with potent curarising properties but then loses potency when converted to a quaternary compound. Muscle paralysis is by competitive antagonism of acetylcholine receptors at the motor-end plate and like tubocurarine, this antagonism can be reversed by anticholinesterases. It is less potent and shorter acting than tubocurarine. Its great virtue is that the compound is completely absorbed from the gastrointestinal tract and is therefore as active after oral administration as it is after injection. The alkaloid was used sporadically for reducing skeletal muscle spasm and for prevention of fractures during convulsive shock therapy, but the advent of newer muscle relaxants has resulted in a reduced interest in this compound. Not much is known of the alkaloidal content of many species of Erythrina e.g. *E. senegalensis, E. excelsa* growing in West Africa. (See Fig. 1.5).

The origins of a few important drugs have been described briefly to emphasise the point that not all compounds which have turned out to be useful drugs were found in traditional herbal remedies. This description should be read with Table 1.2 where other examples are mentioned.

Plants as sources of raw materials for the pharmaceutical industry

So far in this chapter we have discussed plants as potential sources of chemicals with well defined pharmacological activities and which can be used in the treatment of specific diseases. Very importantly, plants are also sources of substances such as oils, starch, flavouring and sweetening agents, gum, wax etc. which can be used, not only in the manufacture of pharmaceuticals, but also in the manufacture of perfumes, foods, and beverages (see Kio & Gbile, 1987). Examples of plants from which some of these products can be obtained are given in Table 1.3.

Fig. 1.5. Structural formulae of d-tubocurarine and β-erythroidine.

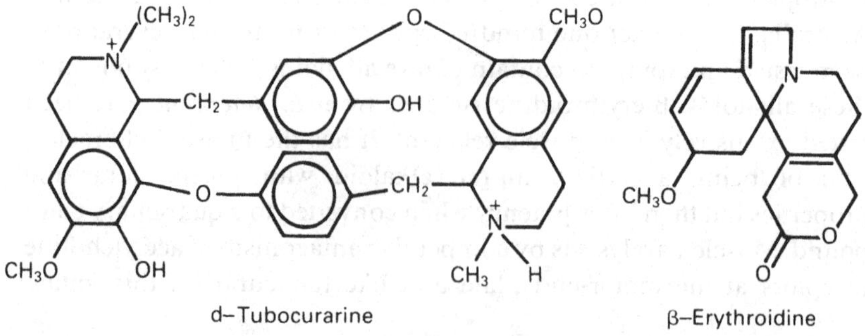

d–Tubocurarine   β–Erythroidine

REFERENCES
Apata, L. (1979). The practice of herbalism in Nigeria. In *African Medicinal Plants*, ed. A. Sofowara, p. 16, University Press, Ile-Ife.
Burn, J.H., (1948). *Background to Therapeutics*. Oxford University Press page 2.
Dale, H.H., Feldberg, W. & Vogt, M. (1936). Release of acetylcholine in voluntary motor nerve ending. *J.Physiol.* (London) **86**, 353–80.
Feldberg, W. & Gaddum, J.H. (1934). The chemical transmitter at synapses in a sympathetic ganglion. *J. Physiol.* (London) **81**, 305–19.
Fraser, T.R. (1863). On the characters, action and therapeutic uses of the ordeal bean of Calabar (*Physostigma venemosum* Belfour). *Edinb. Med. J.* **9**, 36–56; 123–32; 235–48.
Holmstedt, B. (1972). The ordeal bean of Calabar. In *Plants in the Development of Modern Medicine*, ed. T. Swain, Harvard University Press, Cambridge, Mass.
Imperato, P.J. (1977). *African Folk Medicine Practices and beliefs of the Bambara and other peoples*. York Press INC. Baltimore, page 36.
Isaacs-Sodeye, W.A., Sofowora, E.A., Williams, A.O., Marquis, V.O., Adekunle, A.A. & Anderson, C.O. (1975). Extract of *Fagara zanthoxyloides* root in sickle cell anaemia. Toxicology and preliminary trials. *Acta Haematologia*, **53**, 158–84.
Jaroszewski, J.W. (1984). Natural products and drug development. *Pharmacy International*, **5**, 27–8.
Kio, P.R.O. & Gbile, Z.O. (1987). Problems of raw materials in Pharmaceutical Research. Paper presented at the Annual Meeting of the Nigerian Society of Pharmacognosy. University of Ibadan. January 8, 1987.
Lambo, T.A. (1969). Traditional African cultures and Western Medicine. In *Medicine and Culture*, ed. F.N. Poynter, Wellcome Institute of the History of Medicine, London.
Maclean, U. (1971). *Magical Medicine – A Nigerian Case Study*. Allen Lane The Penguin Press, London, page 84.
Odelola, A.O. (1979). Address In *African Medicinal Plants*, ed. A. Sofowora, University of Ife Press, Ile-Ife, page 3.
Osuntokun, B.O. (1975). The traditional basis of neuropsychiatric practice among the Yorubas of Nigeria. *Trop. Geogr. Med.* **27**, 412–30.
Shellard, E.J. (1979). The significance of research into medicinal plants. In *African Medicinal Plants*, ed. A. Sofowora, p. 102, University Press, Ile-Ife.
Turner, V.W. (1981). *The Drums of Affliction. A study of Religious processes among the Ndembu of Zambia*. IAI, Hutchinson, pages 61–2.
World Health Organisation (1976). African Traditional Medicine. Afro. Tech. Rep. Series 1, pages 3–4, WHO Brazzaville.

Further reading
Sofowora, A. (1982). *Medicinal Plants and Traditional Medicine in Africa*. John Wiley and Sons Ltd.
World Health Organisation (1983). *Traditional Medicine and Health Care Coverage*, eds. R.H. Bannerman, J. Burton, C. Wen-Chieh. Geneva.
Turner, V.W. (1981). *The Drums of Affliction. A study of Religious processes among the Ndembu of Zambia*. IAI, Hutchinson.

Table 1.3 *Useful products in the pharmaceutical industry which can be obtained from tropical plants*

Type of substance	Uses/potential uses	Plant source	
		Species	Family
Essential oils			
citriol, thymol	Antiseptic; thymol can be incorporated into toothpaste, mouth washes, etc.	*Citrus spp.* (leaf and peel)	Rutaceae
cineole, citronellol, citronellal	Perfume industry, expectorant and decongestant in cough mixtures	*Ocimum gratissimum* (leaf) *Eucalyptus spp.*	Labiatae Myrtaceae
gingerol, dehydrogingerol	Antiseptic, anti-inflammatory, soft drink industry	*Zingiber officinale* (rhizome)	Zingiberaceae
citral (lemongrass oil)	Lemon flavour in flavourings, perfume application in soaps, antiseptic	*Cymbopogon citratus* (Lemongrass	Gramineae
palm kernel oil	Emollient, in preparation of local cosmetic products, potential substitute for fixed oils and suppository bases	*Elaeis guineensis*	Palmae
Jojoba oil	Hair oil, shampoo, soap, skin cream antiseptic, stabiliser of penicillin products	*Simmondsia chinensis*	Buxaceae

Starches	Disintegrant, filler in tablet formulations	*Manihot esculenta* (cassava)	Euphorbiaceae
		Colocasia esculenta (cocoyam)	Araceae
		Zea mays (maize)	Gramineae
Flavours and sweeteners			
oil of garlic (allylpropyl-disulphide)	Flavour in meat products, soups, sauces and canned goods	*Allium sativum* (fresh bulbs)	Liliaceae
Talin (sweet protein)	Substitute for sugar in pharmaceutical preparations, food, and drinks for the diabetic or the obese	*Thaumatococcus daniellii*	Marantaceae
		Dioscoreophyllum cumminsii	Menispermaceae
Gums and waxes			
Zanthoxylum gum	Emulsifying agent	*Zanthoxylum Fagara zanthoxyloides*	Rutaceae
Liquid wax (Jojoba)	Lubricant, useful in the cosmetic and pharmaceutical industry	*Simmondsia chinensis*	Buxaceae

Maclean, U. (1971). *Magical Medicine – A Nigerian Case Study*. Allen Lane The Penguin Press, London.

Morley, P. & Wallis, R. (1978) (eds.), *Culture and Curing. Anthropological perspectives on traditional medical beliefs and practices*. Peter Owen, London.

2

The problems of availability and quality of modern drugs in the tropics

2.1   INTRODUCTION

Third world countries spend high percentages of their meagre foreign exchange earnings on drugs usually imported from industrialised Western countries. Long term plans for the prevention of so called tropical diseases are frequently frustrated by political instability, natural disasters such as floods and droughts, illiteracy and under-developed economies. Most third world countries are short of foreign exchange to buy drugs, so the quantity imported is highly restricted. Consequently, a very high demand by rapidly expanding populations puts the price of most drugs beyond the reach of all but the few rich. A common criticism of the health services of many countries in tropical Africa is their inability to provide drugs in adequate amounts. It is common for relatives of inpatients to have to buy drugs from outside on the basis of prescriptions written by hospital consultants and then take them to the nurses for administration. This is wrong as the quality of some of these products cannot be guaranteed. The whole issue of modern drugs in third world countries can be considered as problems of (a) quality assurance and drug availability, and (b) stability of drugs in the tropics.

The two problems are closely related. For if an unstable pharma-ceutical preparation loses its potency in the harsh tropical environ-ment, the material is virtually unavailable, if not actually harmful.

2.2   QUALITY ASSURANCE AND DRUG AVAILABILITY

Since third world countries have to spend very large pro-portions of their income on drug importation, it is imperative that what is imported is of good quality. The British guide to 'Good Manu-facturing Practice' (GMP) has taken pains to define quality as the essential nature of a thing and the totality of its attributes and properties which bear upon its fitness for its intended purpose.

Unfortunately, third world countries cannot ensure the quality of the drugs they import, for, quality assurance (QA) is

the sum total of the organised arrangements made with the object of ensuring that products will be of the quality required by their intended use. It is GMP plus other factors such as product design.

The best that a third world importer can do is test samples of the imported product to check a few selected aspects of its quality. It is not possible to check every desirable quality characteristic for every item in a batch. Assurance of quality can only be obtained through intimate knowledge and control of the entire process and conditions of manufacture, which should be conducted according to the principles of good manufacturing practice. Even selected quality control checks cannot be guaranteed in many third world countries.

A survey in the early 1970s of medical stores in West Africa found that most preparations, and in particular liquid antibiotics, were of poor quality. The products were imported and there was widespread belief at that time that drugs imported from Europe did not need testing. Unfortunately, such uncritical trust in the quality of drugs of Europe origin is still prevalent. Some unscrupulous manufacturers abuse this trust by dumping low quality products in third world countries. The issue really is that quality assurance and good manufacturing practice in industrialised societies are designed for products to be used mostly in temperate environments. Shelf lives are calibrated with room temperatures of 25°C in view. So even with high standards of manufacture, the quality of a product cannot be guaranteed once it has been subjected to tropical conditions. The point being made here is not to suggest that quality control spot checks on imported products are of no value. Simple reliable tests are needed which would ensure that the product contained the correct active ingredient and in roughly the right amount. Beckett has suggested that thin layer chromatography (TLC) is such a test. It can be used to check some gross malpractices encountered in third world countries. One dimension of the problem is products coming in labelled as aspirin when they are in fact something else e.g. amphetamine. Simple tests can also be applied to traditional medicines. In many parts of the tropics, so-called traditional medicines have been found to be 'activated' by incorporation of orthodox drugs. In Malaysia, for example, indomethacin and other nonsteroidal anti-inflammatory drugs have been found in 'traditional' remedies. Similar practices have been reported among urban herbalists in Nigeria. Beckett also recommends a simple dissolution test to check for release of active ingredient. This consists of a rotating bottle at controlled temperatures and pH. A simple test of this kind reliably performed would allow us to determine that the product was roughly in good condition while elaborate and more sophisticated quality control facilities are being developed.

Procurement of drugs

Most tropical countries lack the technology to manufacture pharmaceutical products. The United Nations Industrial Development Programme's recent report *Establishment of Drug Industries in Developing Countries* classified less developed countries into five categories in terms of their capacity to manufacture drugs. Brazil, India, Mexico and Egypt are some of the third world countries in Group 5, that is, countries which manufacture most of the intermediates required by the pharmaceutical industry and undertake local research on the development of products and manufacturing processes. Most African countries (including Nigeria) are in Group 1, that is, countries with no pharmaceutical manufacturing facilities and are dependent upon imports of finished products.

Apart from the difficulties which third world countries have in monitoring the quality of finished products, direct importation of pharmaceuticals entails other problems such as bureaucratic delays which can affect the usefulness of the product. Pilfering is another problem at points of entry (sea and airports). The use of shipping containers can reduce pilfering; the problem with containers is that their internal termperatures can go up to 50°C in the tropics. For these and other reasons multinational pharmaceutical companies have established presence in many tropical countries. In most cases, the main function of the organisations is importation and distribution of drugs manufactured in factories in their countries of origin, but many have local small-scale manufacturing facilities. Some governments and local business entrepeneurs have also gone into manufacturing of drugs. The output of locally made drugs (both multinational and indigenous) still constitute a small proportion of what is needed in many countries. In India and Brazil, indigenous drug manufacturing accounts for a substantial proportion of the needs of these countries. In North Africa, Egypt and Libya also produce most of their needs locally. In tropical Africa most countries still rely on drug importation, and local production by multinational firms for their drug requirements. It will be a long time before African countries can be self sufficient in that they will be able to rely for a large part of their drug needs on local manufacture. At present even the local industries rely on basic raw materials imported from abroad, so most of them are little more than packaging industries. As imported raw materials become increasingly dear, more and more industries are looking to locally available raw materials such as essential oils, starches, gums etc for use in drug and cosmetics manufacture (see Table 1.3).

Availability of raw materials should be aided by local petrochemical industries in countries like Nigeria where petroleum is being exploited. What is needed is a firm policy on drug production with targeted objectives built into the framework of national development.

Essential drugs

In order to ease the problem of drug shortage and to ensure to some extent the quality of available drugs (whether these are made locally or imported) the World Health Organisation has formulated the essential drugs concept. This recommends that each third world country should compile a list of drugs which it considers to be the most essential for its health needs. The list will be different for each country since it is compiled on the basis of the particular health needs of the individual countries and the complexity of the health programmes in that country. The idea is based on the fact that for a given class of disease, e.g. rheumatoid arthritis, there is a long list of drugs having basically the same mode of action available for specific treatment. Instead of allowing importation or manufacture of all types of anti-inflammatory drugs, the WHO recommends that each country decides which anti-inflammatory drugs shall be imported or manufactured. Another source of confusion is the existence of *brand* and *generic* preparations of the same drug. For example the drug that goes by the generic name of chloroquine comes in different brand names such as nivaquine, fivaquine, etc. packaged by different manufacturers. In 1981, Olatunde listed 21 brands of chloroquine in the Nigerian drug market each claiming to cure malaria fever fast. Another drug that comes in several brands is aspirin. Several studies have shown that the disintegration profiles of different brands are such that predicted bioavailability (page 144) would vary between a maximum value and zero, suggesting that some manufacturers do not hold to the principles of GMP and QA.

It is partly for this reason that the WHO suggests that the essential drugs list (EDL) should identify drugs by their generic names where appropriate, for example when the drugs become 'orphan' that is, when a patent has expired. Some argue that the use of brand drugs should be encouraged because the manufacturer must protect its reputation by manufacturing to high quality and that encouraging the use of generic drugs would discourage the brand manufacturer from taking further interest in research (e.g. into its pharmacokinetics and the activity of its metabolites) to improve the drug's therapeutic value. The problem with third world countries inundated with numerous brand products is that they would have difficulty in ensuring quality of product.

The WHO has drafted a model EDL (See WHO Technical Report Series No. 685, 1983). Several countries have adopted this model in developing their own lists. Readers of this paragraph should by now have, or have access to, their national EDL. The way the concept of essential drugs can simplify drug administration may be illustrated by reference to Mozambique and Mexico. Before the former adopted the EDL concept, Mozambique used to import annually about 13,000 brand name products. The Mozambique EDL now has about 340 drugs listed. The figures for Mexico are about 10,000 before and 330 after adoption of EDL. EDL is compiled by a national committee, members of which include doctors representing different levels of specialisation, and pharmacists with knowledge of drug formulation, bioavailability, pharmacokinetics and costing policy. The committee must meet regularly to update the list. Each national committee may recommend shorter lists for small health units (See Fig. 2.1). For example, in Malawi, there is a national EDL of 300 items available to teaching and other specialist hospitals, and a shorter list of 140 items recommended for district hospitals. Another list of 24 drugs is avail-

Fig. 2.1. Organisation of Essential Drug List. (a) National List; (b) Teaching Hospital List; (c) District Hospital List; (d) Rural Health Centre List.

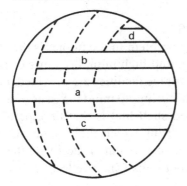

able for rural health centres. Once the national list has been determined, each hospital can use it as a basis to make its own list. It is indeed essential that a teaching hospital should have an essential drugs list. In addition to making procurement of drugs easier to administer, an EDL should cut down the budget on drugs. The rate of turnover of medical consultants in a teaching hospital is high and if each is allowed his preference in drugs without restriction, the hospital pharmacy store is soon full of outdated, unwanted, expensive drugs. It is also recommended that each country should compile a national formulary which lists the essential drugs with brief and concise descriptions of their properties and proper uses.

The existence of an EDL will not erase all the problems faced by third world countries as far as drugs are concerned, but it should do three things:

(a)   Prevent wastage,

(b)   Facilitate quality control, and

(c)   Facilitate the monitoring of abuse and adverse effects of drugs.

As you read this, your country may have produced its own EDL. It is worth noting what the Commonwealth Pharmaceutical Conference had to say in 1987 on GMP and quality control in developing countries in relation to essential drugs.

> Careful considerations should be given to the main stages of establishing essential drugs programmes so that quality assurance and GMP are effected in each step.

The steps enumerated are: (a) health policy, (b) selection of essential drugs, (c) procurement, (d) logistics of supply, (e) dispensing, handling and use of essential drugs, (f) quality control, and (g) training. What this says is that the EDL is only a part of a comprehensive health policy which is designed to make good quality drugs available to the people.

2.3   STABILITY OF DRUGS

Another aspect of the drug problem in the tropics is the effect of the weather on drugs. Heat, light and high humidity cause drugs to deteriorate, so that unless proper storage facilities are provided, many drugs may rapidly lose potency. This brings to mind the issue of expiry dates. The expiry date (also termed shelf life) is that time period as determined by the manufacturer, during which the product remains within its defined specifications. The expiry date is decided after testing the drug for stability under conditions which reflect those under which the drug would be stored in the patient's home, hospital store, pharmacy store or shop shelf. For imported drugs these conditions are often vastly different in the country of origin from those in the tropics. Few European or North American pharmaceutical firms would ensure stability under conditions of light, temperature, humidity and microbial contamination encountered in tropical countries. These conditions accelerate deterioration. In Nigeria there has been much concern in the last few years about the distribution, dispensing and offer for sale of 'expired imported drugs'. It is right that drugs should not be used after their expiry dates, for in the tropics, the expiry dates printed on packages of imported drugs are optimistic, i.e. many drugs probably lose much of their potency sooner. When drugs deteriorate under the impact of harsh tropical conditions, not only do they become therapeutically worthless, but also the products are often also toxic. It is thus imperative in a tropical environment to devote resources to the provision of facilities for proper storage of drugs under conditions which minimise contamination and deterioration in order to enhance shelf-life, guarantee efficacy and prevent waste.

2.4   FACTORS CONTRIBUTING TO RAPID DRUG DETERIORATION

The elements in a tropical environment which contribute to drug spoilage include temperature, humidity, light and the sheer absence of proper storage facilities, not to mention ignorance on the part of patients. Microbiological contamination of drugs, crude drugs and raw materials is another important factor. Mould grows on everything in a hot humid climate. Gross contamination of raw materials with *Aspergillus flavus* can make the material worthless for use in pharmaceutical manufacture. Tablets, capsules, and syrups will support the growth of fungi in this environment.

The sorts of chemical degradation which can occur under the influence of heat, light and humidity have been studied; some examples will now be given.

Temperature

In the temperate countries of Europe and North America, the ambient temperature lies between less than 0°C and about + 10°C for something like 9 months of the year. In tropical countries, the ambient temperatures rarely fall below 20°C and are more often than not as high as 40°C with relative humidities in the region of 95%. Most imported drugs have instructions to 'store in a cool place'. This instruction is given with inhabitants of temperature countries in mind. Outside the cold room or refrigerator, there is virtually no 'cool place' in the tropics. Strictly, drugs for use in the tropics which need to be kept in a cool place should have the categorical statement 'store in the refrigerator'. Manufacturers know that this is not a practical instruction to give to inhabitants of tropical countries, 99% of whom have no access to an air conditioned room or refrigerator. The research has not been done yet, but it would be interesting to determine what potency if any is left in capsules and tablets found on sale in open markets, road side buses etc. all over Nigeria.

Heat causes spoilage in many ways. The most obvious is that sugar coated tablets and gelatin capsules melt and become stuck together and to the container. Less obviously but more significantly, heat accelerates the process of chemical deterioration of drug constituents; rates of hydrolysis, oxidation–reduction, photolysis or racimisation are all accelerated at increased temperatures. Roughly the rate of chemical decomposition increases two-fold with every 10°C rise in temperature. Although this rule of thumb can serve as a fairly accurate basis for predicting stability of certain preparations, it is not of general application in that some deterioration reactions are not measurably influenced over a 10°C temperature range while others undergo rapid degradative changes over narrower temperature ranges. In tests of stability the temperature dependence of the chemical degradation of each product has to be ascertained.

The most satisfactory method for expressing the influence of temperature on reaction velocity is the quantitative relationship proposed by Arrhenius which in its simplified form is

$$\log k = \frac{Ha}{2.303\ R} - \frac{1}{T} + \log S$$

Where
k = rate constant of degradation; R = gas constant (1.987 calories degree mol^{-1}); T = absolute temperature; S = frequency factor (a constant); and Ha = heat of activation (the energy the reacting molecules must acquire in order to undergo reaction).

The higher the value of Ha the more the stability is temperature dependent. A plot of $\log k$ versus $1/T$ gives a straight line. Determinations are done at high temperatures and values of k at low temperatures are determined by extrapolation. Knowing k, the rate of degradation for a given product can be plotted from the equation.

$$t_{10\%} = \frac{0.104}{k}$$

Where $t_{10\%}$ is the time required for 10% of the active constituent of the drug to degrade. $t_{10\%}$ is analogous to $t_{1/2}$ which is described later on page 142 and its determination is also based on the assumption that drug degradation reactions follow first-order kinetics. Figure 2.2 shows diagramatically how temperature would affect the rate of degradation of a given drug; the percentage of drug remaining is plotted on a log scale. The graph shows that $t_{10\%}$ values for a given drug would vary with temperature.

Humidity

Another factor that affects stability of drugs in the tropics is humidity. Absolute humidity is the amount of water vapour (expressed in grams present per unit volume (cubic meter) of air. Relative humidity is the ratio between the actual amount of water vapour in a given volume of air and the amount which would be present if the air were saturated at the same temperature. Relative humidity is usually expressed as a percentage and is a measure of the relative dampness of the atmosphere. Regions of the world with the highest relative humidities are to be found in the tropics. In the tropical rain forests of

Fig. 2.2. The effect of temperature on degradation of a drug.

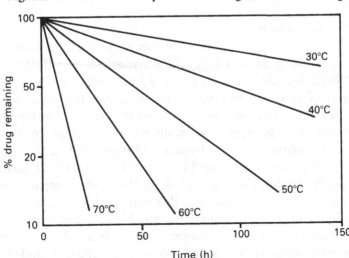

Africa and the Amazon basin in South America, the air is virtually saturated practically all year round.

High relative humidity can damage drugs in several ways. Sugar coated tablets absorb water from the atmosphere (glucose is hygoscopic) and become valueless. High humidity also affects many other reagents and chemicals used in the manufacture of drugs. This underlines the necessity for pharmaceutical industrial warehouses to be humidity and temperature controlled (air conditioned).

Apart from the physical effect which dampness can have on a product, water absorbed from the atmosphere can catalyse the hydrolysis of esters and amides (see below). Another point that is worth noting here is that plastic containers are permeable to water vapour, so the chemical and physical stability of tablet dosage forms can be considerably affected by penetration of water vapour from the atmosphere into the container. Penicillin tablets were found to degrade in polystyrene containers due to penetration of water vapour. Tetracycline suspensions were found to change colour and taste owing to permeation of water vapour through the walls of a polystyrene container. All these problems which have also been observed in temperate climates are exaggerated in a hot humid tropical atmosphere.

2.5   DEGRADATION REACTIONS

All the degradation reactions which normally affect drug stability, namely hydrolysis, oxidation-reduction, photolysis and racemisation are accelerated in the tropics due to high relative humidities and temperatures.

Hydrolysis

Many pharmaceuticals contain ester or amide groups which undergo hydrolysis in solution. The hydrolysis of an ester such as acetylsalicylic acid yields a phenol, salicylic acid and acetic acid. In the case of an amide the product is an acid and an amine. The critical issue for stability of esters and amides in the tropics is the high relative humidity and temperature. Generally it is only the fraction of the drug that is in solution that undergoes hydrolysis and in the dry form, hydrolytic degradation should not occur provided the atmosphere is dry i.e. the relative humidity is low. In the tropics, preparations containing sensitive compounds whether in liquid form or tablets undergo hydrolysis due to high temperature and high relative humidity which enable tablets to absorb moisture from the atmosphere. A notorious example is acetylsalicylic acid (aspirin). This drug is degraded to produce salicylic acid and acetic acid, which gives the degraded product a characteristic odour. Salicylic acid is reputed to be mainly responsible for the stomach upset caused by aspirin. (See Table 2.1 for examples of esters and amides likely to undergo hydrolytic degradation if not properly stored.)

Oxidation – reduction

Oxidative decomposition is responsible for the instability of a large number of drugs. Examples are steroids, antibiotics and adrenaline. The reactions are mediated by free radical or by molecular oxygen. Oxidation often involves the addition of oxygen or removal of hydrogen. The most common form of oxidative decomposition occurring in pharmaceutical preparations is autoxidation which involves a free radical chain reaction. Rancidity in oils and fats is a well known term used to describe deterioration in these products. The distinct odour of a rancid oil is due to volatile compounds that are formed upon oxidation of the oils and fats. The mechanism involves free radicals.

Oxidative degradation can be minimised by decreasing the oxygen content of the water used in the preparation of the medicament or the use of anti-oxidants such as sodium metabisulphite, and ascorbic acid (for aqueous preparations), hydroquinone, propylgallate, and toluene for oily preparations. Trace elements of heavy metals tend to catalyse oxidative degradation of pharmaceutical products, so chelating agents are used to prevent such catalysis. Chelating agents commonly used are ethylenediamine tetraacetic acid derivatives, citric acid, and tartaric acid.

Photolysis

This is the decomposition of pharmaceutical compounds as a result of the absorption of radiant energy in the form of light. Photolysis is an important factor for drug stability in the tropics because of long hours of sunshine in these regions and exposure of drugs at sea and airports, open markets etc. Degradative reactions such as oxidation-reduction, or polymerisation can be initiated by exposure to light at particular wavelengths. Radiation from ultraviolet and violet portions of the light spectrum are more active in initiating chemical reactions than those from the longer wavelengths. Photochemical reactions are complex reactions but usually involve free radicals. Examples of drugs which undergo photodecomposition are chlorpromazine, and hydrocortisone (see Table 2.1).

Table 2.1 *Examples of drugs liable to undergo rapid chemical degradation in a tropical environment*

Degradation reaction	Drug	Mechanism	Increased by
Hydrolysis	Esters: acetylsalicylic acid, benzocaine, atropine, lincomycin	Cleavage of acyl–oxygen linkage	High relative humidity and high temperature (hence store in cool dry place)
	Amides: niacinamide, phenethicillin, barbiturates, choramphenicol	cleavage of amide group	High relative humidity and high temperature (hence store in cool. dry place)
Oxidation–reduction	Various drugs: prednisolone, morphine, adrenaline, amylnitrite, phenothiazines	reaction with molecular oxygen, free radical reactions	Improper storage, air, high temperatures (store in a cool, dry place in well stoppered containers)
	Polyunsaturated vitamin A, compounds: vegetable oils, fats	auto-oxidation, free radical mechanisms	Improper storage, air, high temperatures (store in a cool, dry place in well closed containers)
Photolysis	chlorpromazine, antihistamines, hydrocortisone, prednisolone, methylprednisolene	various degradation reactions initiated by ultraviolet and violet radiation energy	Exposure to sunlight (store in cool, dry place in amber coloured glass containers)
Protein denaturation	vaccines and sera	–	Heat, humidity and microbiological contamination (store in refrigerator)

Racemisation

In this reaction an optically active substance undergoes spontaneous change to lose its optical activity without changing its chemical structure. This reaction is important for the stability of drugs because the laevorotatory form of a drug can be several times more biologically active than the dextrorotatory form. An example is adrenaline whose laevo-form is up to 20 times more active than dextro-adrenaline. Solutions of l-adrenaline undergo racemisation to yield a racemic mixture consisting of equal parts of l- and d-adrenaline which is only about half as active as the pure l-adrenaline.

What has been said in this chapter does not represent a comprehensive treatment of the subject of stability of drugs. Pharmacy students will come across a more detailed treatment including the properties of different containers (metal, glass, plastic) which affect drug stability and formulation strategies to minimise drug deterioration. I hope that enough examples are given here to bring home the point that in the tropics the issue of stability of medicaments is especially important because the degradation reactions are all enhanced by the high relative humidities, high temperatures and sunlight of these regions. What are needed are adequate refrigerated warehouses at sea and airports and awareness that medicaments are liable to lose their usefulness when exposed to the natural atmosphere of the tropics. This means that bureaucratic delays must be minimised in clearing pharmaceuticals from our ports.

PART II
Fundamental Pharmacodynamic Principles

3

Measurement of drug response

3.1   INTRODUCTION

In modern drug therapy, accurate measurements are important. The drug must reach its site of action in an appropriate quantity to do any good. In inadequate amounts, the drug is ineffective, and worse still, bacteria may become resistant to it. Excessive amounts also defeat our purpose since toxic unwanted side-effects may supervene. The aim therefore is to give a quantity of drug such that plasma concentrations are maintained at therapeutic level for long enough to bring relief to the patient. The achievement of this objective calls for accurate measurements of the dose of drug and the corresponding pharmacological response.

There are two basic assumptions behind pharmacological measurements:

(i) the healing power of the drug comes from pharmacological responses which it evokes in the body, and

(ii) the magnitude of the response is directly proportional to the amount of drug.

These assumptions constitute the major difference between modern drug therapy and the use of herbs in other medical systems (see Chapter 1). Much of what the modern pharmacologist does consists in characterising drugs by analysis of dose–response relationships. In this chapter the general properties and uses of different types of dose-response lines are described including their use in biological assays. Statistical procedures commonly used in pharmacological measurements to estimate error are also described.

Units of measurement

All measurements in pharmacology are expressed in the metric system. Inch, foot, yard, ounce, pound, °Fahrenheit, and imprecise measures such as tablespoonful, calabashful, armlength etc., are not accepted units.

3.2   RECORDING DEVICES

A simple system which can be used to demonstrate the relationship between the dose of a drug and the response evoked by it, is the isolated mammalian smooth muscle (guinea-pig or rabbit ileum) suspended in a suitable physiological salt solution. Many pharmacologically active substances cause relaxation or contraction of these muscles. These responses can be recorded isotonically in cm or mm or isometrically in g or mg.

In an isotonic measurement, the muscle alters its length in response to drug. The amount by which the muscle shortens (contraction) or lengthens (relaxation) is recorded. Since only about a 2-cm length of muscle, is used, the alteration in length has to be amplified. A common set up is the frontal writing lever shown diagramatically in Fig. 3.1. Electronic devices are also available for isotonic measurements. With practice, the frontal writing lever recording on smoked paper can be used to obtain good measurements.

In isometric recording, the muscle cannot alter its length. The increase (contraction) or decrease (relaxation) in resting tension is measured electronically by means of a transducer which converts mechanical force to electrical energy which after suitable amplification is pen-recorded. Both methods yield similar results.

3.3   TYPES OF DOSE–RESPONSE CURVES

The dose–response curve describes the relationship between the magnitude of the response and the dose of drug which evokes it. In the type of measurement just described, the response increases with increasing dose until a maximum response (max r) is reached after which an increase in dose no longer produces an increase in response. The response is initiated by activation of receptors or ion channels on the muscle cell membrane. The number of receptors activated is proportional to the dose of drug and the max r is reached when all or sufficient receptors or channels are activated. The submaximal response is therefore assumed to be proportional to the fraction of receptors activated. Hence,

$r = y\text{k}$

where r = submaximal response, y = fraction of receptors activated, and k = constant.

The quantity y is proportional to dose, so that when dose is plotted against response, a hyperbolic curve results (Fig. 3.2), whereas a log dose versus response plot gives a sigmoid curve. A sigmoid curve is also obtained when the plot is made on semilogarithmic paper. Note that the *dose is plotted on a log scale and the response on a linear scale not vice versa.*

The theory that the response, r, is proportional to the fraction of receptors occupied is discussed in more detail on page 83.

Advantages of the log dose–response plot
Plotting the dose on a log scale has a number of advantages:

Fig. 3.1. Frontal writing lever arrangement for recording the isotonic response of isolated muscle.
F = fulcrum about which the shaft of the lever moves when the muscle alters its length. ct = cotton thread attaching the muscle to the lever at P (a blub of plasticine is used for this).
W = weight of plasticine used to adjust the load on the muscle such that the muscle is not stretched initially by more than a few grams (1 to 3 g).
TH = tissue holder which anchors the muscle immovably to the bottom of the organ bath (ob). TH also serves as the aerator for bubbling the physiological salt solution (Pss) with oxygen, air or other gas mixture.
WP = writing point. The ratio of the lengths a/b is the magnification of the response. For example, if the muscle alters its length by 1.0 mm and the ratio $a/b = 10$, a 10.0 mm response is recorded.

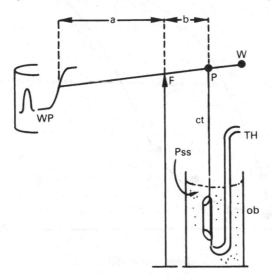

(a) It allows a wide range of doses to be compacted, and
(b) in the region of the graph which lies between about 20–80% of the max *r*, the regression of response on log dose is virtually linear.

A straight line is more convenient for the computation of such quantities as relative potency than a hyperbolic curve.

Fig. 3.2. Graphs of dose versus response. (A), Contractions of isolated guinea-pig ileum to increasing doses of histamine. (B), Data from (A) plotted on a linear scale. (C), Same data on log scale.

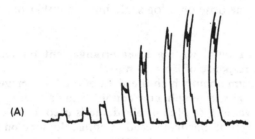

(A)

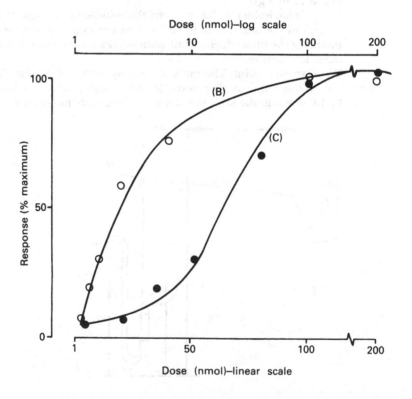

Dose–response curves can also be derived from quantal responses. In this measurement procedure, various doses of drug are given to groups of experimental animals and the proportion of animals in each group responding to the drug is computed. The response may be death of the animal, loss of righting reflex or some other end-point which allows the animals to be classified as responding or not responding. When the results of such an experiment are plotted graphically with the proportion responding (response) on the ordinate and the log dose on the abscissa, a sigmoid curve is obtained (Fig. 3.3). It is useful to convert the quantal response curve to a straight line by rescaling the ordinate. This is done by converting the percentage response to another unit known as probit (probability unit). There are published tables giving probit values for corresponding percentage values. Graph papers with probit scales are also available commercially.

Some uses of dose–response lines
Measurement of relative potency
The relative potencies of drugs can be estimated by analysis of dose–response lines. The drugs must have similar properties and the responses elicited under similar conditions. This applies to graded and quantal responses; for graded measurements responses are determined at, at least, two dose-levels, the doses being chosen in such a way that the responses lie between about 20 and 80% of the maximum. In this portion of the log dose–response curve relatively large changes in

Fig. 3.3. A hypothetical log-dose quantal response curve with responses plotted (A) on a linear scale and (B) on a probit scale.

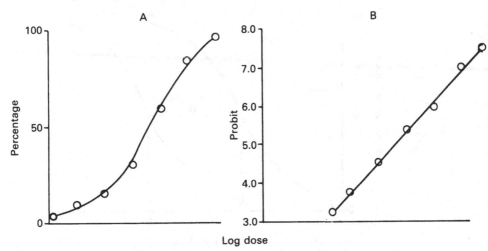

response occur with small changes in dose. Log dose versus response plots then give virtually straight lines. In the case of quantal responses, straight lines are also obtained when probit values are plotted against log dose. Using two drugs with different potencies (such as members of a homologous series) two parallel lines are obtained. The horizontal distance between the lines is a measure of the relative potencies of the two drugs, the lines for the weaker drug being to the right of the line for the more potent drug. (See Fig. 3.4 and also page 75 for analysis of M). Another application of this procedure is in the determination of the active drug in an extract. In this case, one of the two lines is constructed using a solution containing a known amount of active drug (standard) and the other with graded amounts of the preparation with unknown amounts of the active principle (test). The amount of active drug in the test preparation is determined from M (see page 75 for a further discussion of this procedure).

Therapeutic index (TI)

The therapeutic index is a measure of drug safety. It was first formulated by Ehrlich as *Chemotherapeutic index*. It applied originally to the measurement of the safety of anti-parasitic drugs. The index is a ratio of the dose of drug needed to cause *a toxic effect in or kill*, a certain

Fig. 3.4. Relative potency determination from log-dose–response lines. Drug A is more potent than drug B. Antilog M is the relative potency of drug B. This can be directly estimated by comparing doses D_1 and D_2 which produce 50% of the max r for each drug.

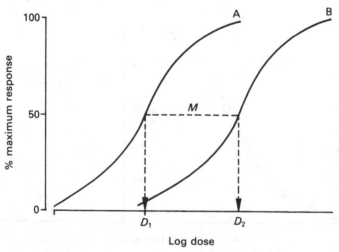

proportion of the population (lethal dose or LD) to the dose needed to effect cure in a certain proportion of the population (effective dose or ED). TI can be defined as LD_{50}/ED_{50}, that is the dose to kill 50% of the population divided by the dose to cure 50% of the population. Obviously the bigger the value of TI the safer is the drug. Drugs such as digitalis have small TI values, indicating that they must be used with great care and only under supervision. If the recommended dose is slightly exceeded, toxic symptoms may occur. TI can be estimated from quantal log dose–response or log dose–probit lines (see Fig. 3.5). TI is not always sufficient to express the safety of drug. Some investigators use the ratio LD_1/ED_{99}, also called the certain safety factor (CSF).

Qualitative use of dose–response lines

Dose–response lines can be used to determine the nature of drug action. They may be used to differentiate drugs as *full* or *partial* agonists (see page 85). Partial agonists have lower maxima than full agonists when acting on the same receptors. On the other hand, *competitive* antagonists shift the log dose–response curve of the agonist to the right of control curves whereas *non-competitive antagonists* may

Fig. 3.5. Determination of TI from log-dose response lines. (A), Log-dose-response line for the desired effect, e.g. hypnosis, anaesthesia, analgesia. (B), Log-dose-response line for the toxicity or lethality of the same drug.

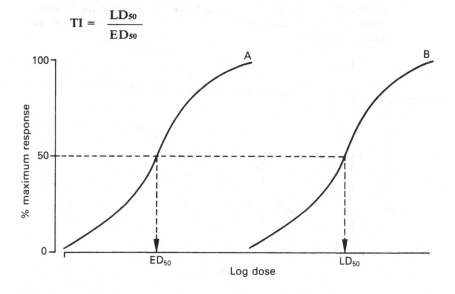

depress the maximum without much change in threshold dose (see Fig. 3.6). A more detailed treatment of the quantitative measurement of competitive antagonism is given in Chapter 4.

3.4   BIOASSAY

Bioassay is the assessment of a drug in terms of its biological activity. It can be qualitative or quantitative. The following statement attributed to Gaddum is widely quoted:

> the pharmacologist has been a Jack of all trades, borrowing from physiology, biochemistry, pathology, microbiology and statistics – but he has developed one technique of his own and that is the technique of bioassay.

In qualitative bioassay, the objective is to determine what type of action a drug produces by comparing its action with those of other substances of known activity. It can be used to detect small amounts of biologically active substances present at disease sites or released in pathology. An adaptation of bioassay used extensively by Vane in his research on prostaglandins consists of superfusing several isolated smooth muscle preparations in cascade (Fig. 3.7). When the extract containing the substance to be detected is introduced into the circuit, it causes contractions or relaxations of all or some of the muscles. By comparing the responses of the muscles in the circuit to known com-

Fig. 3.6. The log-dose–response curve (A) is shifted in a parallel fashion to the right (B) by a competitive antagonist drug. In noncompetitive antagonism (C) the curve is not shifted, but the maximum is depressed.

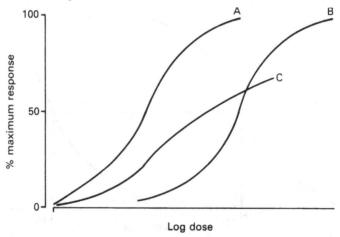

pounds and to the extract, the type of activity in the extract is determined. For example three smooth muscles commonly used to detect prostaglandins are rat colon (RC), rat stomach strip (RSS) and chick rectum (CR). These three tissues are relaxed by adrenaline and noradrenaline, are contracted by prostaglandins E_2, F_{2a}, acetylcholine, and 5-HT, but do not react to low doses of histamine, angiotensin, bradykinin or other substances commonly found in biological fluids. Therefore if an extract contracts all three tissues in the presence of a cocktail of conventional antagonists (mepyramine, lysergic acid, diethylamide, atropine and adrenoceptor blockers) the activity in the extract is most probably that of a prostaglandin.

The superfusion fluid may be a physiological salt solution or blood taken from an artery of an anaesthetised animal which is used to superfuse the tissues and then returned to the animal through a vein. Superfusion techniques allow very small quantities of active sub-

Fig. 3.7. A superfusion bioassay assembly. T, transducer (recording device); PP, peristaltic pump; Pss, physiological salt solution; B, bubbler; M, muscle strip.

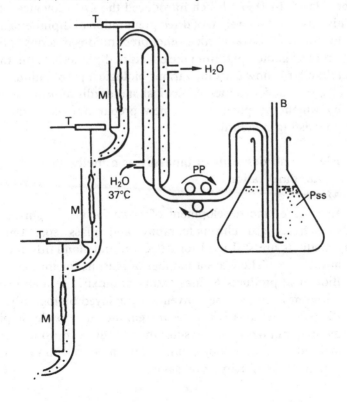

stances to be detected without prior extraction. Substances which might lose their activity during extraction can thus be detected. For example, Vane used this procedure to detect short-lived but highly active intermediate products of arachidonic acid metabolism e.g. thromboxanes and prostacyclin.

Quantitative bioassay

In quantitative bioassay, the object is to determine the amount of active constituent in a drug preparation. For this purpose another preparation containing a known amount of the active constituent is used as a standard.

Biological standards

The major initial difficulty encountered with biological preparations used in medicine was the wide variability in potency of preparations made in different laboratories. In the case of crude drugs (leaves, bark, crude extracts etc.), the potencies varied with season or even time of day of collection. It therefore became necessary to have some sort of standard unit of potency to which other preparations could be related. In 1897 Ehrlich introduced the first biological standard. This was a certain weight of dried preparation of diphtheria antitoxin. This was used to standardise other preparations in terms of their ability to protect guinea-pigs from the effects of diphtheria toxin. International Standards now exist for various biological preparations such as digitalis, sera and vaccines. Biological standardisation is the procedure by which the potency of a new preparation is established against an existing standard.

Merits and demerits of bioassay as a method of standardisation
Merits

In spite of the development of powerful and sophisticated methods such as gas chromatography and mass spectrometry, bioassay methods are still used for detection and standardisation of biological materials. There are a number of reasons for this:

(a) Biological products such as toxins, antitoxins, sera and some hormones can only be conveniently assayed biologically.
(b) Bioassay methods can measure minute (nanomole or picomole) quantities of active substance. Until the introduction of methods such as radioimmunoassay, there was no method to match the sensitivity of bioassays.

(c) Bioassay methods can detect active substances without prior extraction or other treatment. It is doubtful whether the thromboxanes and prostacyclin with biological half-lives of a few minutes could have been discovered in any other way except by Vane's superfusion bioassay at the time they *were* discovered.

Demerits

The key problem with bioassay is the variability in responses. This is an inherent property of biological materials. Therefore, to obtain a reliable estimate of potency, the measurement has to be repeated a number of times or a large number of experimental animals must be used. Expertise in experimental design, execution of the assay and analysis of data is required. What all this means is that bioassays are expensive and time consuming, and are not as accurate as other procedures. Some other factors which may complicate matters are the presence in the material to be assayed, of interfering substances (this can be minimised by the use of specific antagonists if the interfering substances are known), time-related changes in the sensitivity of the test organ, or tachyphylactic response to the substance being assayed.

Types of bioassay
Direct comparison assay

In this type of assay, responses to standard and test solutions are measured in the same preparation. This may be an anaesthetised whole animal (e.g. a cat for blood pressure measurements), isolated muscle preparation or isolated perfused organ. An example is the assay of posterior pituitary extract (oxytocin) by its contraction of the rat isolated uterus. Direct comparison assay is commonly used to demonstrate the principles of bioassay in class experiments. The statistical treatment of the data from such an assay is given on page 69.

The measurement of a particular response in separate animals

An example of this type is the assay of protamine Zinc Insulin (PZI). Four groups of rabbits are used; two groups receive a low and high dose of standard PZI and two groups receive low and high dose of the test preparation. A fall in blood sugar is measured in each rabbit. The average fall in each group is computed and from log dose-response lines the potency of the test preparation is determined. The rabbits survive the assay and they can be used again in a socalled crossover design (see page 63).

Quantal assay

The percentage of animals in a group responding to different doses of test and standard is determined. An example of this is the assay of soluble insulin. Different doses of the drug are injected intravenously into different groups of mice. The numbers of animals responding (death, convulsion or loss of righting reflex) are determined.

Threshold assay or measurement of minimal effective dose

Tincture of digitalis is assayed by this method. Dilutions of the standard and unknown are infused into anaesthetised guinea-pigs at a standard rate. The smallest volume of tincture (measured in terms of the animal's body weight) causing arrest of the heart is determined for standard and test preparations. This is repeated in different animals using at least two different dilutions of standard and test solutions.

Points to note about the design of an assay

Replication

This is the repetition of the measurement so that enough data are generated from which an average value is calculated and an estimate of the error or reliability of the assay is made by statistical analysis.

Use of more than one dose of test and standard

Most assays employ two doses of standard (low, ds_1 and high ds_2) and two doses of test (dt_1 and dt_2). The doses are chosen in such a way that the ratio d_2/d_1 is the same for standard as it is for test, that is

$$ds_2/ds_1 = dt_2/dt_1$$

Also where applicable, doses must give responses which lie between about 20% and 80% of the maximum response. These conditions need preliminary experiments to be carried out to determine the approximate potency of the test preparation.

Randomisation

In assays where responses to standard and unknown are determined in the same preparation, doses must be randomised so that any changes in sensitivity of the test preparation during the course of the assay should affect test and standard responses equally. Randomisation is achieved by a Latin Square Design, which is *an arrangement of n symbols in n rows and n columns in such a way that no symbol occurs twice in the same column or the same row.* In a 2 x 2 assay where the doses are ds_1, ds_2, dt_1, dt_2, the order of injection in a Latin square design would be as shown below.

ds_1	ds_2	dt_1	dt_2
ds_2	ds_1	dt_2	dt_1
dt_2	dt_1	ds_1	ds_2
dt_1	dt_2	ds_2	ds_1

There are thus four responses measured for each dose. This sort of assay can be subjected to statistical analysis.

Miscellaneous matters

When an assay is performed on groups of animals, steps should be taken to minimise variability in responses due to differences in the environmental and nutritional conditions of the animals. Determinations of the responses to standard and test should be done as nearly as possible at the same time to minimise error due to diurnal variation in animal response to drugs. No accuracy can be expected if the test responses were determined in the morning and the standard responses at night.

If the effect is not lethal, e.g. the assay of protamine zinc insulin in rabbits, a 'crossover' assay should be done to minimise error due to variability in the response of individual rabbits. In 'crossover' (Fig. 3.8), the test is performed twice on the same animals after allowing a period of time for recovery. At the second trial, the animals are switched, so that those initially receiving the standard, now receive the test preparation, and, those initially receiving the low dose now receive the high dose.

Fig. 3.8. A cross-over assay (see text).

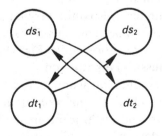

Alternative procedures in toxicological tests and bioassays

Animal rights supporters argue that LD_{50} tests and bioassays involve unnecessary killing of animals. They argue that since these tests are neither accurate nor 100% predictive of drug action in man, the death of animals is not entirely justified. These groups and many scientists advocate alternative procedures involving fewer animals or *in vitro* tests using cultured human cells. An alternative to the LD_{50} test is the fixed dose procedure devised by the British Toxicological Society. It avoids death of animals as the end point. Three doses of the substance under test are chosen and one dose (say the middle dose) is administered to only five animals. If signs of toxicity are observed, the animals are killed and examined in detail. From this the substance is assigned a particular category of toxicity, depending on which the substance may not be tested further. Alternative procedures are also being developed for bioassays. For example, high performance liquid chromatography (hplc) is replacing chicken blood pressure in the assay of oxytocin.

3.5   STATISTICAL ANALYSIS OF DATA

The problem of variability in biological measurements is dealt with by use of statistical methods. In this section, some of the statistical procedures commonly employed to analyse pharmacological data are described. No attempt is made to be exhaustive or to offer proof of the procedures described. Some useful texts on biostatistics from which more detailed information can be gained are listed at the end of the Chapter. The objective here is to explain some common statistical ideas and how to use them to analyse the sort of data which a student is likely to generate in the laboratory.

Normal distribution

When a certain dilution of digitalis tincture is infused into anaesthetised guinea-pigs, some animals' hearts will stop after infusion of a small volume; a small number will require very large volumes. The majority will require intermediate amounts. This sort of result can be presented as a frequency distribution curve (Fig. 3.9). The data are said to follow a normal (Gaussian) distribution.

In a normal distribution, the individual measurements are distributed equally on either side of a hypothetical 'true' mean or *average*. The majority of values are clustered around the 'true' mean, but a few will deviate greatly from it; 68% of the data in a normal distribution fall within plus or minus one standard deviation (see below), 95% within 2 and 99.7% within 3 standard deviations. Pharmacological data are assumed to be normally distributed and the methods used to estimate the error of measurements are based on this assumption. Error is technically defined as variability in experimental observations due to the operation of chance factors. The usual approach in estimating the error of a set of measurements is to take the mean of several observations. It is assumed that the mean of several measurements is more representative of the hypothetical true mean. Error is inversely related to the number of observations. Therefore, the larger the number of observations from which the mean is taken, the smaller is the error, i.e. the mean is then truly representative of the true mean. However, the number of observations that can be made in a given experiment is limited by time and expense. Therefore, the small numbers of data usually available are statistically treated so that the variability of the individual observations from which the mean is calculated, and hence the reliability of the assay, can be inferred. Consider two experiments in which 50 ng of histamine were added at regular intervals to an isolated length of guinea-pig ileum in a 10-ml organ bath and the following heights of contractions were recorded in cm (Table 3.1). The mean or average contraction is given by: $\sigma X/N$ where σX is the sum and N is the number of observations. In both experiments the mean is 4.8. Obviously the individual results in experiment 2 are more different from one another and from the mean than they are in experiment 1. Statistical analysis will show that the error in experiment 2 is greater than in experiment 1.

The following quantities are used to estimate the error.

Fig. 3.9. A normal distribution curve, showing digitalis action.

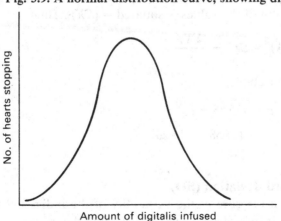

Amount of digitalis infused

Table 3.1 *Heights of contractions (cm) induced by 50 ng of histamine in isolated guinea-pig ileum*

Experiment 1	Experiment 2
4.5	3.6
4.5	4.8
5.0	3.2
4.7	7.2
5.3	5.2

Variance (V)

This is defined as the sum of the squares of the deviations of the individual values from the mean divided by the number of observations less one. If the individual measurements are designated X and the mean value $\overline{X}$, then variance, is

$$V = \frac{(X_1 - \overline{X})^2 + (X_2 - \overline{X})^2 \ldots}{N - 1} \tag{3.2}$$

$$= \frac{\Sigma(X - \overline{X})^2}{N - 1} \tag{3.3}$$

The quantity $N - 1$ used in the calculation of the variance is *the number of degrees of freedom*. If from a total of five values, the mean is calculated, that is said to use up one degree of freedom. Hence the number of degrees of freedom is 4. For example, to calculate the variance from the guinea-pig ileum experiment the data are arranged as follows (Table 3.2): The sum of squares of the deviation of individual values from the mean $\Sigma(X - \overline{X})^2$, can be calculated more directly as follows: each individual value is squared, the squared values are summed = ΣX^2. Next the sum of the values is squared = $(\Sigma X)^2$. Then

$$\Sigma(X - \overline{X})^2 = \Sigma X^2 - \frac{(\Sigma X)^2}{N}$$

For experiment 1 above,

$$\Sigma(X - \overline{X})^2 = 115.58 - \frac{576}{5}$$

$$= 115.58 - 115.20$$

$$= 0.38$$

Standard deviation (SD)

This is a measure of the variability of the individual values from the mean. It indicates how widely scattered the values are about

Table 3.2 *Analysis of data in Table 3.1*

	Experiment 1			Experiment 2	
X	$X - \bar{X}$	$(X - \bar{X})^2$	X	$X - \bar{X}$	$(X - \bar{X})^2$
4.5	−0.3	0.09	3.6	−1.2	1.44
4.5	−0.3	0.09	4.8	0	0
5.0	+0.2	0.04	3.2	−1.6	2.56
4.8	0	0	7.2	+2.4	5.76
5.2	+0.4	0.16	5.2	+0.4	0.16
Total:		0.38	24		9.92

$$V = \frac{\Sigma(X - \bar{X})^2}{N - 1}$$

$$= \frac{0.38}{4}$$

$$= 0.095$$

$$V = \frac{\Sigma(X - \bar{X})^2}{N - 1}$$

$$= \frac{9.92}{4}$$

$$= 2.28$$

the mean and to what extent the mean result can be accepted as representing the true event. SD is the square root of the variance, i.e.

$$SD = \left(\frac{(\Sigma X - \bar{X})^2}{N - 1} \right)^{1/2} \tag{3.4}$$

Being a square root, SD can be both a positive and a negative number. The standard deviation from experiment 1 is 0.31, so that the mean ± standard deviation are written as 4.8 ± 0.31. Similarly the values from experiment 2 are 4.8 ± 1.57.

From the large SD of experiment 2 (relative to the SD of experiment 1), it can be inferred that the individual values from which the mean was calculated were more widely scattered than those of experiment 1, even without seeing the individual values. Various factors can account for such a situation, some of which are (a) the organ bath was not filled exactly to the same level each time, or the volume of drug delivered was not accurately measured, so that the final concentration of drug varied with each dose application, (b) the dosing sequence was not strictly adhered to, so that there were different rest periods between doses, (c) the physiological salt solution in experiment 2 was inaccurately made up, or (d) aeration was inadequate, irregular or excessive. These are some of the reasons why there are now automated devices for this sort of assay to minimise human errors.

The standard error of the mean (SEM)

The standard error of the mean is an estimate of the variability of the mean. The mean value from a set of measurements is one possible mean out of several normally distributed values which could be obtained if the experiment were repeated under similar conditions. The standard error describes how likely it is that a mean value similar to the one obtained in an experiment would be obtained should the experiment be repeated. The standard error is the standard deviation divided by the square root of the number of observations.

$$SE = \frac{SD}{N^{\frac{1}{2}}} \tag{3.5}$$

The standard error of the mean from experiment $1 = \dfrac{0.31}{5^{\frac{1}{2}}}$

$$= 0.14$$

The result is stated as 4.8 ± 0.14 (SEM).
Similarly the result of experiment 2 is stated as 4.8 ± 0.70 (SEM).

Confidence limits or fiducial limits

The confidence limit is a more exacting statement of the error of the measurement. It states the probability at which the mean value from a set of measurements will lie within a certain stated range, if the experiment was repeated. To determine the confidence limits of a mean proceed as follows: The mean value and standard error of the mean are calculated: the value of a quantity called 't' corresponding to a certain level of probability, usually 95%, is read from published tables. Then the limits of the mean are given by:

$$\pm SE \times t$$

In our example (experiment 1), the value of t (4 degrees of freedom) at a probability of 0.95 (95%) = 2.78. The limits for the mean in experiment 1 are therefore $\pm 0.14 \times 2.78 (\pm 0.39)$. The mean value therefore lies between $4.8 - 0.39$ and $4.8 + 0.39$ i.e. 4.41 and 5.19. The mean result is stated as: 4.8 (4.41 − 5.19) 95% confidence limits in brackets. These limits are 92 and 108% respectively of the mean. The corresponding limits for the mean in experiment 2 are $\pm 0.70 \times 2.78 (\pm 1.95)$, and the result is 4.8 (2.85 − 6.75) 95% confidence limits in brackets. These limits are 59 and 141% respectively of the mean, confirming again that although the mean values from the two experiments are identical experiment 2 is much less reliable than experiment 1.

The Student's '*t*' test and the null hypothesis

In pharmacology we frequently have to compare two mean values to see whether some experimental treatment has had a real effect on one set of measurements.

Example

Log–dose response curves were constructed for carbachol from its contractions of the isolated rectal muscle of the rainbow lizard (*Agama agama*). (This preparation has been studied in our laboratory as a muscarinic receptor tissue for the assay of acetylcholine). From the parallel curves produced by different molar concentrations of pirenzepine, pA_2 values for this antagonist were determined by the Schild method at 26°C and at 37°C. The values for each of 7 determinations at each temperature and the necessary calculations are shown below (see Table 3.3).

The mean pA_2 value at 37°C (7.93 ± 0.13) is greater than the value at 26°C (7.42 ± 0.16). The question is whether this difference is due to the influence of temperature or is it the sort of difference that would be expected to occur by chance. To settle the issue, the Null hypothesis is assumed, that is, *temperature has no real effect on the nature of the muscarinic receptor in lizard smooth muscle; the difference could have occurred by chance as a result of error in the measurements.* If the difference of that magnitude was due to chance alone, then we should expect the difference not to occur every time the experiment is repeated. Therefore what the question boils down to is, with what certainty (*probability*) can we assert that such a difference will occur every time the measurements are repeated. *Probability* is a statistical term, on a numerical scale, 0 to 1 or 0 to 100. A zero probability means that the assertion (e.g. that the difference is due to chance alone) is completely unjustified whereas 100% probability, means that the assertion is definitely true. To test the assertion (the Null hypothesis) we make calculations which enable us to say how frequently the observed difference would occur if it arose by chance alone. By convention, if the calculations show that a chance occurrence is likely only in 5 or fewer tests out of 100 (i.e. 5% or 0.05 and less probability) the hypothesis is rejected and the difference is described as statistically significant. On the other hand if the calculations show that the difference would occur more frequently than 5 in 100 measurements (5% or 0.05 and greater

Table 3.3   *Interaction of carbachol and pirenzepine at two temperatures in isolated Lizard rectum*

Experiment	pA₂ values at 37 °C		Experiment	pA₂ values at 26 °C	
	X_1	X_1^2		X_2	X_2^2
1	8.20	67.24	1	7.70	59.29
2	7.66	58.68	2	7.65	58.52
3	8.40	70.56	3	7.10	50.41
4	8.15	66.42	4	7.00	49.00
5	7.54	56.85	5	7.40	54.76
6	7.90	62.41	6	8.10	65.61
7	7.66	58.68	7	7.00	49.00
ΣX_1	55.51	ΣX_1^2 440.84	ΣX_2	51.95	ΣX_2^2 386.59

$$\bar{X}_1 = 7.93 \qquad\qquad \bar{X}_2 = 7.42$$

$$V = \frac{\Sigma X_1^2 - \dfrac{(\Sigma X_1)^2}{N}}{N-1} \qquad\qquad V = \frac{\Sigma X_2^2 - \dfrac{(\Sigma X_2)^2}{N}}{N-1}$$

$$= \frac{440.84 - 440.19}{6} \qquad\qquad = \frac{386.59 - 385.54}{6}$$

$$= \frac{0.65}{6} = 0.11 \qquad\qquad = \frac{1.05}{6} = 0.18$$

Standard Deviation (SD) $\qquad$ SD $= (0.18)^{\frac{1}{2}}$
$= (0.11)^{\frac{1}{2}}$ $\qquad\qquad\qquad$ $= 0.42$
$= 0.33$

Standard Error (SE)

$$= \frac{0.33}{7^{\frac{1}{2}}} \qquad\qquad\qquad SE = \frac{0.42}{7^{\frac{1}{2}}}$$

$$= \frac{0.33}{2.64} \qquad\qquad\qquad = \frac{0.42}{2.64}$$

$$= 0.13 \qquad\qquad\qquad\quad = 0.16$$

probability), the hypothesis is upheld and the difference is said to be not statistically significant. To turn to our example, the assertion that the difference in pirenzepine pA_2 values arose by chance alone is tested as follows: first the value of 't' is calculated from the formula,

$$t = \frac{\bar{X}_1 - \bar{X}_2}{SD} \left(\frac{N_1 N_2}{N_1 + N_2}\right)^{\frac{1}{2}} \qquad (3.7)$$

the standard deviation to be used in this formula is calculated as

$$SD = \left(\frac{(X_1 - \bar{X}_1)^2 + (X_2 - \bar{X}_2)^2}{N_1 + N_2 - 2}\right)^{\frac{1}{2}} \qquad (3.8)$$

Notice that the formula combines the sums of the squares of the deviations of individual values from the mean for measurements at 25 and 37°C. This is because the samples are small (7); a better estimate of the variability of pA_2 values for pirenzepine among the universe of lizard rectal muscles, is secured by pooling the variations in the two samples. So, now,

$$SD = \left(\frac{0.65 + 1.05}{12}\right)^{\frac{1}{2}}$$
$$= 0.38$$

Hence $t = \dfrac{7.93 - 7.42}{0.38} \left(\dfrac{49}{14}\right)^{\frac{1}{2}}$

$$= \frac{0.51 \times 1.87}{0.38}$$
$$= 2.51$$

From the 't' table, the value of 't' (at 12 degrees of freedom) is 2.18 for a probability of 0.05, and 3.05 for a probability of 0.01. The calculated 't' falls between these values. This means that a difference between pA_2 values as great or greater would occur by chance only between 5 in 100 and 1 in 100 similar determinations if temperature had no effect on the nature of the muscarinic receptors in lizard rectal muscle. The null hypothesis is rejected and the difference between pirenzepine pA_2 values at 26°C and 37°C is described as statistically significant. The result is stated as follows: In the isolated rectal muscle preparation of the rainbow lizard, the pA_2 of pirenzepine is significantly greater at 37°C than at 26°C (Student's 't' test. P<0.05).

While this level of significance is good enough to encourage investigations into the way temperature changes may modify muscarinic receptors in the rectal muscle of this reptile, a higher level of significance would enable the experimenter to reach a firmer conclusion. A level of significance with P<0.01 is said to be *statistically highly significant* and P<0.001 is *statistically very highly significant*.

Test of significance of difference between means from large samples

The '*t*' test just described is adequate for most tests of significance in pharmacology in which the sample from which the means are calculated is usually less than 20. For samples of the size of 30 or more the '*t*' value is calculated from the formula

$$t = \frac{\bar{X}_1 - \bar{X}_2}{[(SE_1)^2 + (SE_2)^2]^{1/2}} \tag{3.9}$$

where $\bar{X}_1$ and $\bar{X}_2$ represent the higher and lower means respectively and SE_1 and SE_2 are their respective standard errors. In this case since the samples are large, the separate errors are good estimates of the variability of individual values in the population from which the samples are taken.

Paired test

Many measurements in pharmacology are of the 'before and after' type. The following example illustrates this sort of measurement. The aim of this particular experiment was to find out whether the antihypertensive drug guanfacine lowered plasma noradrenaline. If it did, the fact would be evidence that the drug interfered with sympathetic nerve activity as its mechanism of action. Guanfacine is an alpha2-(prejunctional) agonist. Five patients suffering from essential hypertension were hospitalised for six days and plasma noradrenaline was measured in each patient daily for three days before the onset of treatment with guanfacine and for three further days during the treatment. The data shown in Table 3.4 are for day 3 before the commencement of treatment and day 6 (three days after the start of treatment). In this study, the experimental group served as its own control. In such cases, the test for the significance of the difference between the means of the 'before' and 'after' treatment values is somewhat complicated due to possible correlation between the measurements. For example, patient 4 with the highest plasma noradrenaline before treatment also had the highest level after treatment. Because of the existence of this factor in this kind of measurement the test of significance of difference

Table 3.4 *Plasma noradrenaline in patients with essential hypertension before and after three days of treatment with guanfacine*

Subject	Plasma noradrenaline $(nmol\ L^{-1})$	
	Before treatment	After treatment
1	1.89	0.54
2	1.50	0.63
3	2.47	1.70
4	7.39	2.11
5	4.14	0.66

Data taken with permission from Manhem & Hökfelt, *Br. J. Clin. Pharmac.*, **10** suppl. 1, 109s–114s (1980).

between the means is slightly different from the one we have just described and is called the paired test. This test is actually an analysis of the differences ($\bar{d}$) between the 'before' and 'after' measurements. The average of the differences ($\bar{d}$) is obtained and tested to see if it is significantly different from zero. Clearly, if the treatment has had no effect, the average difference should be not significantly different from zero. The procedure for this is shown below (see Table 3.5) using the guanfacine/plasma noradrenaline data.

At 4 degrees of freedom, a 't' value of 2.78 represents a probability (P) of 0.05. The calculated 't' (2.52) is less which means that there is a greater than 5% probability that the 'before' and 'after' difference in plasma noradrenaline can occur by chance alone. The Null hypothesis is upheld and the conclusion is that the difference in plasma noradrenaline before and after treatment with guanfacine is not statistically significant (paired 't' test, P$>$0.05). This should not be taken as the last word on the effect of guanfacine on plasma noradrenaline. The lack of significance in this particular set of measurements does not prove that guanfacine does not reduce plasma noradrenaline in patients with essential hypertension. The problem is that encountered with small samples. The interested reader may consult the original paper where the authors in fact conclude that guanfacine reduces plasma noradrenaline after considering other data.

Table 3.5   *Analysis of data in Table 3.4*

Subject no.	Noradrenaline (nmol l⁻¹) Before treatment	After treatment	d	$d - \bar{d}$	$(d - \bar{d})^2$
1	1.89	0.54	+1.35	−0.4	0.16
2	1.50	0.63	+0.87	−0.88	0.77
3	2.47	1.70	+0.77	−0.98	0.96
4	7.39	2.11	+5.28	+3.53	12.46
5	4.14	0.66	+3.48	+1.73	2.99
Total	17.39	5.64	11.75		17.34
Mean	3.48	1.13	2.35($\bar{d}$)		

The standard deviation of the differences is

$$SD = \left(\frac{\Sigma(d - \bar{d})^2}{N - 1} \right)^{1/2}$$

$$= \left(\frac{17.34}{4} \right)^{1/2}$$

$$= 2.08$$

The standard error of the mean difference

$$SE_{\bar{d}} = \frac{SD}{N^{1/2}}$$

$$= \frac{2.08}{2.23}$$

$$= 0.93$$

$$t = \frac{\bar{d}}{SE_{\bar{d}}} \qquad \text{(where } \bar{d} = d/N = 2.35)$$

$$= \frac{2.35}{0.93}$$

$$= 2.52$$

Statistical analysis of a 2 × 2 assay

It was pointed out earlier that in the design of a 2 × 2 assay, the doses of test and standard should be chosen such that the responses are within about 20 to 80% of the maximum. The ratio of high to low dose (d_2/d_1) should be same for test and standard and the test must be compared with a standard of identical pharmacological activity. Then plots of log dose (volume) versus mean response for standard and test should produce two straight lines which should be parallel as in Fig. 3.4. Assuming the mean response ($\bar{X}$) to a dose d_1 of drug is a linear function of log d_1, then

$$\bar{X} = b \log d_1 + a \tag{3.10}$$

where b is the slope of the line and a is a constant.

Two tests are important in this sort of assay, namely, a test for parallelism and determination of the limits of the relative potency (M).

Test for parallelism

For M (Fig. 3.4) to be a valid measure of the relative potencies of standard and test, the slopes of the two lines must be identical or differ by not more than can be expected from chance error in the mean responses. If they do, the assay is not valid and there are many practical reasons why this can happen. To test for parallelism the value of b in equation (3.10) is calculated for standard and test.

$$b = \frac{T_2 - T_1}{\log (d_2/d_1)} \tag{3.11}$$

where T_2 and T_1 are mean responses to high and low doses of test, and for the standard,

$$b = \frac{S_2 - S_1}{\log (d_2/d_1)} \tag{3.12}$$

The British Pharmacopoeia represents log (d_2/d_1) with the letter I and the best estimate of b is the arithmetic mean of the b values for standard and test. Hence

$$b = \frac{1}{2} \left(\frac{S_2 - S_1}{I} + \frac{T_2 - T_1}{I} \right) \tag{3.13}$$

$$= \frac{T_2 - T_1 + S_2 - S_1}{2I}$$

The next quantity we have to calculate is M, the logarithm of the potency ratio.

$$M = \frac{T_1 + T_2 - S_1 - S_2}{2b} \qquad (3.14)$$

The slopes of the two lines are now compred by a 't' test of significance.

$$t = \frac{T_2 - T_1 - S_2 + S_1}{2V^{\frac{1}{2}}} \qquad (3.15)$$

where

$$V = \frac{e_1{}^2 + e_2{}^2 + e_3{}^2 + e_4{}^2}{4}$$

and e is the standard error of the mean response to each of the four doses. Finally the 95% confidence limits of M are given by

$$\pm \frac{t}{b} (V + VM^2/I^2)^{\frac{1}{2}} \qquad (3.16)$$

where t = theoretical value for P = 0.95 at $N - 4$ degrees of freedom (four doses are involved as one degree of freedom is used in the calculation of the mean of the responses to each dose).

The B.P. further recommends that an index of significance (g) be calculated:

$$g = Vt^2/I^2 \, b^2$$

where t = theoretical value for P = 0.95 at $N - 4$ degrees of freedom. If the value of g exceeds 0.1, the formula (3.16) cannot be used for calculation of the limits of M. The experiment may be repeated with a larger N or a more complicated method can be used to calculate the error limits of M. An easily understandable proof of these principles can be found in Saunders & Fleming (1971).

Example

In an assay of acetylcholine on the eserinised isolated rectal muscle of the rainbow lizard, the standard solutions used in the assay were 0.2 ml and 0.4 ml and the test doses were 0.3 ml and 0.6 ml. These doses were applied in a Latin square sequence to the muscle mounted in a 20-ml organ bath until 4 responses to each dose had been recorded on smoked paper. The following results were obtained:

Symbol		Dose (ml)	Contraction heights (mm)			
Test	T_2	0.6	35	24	40	33
	T_1	0.3	13	19	17	19

Standard	S_2	0.4		22	27	39	29
	S_1	0.2		11	16	14	17

What is the potency of the test solution?

The mean and standard errors of the responses to each dose are calculated.

Dose	Mean response	SEM (e)	(e²)
T_2	33	3.34	11.15
T_1	17	1.41	1.98
S_2	29.25	3.56	12.67
S_1	14.5	1.32	1.74

$$I = \log(2) = 0.30$$

$$
b = \frac{T_2 - T_1 + S_2 - S_1}{21}
$$

$$
= \frac{33 - 17 + 29.25 - 14.5}{0.60}
$$

$$
= \frac{51.25}{2}
$$

$$
= 25.6
$$

$$
V = \frac{e_1^2 + e_2^2 + e_3^2 + e_4^2}{4}
$$

$$
= \frac{11.15 + 1.98 + 12.67 + 1.74}{4}
$$

$$
= 6.88
$$

To test the significance of b, that is whether the lines are parallel, t is calculated

$$
t = \frac{T_2 - T_1 - S_2 + S_1}{2V^{\frac{1}{2}}}
$$

$$
= \frac{1.25}{5.25}
$$

$$
= 0.24
$$

At 12 degrees of freedom, the value of t for a probability of 0.05 is 2.18. The calculated t is much smaller than this. Therefore the slopes of the two lines are not significantly different. The assay is valid and M represents the log relative potency of the test solution. Now,

$$M = \frac{T_1 + T_2 - S_1 - S_2}{2b}$$

$$= \frac{6.25}{102.5}$$

$$= 0.06$$

The relative potency is antilog M

$$= \text{antilog } 0.06$$

$$= 1.14$$

The index of significance g is now calculated:

$$g = \frac{Vt^2}{I^2 b^2}$$

$$= \frac{6.88 \times (2.18)^2}{(0.3)^2 \times (51.25)^2}$$

$$= \frac{32.69}{236.39}$$

$$= 0.14$$

Since g is greater than 0.1, the formula (3.16) cannot be used to determine the limits of M. The more complicated formula must be used. This is

$$\frac{gN}{1-g} \pm \frac{t}{b(1-g)} \, (V(1-g) + VM^2/I^2)^{\frac{1}{2}} \tag{3.17}$$

Substituting in (3.17), the 95% confidence limits are

$$\frac{0.14 \times 0.06}{0.86} \pm \frac{2.18}{51.25 \times 0.86} \, (6.88 \times 0.86 + 6.88 \, M^2/0.09)^{\frac{1}{2}}$$

$$= \frac{0.0084}{0.86} \pm 0.049 \, (5.91 + 0.27)^{\frac{1}{2}}$$

$$= 0.0097 \pm 0.12$$

The limits of M are $0.0097 + 0.12$ and $0.0097 - 0.12$, that is
  0.13 and -0.11

Taking antilogarithms, antilog $0.13 = 1.34$ and antilog $- 0.11 = 0.7762$
Since the standard solution contained 100 ng ml^{-1}, the test solution
contains

$$1.14 \times 100 \text{ ng ml}^{-1}$$
$$= 114 \text{ ng ml}^{-1} (77.62 - 134)$$

95% confidence limits are given in parentheses.

FURTHER READING

Colquhoun, D. (1971). *Lectures in Biostatistics. An introduction to statistics with application in biology and medicine.* Clarendon Press, Oxford.
Fisher, R.A. & Yates, F. (1963). *Statistical Tables for Biological, Agricultural and Medical Research*, 6th edn. Oliver & Boyd, Edinburgh.
Saunders, L. & Fleming, R. (1971). *Mathematics and Statistics for Use in the Biological and Pharmaceutical Sciences.* The Pharmaceutical Press, London.

4

Receptors and drug response

4.1 INTRODUCTION

The objective in this chapter is to enable the reader to acquire some understanding of:

(a) the theoretical and experimental bases for different forms of receptor theory.

(b) the important parameters which are derived from receptor theory and which are frequently used to describe pharmacological properties of drugs and some of the problems which can be encountered in such studies, and

(c) the way in which receptor theory has been applied in receptor classification and drug development.

4.2 AGONISTS AND ANTAGONISTS

The most widely accepted principle in pharmacology is that drugs produce effects by first combining with specific components of the living cell, called receptors, and for different drugs there are different receptors. Figure 4.1 is a simple illustration of the idea. Acetylcholine (ACH) and histamine combine with their respective receptors to contract the isolated guinea-pig ileum. Atropine and mepyramine also combine with these receptors: however, these drugs do not contract the ileum, but while they occupy the receptors, ACH and histamine are prevented from causing the usual contractions. Atropine and mepyramine can be said to behave like the proverbial dog in the manger! Such drugs are called competitive *antagonists*. Those drugs which combine with the receptor and cause the cell to respond (contraction or relaxation of muscle or glandular secretion) are called *agonists*.

4.3 FACTS WHICH SUPPORT THE NOTION OF RECEPTORS

Receptors for most drugs are known only by their pharmacological properties. Very little is known about their physicochemical properties. Nevertheless several facts support the notion of receptors. For example, many drugs act at very high dilutions, e.g. in nanomole concentrations or less. At such low concentrations, we assume that the drug evokes cellular responses by combining with highly sensitive recognition sites on the cell membrane. Furthermore, small changes in chemical structure can lead to profound changes (quantitative and qualitative) in biological activity (Table 4.1a,b), and optical, isomers of

Fig. 4.1. Specificity of drug action. Isometric contractions were elicited in two isolated segments of guinea-pig ileum with 400 ng each of histamine (H) and acetylcholine (ACH). At the arrows, atropine (A, upper trace) or mepyramine (M, lower trace), each $10^{-9}M$, was included in the physiological salt solution. Atropine considerably reduced ACH contractions, but left H contractions unaffected. Mepyramine did the reverse. Calibrations: Vertical, 1 g tension; horizontal, time 30 s.

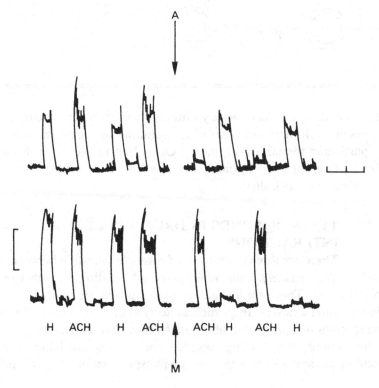

Table 4.1a   *Structure – activity relationships – catecholamines*

Drug	Activity	
	Vasoconstriction	Bronchodilation
Noradrenaline	high	low

HO—(ring)—CH–CH$_2$NH$_2$ / OH ; HO

Adrenaline	intermediate	intermediate

HO—(ring)—CH–CH$_2$–NH · CH$_3$ / OH ; HO

Isoprenaline	low	high

HO—(ring)—CH–CH$_2$–NH–CH(CH$_3$)CH$_3$ / OH ; HO

the same drug can have widely different potencies. The theory therefore is that cells have receptors which contain specific chemical groups
in particular spatial arrangements. Only drug molecules with complementary groups appropriately arranged can react with the receptors
to activate or block them.

4.4   TYPES OF BONDS IN DRUG – RECEPTOR INTERACTIONS

There are three main types of reversible binding between drug
and receptor, namely, ionic, ion-dipole and bonding through Van der
Waals forces. These are low-energy bonds which are easily broken so
that the interaction of drugs such as acetylcholine and histamine with
the receptor is rapidly reversible. On the other hand, a covalent bond is
a high-energy bond. Drug–receptor interactions involving covalent
bonding are irreversible. Examples are phosphorylation of acetylcholine-

Table 4.1b *Structure – activity relationships – cholinergics*

Drug	Activity	
	Agonist or antagonist	Relative agonist potency
Acetylcholine $CH_3 \cdot \underset{\underset{O}{\|\|}}{C}-O \cdot CH_2 \cdot CH_2 \cdot \overset{+}{N}(CH_3)_3$	Agonist	100
Propionylcholine $CH_3 \cdot CH_2 \cdot \underset{\underset{O}{\|\|}}{C}-O \cdot CH_2 \cdot CH_2 \cdot \overset{+}{N}(CH_3)_3$	Agonist	5
Butyrylcholine $CH_3 \cdot CH_2 \cdot CH_2 \cdot \underset{\underset{O}{\|\|}}{C}-O \cdot CH_2 \cdot CH_2 \cdot \overset{+}{N}(CH_3)_3$	Partial agonist	0.5
Valerylcholine $CH_3 \cdot CH_2 \cdot CH_2 \cdot CH_2 \cdot \underset{\underset{O}{\|\|}}{C}-O \cdot CH_2 \cdot CH_2 \cdot \overset{+}{N}(CH_3)_3$	Antagonist	0

sterase by organophosphorus compounds or the alkylation of alpha-adrenoceptors by haloalkylamines (phenoxybenzamine and dibenamine).

4.5 OCCUPATION THEORY OF DRUG–RECEPTOR INTERACTION

In 1937, Clark formulated the theory that the response evoked by an agonist is proportional to the fraction of receptors occupied by agonist molecules. This has become known as *occupation theory*. The occupation of the receptor by a drug molecule is supposed to activate the receptor. When the molecule dissociates from the receptor, the action ceases. The interaction is supposed to be biomolecular and to obey the mass action law. At equilibrium, the fraction of receptors occupied by a given concentration of drug is:

$$p = \frac{1}{1 + 1/K_{aff} d} \tag{4.1}$$

where p = fraction of receptors occupied (proportion of receptors occupied, or the occupancy), K_{aff} = affinity constant for the agonist, and d = molar concentration of drug.

This equation is similar to the Langmuir equation for the absorption of gases onto a monolayer. A graph of occupancy, p, versus d is hyperbolic and a graph of p versus $\log_{10} d$ is sigmoid. In many instances experimental observations are consistent with the theory. Usually, plots of dose or log dose versus response (proportional to occupancy) give a curve of the expected shape. In exceptional cases, dose–response curves are sigmoid; examples of these are given later.

The affinity constant K_{aff}, and pD_2

The affinity constant (K_{aff}) is a measure of how well an agonist binds to the receptor. It is the reciprocal of the dissociation rate constant. It can be described as follows: For a given concentration of agonist, the response, r, is proportional to occupancy, p. If all the receptors are occupied, then $p = 1$, and the response is maximum (r_{max}). Since r is proportional to p, the latter can be estimated by relating r to r_{max}. Thus:

$$p = \frac{r}{r_{max}} \qquad (4.2)$$

For a response equal to 50% of the maximum $p = 0.5$ and $d = d_{50}$ (molar concentration of agonist causing 50% of the maximum response). Substituting these values in equation (4.1) we have

$$1 + K_{aff} d_{50} = 2 \qquad (4.3)$$

and $$K_{aff} = 1/d_{50} \qquad (4.4)$$

The units of K_{aff} are litres per mole, e.g. if d_{50} is 10^{-7} M L^{-1} then K_{aff} is 10^7 L M^{-1}. The affinity constant of an agonist can thus simply be derived from a log dose–response curve. *But this is valid only if the maximum response is equivalent to 100% receptor occupancy.* As will be seen in the section following, some agonists can cause the maximum response by occupying less than the total population of receptors. Therefore this method is not applicable to the measurement of K_{aff} for all agonists.

Furchgott devised a measurement of K_{aff} for agonists in which irreversible antagonists (benzilylcholine mustard (BCM) for muscarinic receptors and haloalkylamines for alpha-adrenoceptors) are used to progressively reduce the population of receptors. The value of d_{50} used in the calculation of K_{aff} is then the limiting value as r_{max} tends to zero.

p^D2

Another quantity frequently encountered in the literature is the *pD2, defined as, the negative logarithm of the molar concentration of agonist causing 50% of the maximum response.* Some investigators use pD2 as a measure of the relative potency of agonists acting at a given receptor but it should be distinguished from affinity constant.

Some difficulties with occupation theory

In general, the theory is adequate in explaining many observations in pharmacology. For example, the response is usually found to increase with increasing dose, up to a maximum, and dose–response or log dose–response plots are usually hyperbolic or sigmoidal. However some other observations are not consistent with this theory.

Full agonists and partial agonists

Not all agonists acting on a given set of receptors can elicit the full maximum response of which the tissue is capable; the maximum response elicited by some agonists is less than that produced by others, even when the dose of the 'weaker' agonist is large enough for 100% receptor occupancy to be presumed to occur. Thus in the guinea-pig ileum, the r_{max} for butyrylcholine is less than the r_{max} for acetylcholine even though both drugs act at muscarinic receptors (see Table 4.1b, p. 83). Acetylcholine is referred to as a full agonist and butyrylcholine as a partial agonist at muscarinic receptors. Another example of a full agonist/partial agonist pair is morphine (full agonist) and nalorphine (partial agonist) at opiate receptors.

Spare receptors

If we construct log dose–response curves to acetylcholine alone and to acetylcholine in the presence of atropine, we find that the line in the presence of atropine is shifted to the right of the line for acetylcholine alone (see Fig. 4.2).

Provided the concentration of atropine is not excessively high, the r_{max} in the presence of the antagonist is of the same magnitude as the r_{max} for acetylcholine alone; the lines are parallel. The agonist line is shifted to the right by the antagonist because the latter occupies some of the receptors, so that the number available to the agonist is reduced and a higher dose of the agonist is now required to produce the same response. This implies that an agonist can produce the maximum response by occupying less than the total number of receptors. Those receptors not occupied by the agonist when producing a maximum response are called *spare receptors.* To make the point even more emphatically, a proportion of muscarinic receptors can be irreversibly inactivated by a drug such as benzilylcholine mustard (BCM) after which acetylcholine can still evoke a maximum response of the same magnitude as before. If the dose of BCM is large or if the period of incubation with the tissue is long, then of course so many more receptors are inactivated that the acetylcholine maximum is now depressed (Fig. 4.3) (Taylor, Cuthbert & Young, 1975).

Dose-response plots are not always hyperbolic

In some instances dose–response curves are sigmoidal rather than hyperbolic. Non-hyperbolic curves have been observed when events close to receptor occupation such as membrane potential change or ionic conductance change are measured. The responses most commonly measured in pharmacology such as muscle contraction are distantly separated from receptor occupation by membrane and biochemical events triggered by drugreceptor combination. A response such as ionic conductance change is directly proportional to the number of ion channels opened and therefore more truly reflects drugreceptor interaction than does muscle tension.

Sigmoidal dose–response curves suggest *cooperative* interactions between drug molecules and the receptor. Cooperativity occurs when the combination of some receptors with drug increases its affinity for other nearby receptors. The best known example of cooperativity is oxygen interaction with haemoglobin.

Fig. 4.2. Effects of atropine on ACH responses in guinea-pig ileum. 0, control DRC; a.b,c. are DRCs in the presence of increasing concentrations of atropine.

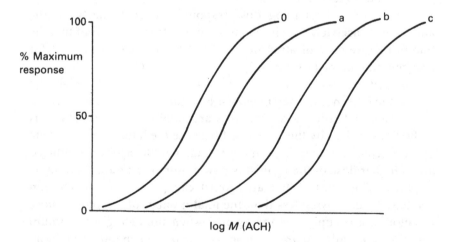

Why are some drugs antagonists?

The theory does not adequately explain why some drugs are agonists, while some others which combine with the same receptors are antagonists, or why some drugs such as nicotine can act as agonists at low concentrations, and as antagonists at high concentrations.

Modifications to occupation theory
Intrinsic activity

In order to explain why some agonists do not produce the full maximum of which the tissue is capable, Ariens introduced the idea of intrinsic activity (α) which he defined as a 'substance constant determining the effect per unit of drug–receptor complex'. Agonists are supposed to have varying capacities to evoke a response after combining with receptor. Agonists capable of producing large effects per unit of drug–receptor complex give rise to the largest maximum response

Fig. 4.3. Progressive inhibition of the contractile response of isolated rat intestine to carbachol after repeated exposure to propylbenzilycholine mustard (Pr BCM). The curve on the left marked 0 was established in the absence of Pr BCM. The muscle strip was thereafter exposed to Pr BCM for 10 min and then washed until a stable DRC could be obtained. Successive 10-min treatments with Pr BCM are shown: (a) 19 nM; (b) 38 nM; (c) 38 nM; (d) 38 nM; (e) 76 nM; (f) 76 nM. The first five curves are parallel. The first *flattened* curve is at a dose-ratio of 700. The last *parallel* curve is at a dose-ratio of 200. Thus the agonist needs to occupy only 0.15 – 0.5% of the available receptors in order to produce a maximum response. (Data redrawn from Taylor, Cuthbert & Young, 1975, with permission.)

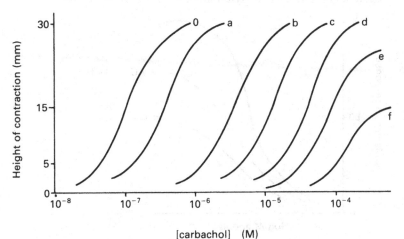

which the tissue can produce. These are called full agonists and have α = 1. Some other agonists acting at the same receptors may evoke lower effects per unit of drug receptor complex and hence have lower r_{max} than the r_{max} for full agonists. These have α<1. The intrinsic activity of a partial agonist is defined as:

$$(r_{max} \text{ of partial agonist})/(r_{max} \text{ of full agonist})$$

Partial agonists reduce the r_{max} of a full agonist and are therefore also called dualists (Fig. 4.4). Drugs which produce no effect per unit of drug–receptor complex and therefore do not give rise to a measurable response while combining with the receptor are antagonists with α = 0. Since it is assumed that the maximum response is equivalent to 100% receptor occupancy, *full agonists* are thus those drugs which can produce the maximum response of which the tissue is capable when occupying *all the receptors* while partial agonists are those which produce a maximum response of lower magnitude when also occupying *all the receptors*.

Efficacy

The main objection to the idea of intrinsic activity is that the maximum response is supposed to involve all the receptors. It means that every agonist producing the highest maximum response must have an intrinsic activity of unity. If it happened that agonists could produce the maximum response of the highest magnitude by occupy-

Fig. 4.4. Interaction of acetylcholine (ACH) and butyrylcholine (BCH) in isolated guinea-pig ileum. Butyrylcholine is a partial agonist compared to acetylcholine.

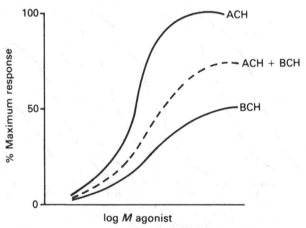

ing different fractions of the receptor population, they could not on Ariens' theory be differentiated from one another. Moreover, the idea that all receptors must be occupied for the maximum response to occur is not consistent with observations that with some agonists, the maximum response is unchanged in the presence of a competitive or irreversible antagonist. To overcome some of these objections, Stephenson introduced the concept of efficacy. Efficacy is a measure of the capacity of the agonist–receptor complex to produce a response. In that respect, efficacy is similar to intrinsic activity conceptually. The critical difference is that in formulating efficacy, it is proposed that full agonists may produce the maximum response by occupying different fractions of the receptor population depending on the efficacy of the agonist. The unit effect of agonist–receptor combination is the biological stimulus (S), defined as:

$$S = ep \qquad (4.5)$$

where e = efficacy, and p = fraction of receptors occupied by the agonist in producing the biological stimulus S.

For a given response, S is constant, and e and p are inversely related. When efficacy is high, p is small, i.e. agonists with a high efficacy need only a small fraction of the receptor population to evoke a maximum response. On the other hand, low efficacy agonists need a large fraction of the receptors to evoke the maximum response. In the rat intestine or guinea-pig ileum for example, carbachol can produce the r_{max} by occupying less than 1% of the muscarinic receptors – 99% of the receptors are spare. The maximum response to butyrylcholine (of lower magnitude than the acetylcholine r_{max} involves 100% occupation of the muscarinic receptors. Agonists which produce low r_{max} when occupying all the receptors are partial agonists, and antagonists are drugs with zero efficacy.

The idea of efficacy allows socalled full agonists to be differentiated on the basis of the fraction of receptors needed for the maximum response. Secondly, we see that the response is determined by two sets of characteristics, namely the ability of the agonist–receptor complex to evoke a stimulus which is a property of the agonist, and the receptor population of the responding tissue. This distinction allows us to account for inter-tissue differences in agonist action.

4.6   RATE THEORY

In 1961, Sir William Paton proposed the theory that the response of a given organ to a drug is proportional to the rate of drugreceptor combination. The basic elements of the theory are: The combination of a drug molecule with the receptor gives rise to a 'quantum' of excitation. The observed response is a summation of the 'quanta of excitations' produced by many drug–receptor combinations. The excitation is short-lived, even though the drug may remain combined with the receptor after expiry of the excitation. The peak of the excitation therefore occurs at the moment when the drug molecule first 'hits' the receptor, after which the excitation fades; much the same way as the note produced by striking the key of a piano might fade from its highest peak even though the key remains depressed. The response to an agonist is thus dependent on the number of drug–receptor combinations occurring in unit time, i.e. the response is proportional to the rate of drug–receptor combination. Paton showed from considerations of the mass action law that the rate of drug–receptor combination is directly proportional to the dissociation rate constant. What this means is that the chances of a drug molecule 'hitting' a free receptor are high if the drug also dissociates rapidly from the receptor after combination. Drugs are thus described as full agonists, partial agonists or antagonists in terms of their dissociation rate constants at a given receptor. Full agonists have high dissociation rate constants, partial agonists have intermediate rates, and antagonists have low rates of dissociation.

Experimental observations

The experimental observation that the action of agonists is quickly terminated by washing out the drug whereas antagonist action often persists long after the drug is removed from the surrounding fluid, is consistent with the theory. Another observation which supports the theory is that in general, antagonist molecules are larger than agonist molecules (see Fig. 4.5). Also by increasing the length of the acetyl moiety in the ACH molecule, the agonist activity of the molecule diminishes and the antagonistic tendency increases as the substituent groups become bulkier (see Table 4.1). The interaction of the large molecule with the receptor involves more different types of bonds than the receptor interaction with the agonist and this may decrease antagonist rate of dissociation.

4.7   COOPERATIVE MODELS OF DRUG–RECEPTOR INTERACTIONS

Classical receptor theories do not account adequately for the observations that when a response such as ionic conductance is measured, the relationship between drug concentration and response may be sigmoidal rather than hyperbolic. The latter is what would be expected if each receptor was separate and reacted independently with a drug molecule, whereas a sigmoid curve implies that cooperative mechanisms may be operating. The way to test for cooperativity is to construct what is known as a Hill plot, the equation for which may be written as:

$$\log \frac{r}{r_{max} - r} = n \log d - \log k$$

Fig. 4.5. Molecular structures of some agonists and their specific antagonists.

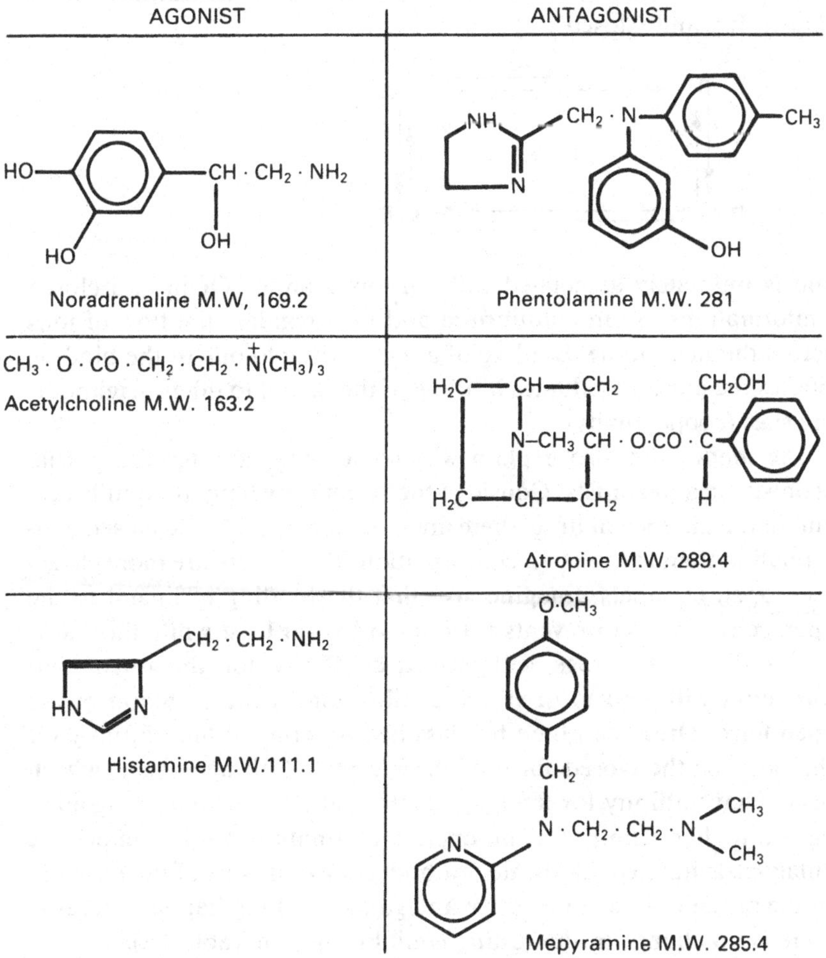
AGONIST
ANTAGONIST
Noradrenaline M.W, 169.2
Phentolamine M.W. 281
CH3 · O · CO · CH2 · CH2 · N(CH3)3
Acetylcholine M.W. 163.2
Atropine M.W. 289.4
Histamine M.W.111.1
Mepyramine M.W. 285.4

where r = response, d = molar concentration of agonist, r_{max} = maximum response, n = number of receptor sites activated by one agonist molecule, and k = a constant. To test for cooperative interactions,

$$\log\left(r/r_{max} - r\right) \text{ is plotted against } \log d.$$

The slope (Hill slope or Hill coefficient) is equal to n. When the Hill slope is 1, the receptors are separate, independent and no mutual interaction takes place between them. Hill slopes of greater than 1 suggest cooperativity. Sigmoid ionic conductance curves usually give Hill slopes of about 2 rather than 1.

To explain the experimental observations, cooperative models have been proposed. One such model views the receptor protein macromolecule as consisting of subunits (drug binding sites) symmetrically disposed in a cluster. The cluster exists in one of two conformations (Open, Ro, and Closed Rc)

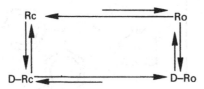

and is intimately associated with an ion channel. Open and closed conformations are in equilibrium and they regulate the flow of ions across the membrane. Binding of a ligand drug to one of the binding sites in the cluster facilitates binding of the ligand to other neighbouring sites (cooperativity).

The model can also explain why some drugs are agonist, partial agonists or antagonists. Consider the situation where at equilibrium and in the absence of drug, there are more receptors in the closed conformation than in the open conformation. Then, there are more closed than open channels. Imagine also that the binding of ligand to the open conformation prevents it from closing (at least while the site is occupied). Then, drugs with selective affinity for the open conformation will tend to drive the equilibrium in the direction of the open form. Drugs can then be classified in terms of their affinity for the open or the closed form of the receptor. Full agonists (high efficacy) have affinity for the open conformation only, partial agonists have a higher affinity for the open conformation, while competitive antagonists have equal affinity for both conformations of the receptor. In the presence of a competitive antagonist, nothing happens because there is no change in the resting equilibrium (see Table 4.2).

Table 4.2 *Classification of drugs in a cooperative allosteric model in which open (Ro) and closed (Rc) forms of the receptor are in equilibrium*

Drug type	Affinity for receptor (K)	Efficacy
Full agonist	Selective affinity for Ro	High
Partial agonist	$K_{Ro} > K_{Rc}$	Intermediate
Antagonist	$K_{Ro} = K_{Rc}$	Nil

4.8 MEASUREMENT OF DRUG ANTAGONISM BY THE NULL METHOD

The following method used in the quantitative measurement of drug antagonism was devised by Schild. It is referred to as the Null Method because it utilises ratios of submaximal responses produced by agonist before and in the presence of competitive antagonist; no assumption is made about the quantitative relationship of response to receptor activation; only that equal submaximal responses with or without antagonist must involve the same numbers of receptors.

In competitive antagonism (that is where the antagonist does nothing more than occlude the receptor) the antagonist reduces the agonist response, but a response of the same size can be produced by increasing the agonist concentration. Thus, competitive antagonism is also called surmountable antagonism. Suppose at a molar concentration d, an agonist produces the response, r; we have seen that the fraction p, of receptors occupied in doing so is given by:

$$p = \frac{1}{1 + 1/K_{aff}\, d}$$

Suppose, a competitive antagonist is added at a concentration b. The concentration of agonist needed to produce the same response, r, must now be increased to d_1. At this new concentration, the fraction of receptors occupied by agonist molecules is now

$$p_1 = \frac{1}{1 + 1/K_{aff}d + K_B\, b/K_{aff}d_1} \tag{4.6}$$

where K_B = affinity constant for the antagonist and b = antagonist molar concentration. It helps to point out that K_B and b on the right-hand side of the equation will tend to reduce p_1 as their values increase.

A submaximal response has to be a function of the number of receptors occupied by the agonist even though we may not all agree on the precise relationship between response and p. If two different concentrations, d and d_1, of the agonist produce identical submaximal responses without and with antagonist present, the responses can be presumed to involve the same numbers of receptors, and hence the same fraction of the population of receptors. Then, $p = p_1$, and

$$\frac{1}{1 + 1/K_{aff}d} = \frac{1}{1 + 1/K_{aff}\,d_1 + K_B b/K_{aff}\,d_1} \tag{4.7}$$

and

$$1 + 1/K_{aff}\,d = 1 + 1/K_{aff}\,d_1 + K_B b/K_{aff}\,d_1 \tag{4.8}$$

From which

$$\frac{1}{d} = \frac{1}{d_1}(1 + K_B b) \tag{4.9}$$

and

$$d_1/d = 1 + K_B b \tag{4.10}$$

Where d_1/d is the *dose ratio*, usually denoted by x. For all effective concentrations of antagonist $x>1$.

From equation (4.10)

$$K_B b = x - 1$$

$$b = \frac{x - 1}{K_B}$$

and

$$\log b = \log (x - 1) - \log K_B \tag{4.11}$$

and

$$-\log b = \log K_B - \log (x - 1) \tag{4.12}$$

Schild defined the quantity pA_x as equal to $-\log b$; *that is the pA_x is the negative logarithm of the molar concentration of antagonist which causes the agonist concentration to be increased x-fold in order that the agonist may produce the same submaximal response as it did without the antagonist.* Substituting pA_x in equation (4.11) and rearranging terms we have

$$pA_x = \log K_B - \log (x - 1) \tag{4.13}$$

What is frequently measured is pA_2, where $x = 2$

Then, $pA_2 = K_B \tag{4.14}$

That is, in a simple competitive antagonism, the pA_2 gives a measure of the affinity constant of the antagonist.

When $x = 10$, $pA_{10} = \log K_B - \log 9$ (4.15)
Since $pA_2 = \log K_B$,
    $pA_{10} = pA_2 - \log 9$ and
    $pA_2 - pA_{10} = \log 9$ or 0.95 (4.16)

The relationship in (4.16) is sometimes applied as a test of competitive antagonism.

The Schild plot and uses of pA_2

A log dose–response curve is constructed in the absence of antagonist and parallel curves are constructed in the presence of increasing concentrations of competitive antagonist (Fig. 4.6). The dose ratio values (x) obtained with different antagonist concentrations (b) are then used. A plot of $-\log b$ on the abscissa and $\log (x - 1)$ on the ordinate gives a straight line whose intercept on the abscissa corresponds to the pA_2 of the antagonist. This is known as the Schild plot. This method is widely used in the quantitative measurement of relative strengths of different antagonists at a given receptor. Where the antagonism is known to be of simple competitive type, an estimate of the pA_2 can be made from one dose ratio since in that case

$$pA_2 = \log (x - 1) - \log b \qquad (4.17)$$

The pA_2 value has the following properties:

(a) It is a measure of the antagonist potency of a drug. For instance, at histamine H_1-receptors, pA_2 for mepyramine, diphenhydramine and atropine are 9.5, 8.5 and 5.5 respectively. Mepyramine is 10 times more potent than diphenhydramine and 10,000 times more potent than atropine at these receptors.

(b) The measurement uses the ratios of agonist doses for equal responses in the presence and in the absence of antagonist. Therefore the antagonist pA_2 is independent of the agonist potency (see Table 4.3).

The Schild method is suitable for measurements of *competitive reversible antagonism*, where, in the presence of antagonist, the log dose–response curve is shifted to the right in parallel to the control curve. The antagonist reversibly binds the site with which the agonist interacts and the latter is occluded. There are other types of antagonistic interactions, for instance *competitive irreversible* in which the antagonist, e.g. benzilylcholine mustard at muscarinic receptors or phenoxybenzamine at alpha-adrenoceptors, covalently binds the receptor and therefore inactivates it. In this instance, parallel shifts can be obtained

Fig. 4.6. Schild Plots.

(A) Log dose–response curves for agonist alone (0) and in the presence of increasing concentrations of antagonist (a, b, c, d). The dose ratios (x) at 50% maximum response for each antagonist concentration are $\dfrac{d_a}{d_o}$, $\dfrac{d_b}{d_o}$ etc.

(B) The plot of log (x-1) versus the negative log of the molar concentration of antagonist (-log b) corresponding to the x value, gives a straight line with intercept on the -log b axis = pA_2 of the antagonist and a slope = 1 (see text).

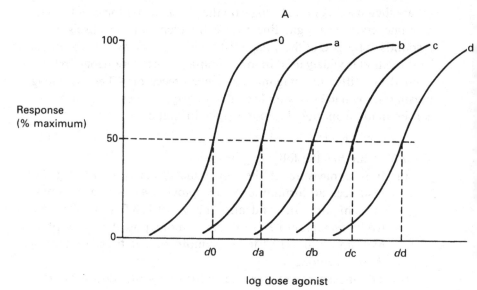

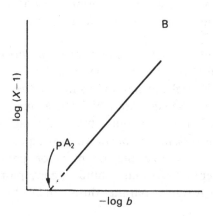

Table 4.3 *pA₂ values of mepyramine in guinea-pig ileum*

Histamine analogue	Relative activity at H_1- receptors (Histamine = 100)	pA_2	
		Analogue	Histamine
N-Benzylhistamine	10	9.3	9.3
N-N-Diethylhistamine	1	9.3	9.3
Pyrazoleethylamine	0.06	9.8	9.7
2-Pyridylethylamine	3.00	9.7	9.7
4-Pyridylethylamine	0.01	9.7	9.8

Data from Schild (1968), p. 265 with permission.

Note that although the histamine analogues were several times less potent than histamine, the pA_2 values for mepyramine determined with these compounds were the same as those determined with histamine.

with low doses of antagonist interacting briefly with the tissue, but with high doses or prolonged contact, sufficient numbers of receptors are inactivated to cut down the agonist r_{max} so that the curves are no longer parallel to the control (see page 87). In *non-competitive antagonism*, the antagonist does not interact directly with the agonist receptor, but with an adjacent site (allosteric site) in such a way that a fruitful agonist-receptor interaction is prevented. A parallel shift of the curve is not observed. Rather, there is a depression of the r_{max}.

Competitive and non-competitive antagonism may also be differentiated by doing a double reciprocal plot on the dose–response curve data. This is analogous to a Lineweaver - Burke plot in enzyme kinetics. The reciprocals of the responses are plotted against the reciprocals of the corresponding doses (not the log dose) (see Fig. 4.7). If the graphs intercept on the ordinate (y axis) the antagonism is competitive. Competitive irreversible antagonists may not obey this rule. If the graphs intercept on the abscissa (x axis) the antagonism is non-competitive.

4.9   LABELLING RECEPTORS

Much of what we know about receptors comes from indirect pharmacological measurements. In recent years, methods have been developed by which the receptor may be studied directly. One approach is to bind a radioactive ligand to the receptor in whole tissue, tissue slices or membrane fragments. This allows the amount of receptor material and the affinity of ligand for the receptor to be determined. The location of the receptor in whole organ can also be determined by autoradiography.

The first experiment of this sort done by Paton & Rang (1965) used radioactive atropine to bind muscarinic receptors in longitudinal muscle strips of the guinea-pig ileum. They identified specific binding to muscarinic receptors at low atropine concentrations. Specific saturation (maximum uptake) was 180 pmol/g wet weight of muscle. This was equivalent to the total amount of receptor material present in the tissue. The affinity constant for atropine (reciprocal of molar concentration for 50% saturation of receptor sites) was about 10^9 L M^{-1}. Since this was similar to values for affinity constant obtained from measurements of pharmacological antagonism, this was evidence that atropine indeed bound specifically to muscarinic receptors. Moreover, uptake of atropine was inhibited by low concentrations of other muscarinic receptor antagonists but not by antagonists of other receptors. Radio ligand binding is now a routine technique in receptor studies.

If the aim is to isolate the receptor material, then the radioactive ligand should bind irreversibly with the receptor, so that homogenisation, centrifugation and fractionation processes do not dislodge the ligand from its binding site. The most successful irreversible ligands so far used for this purpose are benzilylcholine mustard (Fig. 4.8), for the iso-

Fig. 4.7. Double reciprocal plots of agonist dose versus responses in the absense (0) and presence (a) of antagonist. (A) competitive antagonism; (B) non-competitive antagonism. In either case, the affinity constant of the agonist (K_{aff}) is as shown.

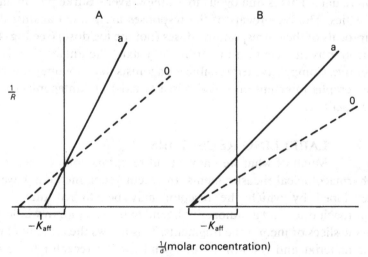

lation of muscarinic receptor material from smooth muscle and alphabungarotoxin for nicotinic receptors in skeletal muscle and electric fish organs. From such studies it is deduced that the nicotinic receptors in skeletal muscle and electric fish organs are similar proteins with molecular weights of about 250000. Other membrane receptors are probably also protein-like molecules.

4.10   RECEPTOR ACTIVATION AND CELL RESPONSE

The events following receptor activation are complex but usually involve a change in permeability of the cell membrane to ions. The most widely studied membrane in this regard is the motor endplate where stimulation of the nicotinic receptor causes a large increase in permeability to potassium and sodium ions. Katz has estimated that the ion channels open for approximately 1 ms and permit the net influx of 50000 univalent ions per channel. The nicotinic receptor thus appears to be directly coupled to an ion channel or a permease whose properties change when acetylcholine combines with the receptor. On the other hand, adrenoceptors appear to be coupled directly to the membrane enzymes, adenylcyclase or guanyl cyclase which become activated when the receptor interacts with agonist. Cyclic nucleotides formed from ATP then control subsequent ion movements. Calcium movement is triggered by agonist receptor interaction in, for example, blood vessels and myocardium.

4.11   RECEPTOR TYPING AND SUBTYPING

It was known from the classical experiments of Dale that the pressor response to adrenaline in the anaesthetised cat can be reversed to a depressor response by prior administration of ergot extract (see Fig. 4.9). The pressor effect of adrenaline is due to stimulation of alpha

Fig. 4.8. Benzilylcholine mustard.

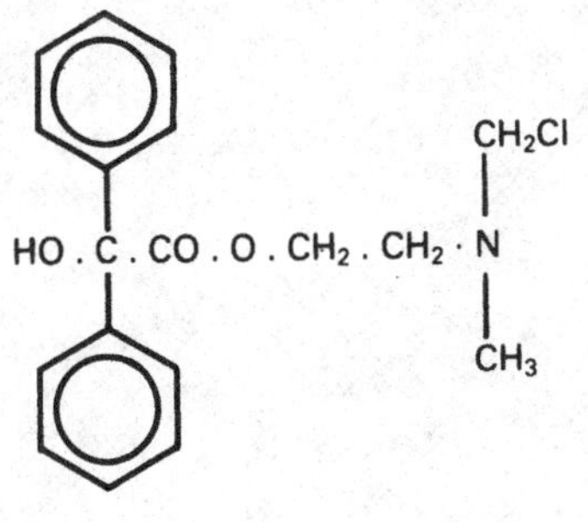

$$\text{HO . C . CO . O . CH}_2\text{ . CH}_2 \cdot \text{N}$$

with attached CH_2Cl and CH_3 groups on the nitrogen.

Fig. 4.9. Pithed cat, carotid blood pressure. Upper trace 0.025 mg adrenaline before, and lower trace, 0.1 mg adrenaline after, 10 mg ergotoxine, (Taken from Dale, H.H. , 1913, *J. Physiol.* XLVI, 291–300, with permission of the publishers).

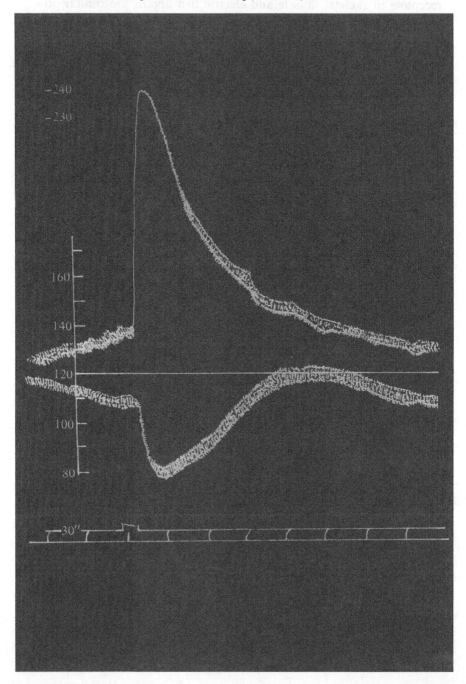

adrenoceptors present in resistance blood vessels in the skin, and in the viscera. The depressor effect is due to stimulation of beta-adrenoceptors present in blood vessels of skeletal muscles, coronary circulation and pulmonary circulation. Both types of receptors are always stimulated when adrenaline is injected into the blood stream, but in the absence of a drug like ergotoxine, the pressor effect overrides the depressor effect. Ergotoxine blocks the alpha adrenoceptors and the depressor effect is then unmasked.

The idea that one agonist can stimulate different types of receptors to produce different types of responses is useful in the development of highly selective drugs. Being able to tell what type of receptor is involved in a tissue or organ response, or what type of receptor is being activated or blocked by a given agonist or antagonist is an important aspect of pharmacological knowledge. There are two major approaches to receptor typing or classification.

The use of agonists

The first study which showed clearly that adrenaline has effects at two distinct types of receptors was by Ahlquist (1948) and he used agonist drugs. The theoretical basis for using agonists to classify receptors can be stated as follows:

If you take a number of compounds structurally related to adrenaline and measure their individual activities in different organs, the drugs should have the same rank order of potency in these organs, if the responses are mediated by the same receptor. If the receptors mediating the response in one organ are different from those in another, then there should be wide inter-organ differences in rank orders of potency. It is supposed that agonist potency is a reflection of how well the molecule interacts with the receptor. If the structural modification decreases the agonist potency for one response and increases it for another, then the two responses must be mediated by different receptors.

Ahlquist's classification of adrenoceptors

The point is illustrated by Ahlquist's work. He measured the activity ratios of dl-noradrenaline, dl-methylnoradrenaline, l-adrenaline, dl-adrenaline, dl-methyladrenaline and dl-isoprenaline in tissues from cats, dogs, rats and rabbits. When he measured vasocontriction, uterine contraction, nictitating membrane contraction, dilator pupillae contraction, urethral contraction, and relaxation of intestinal muscle, the rank order of potency was: l-adrenaline, dl-adrenaline, dl-noradrenaline, dl-methylnoradrenaline, dl-methyladrenaline, dl-iso-prenaline.

But when he measured vasodilation, uterine relaxation, and myo-cardial stimulation he found the rank order of potency to be different. Isoprenaline was now the most potent: isoprenaline, l-adrenaline, methyladrenaline, dl-adrenaline, methylnoradrenaline, noradrenaline.

Ahlquist named the receptors for the first set of responses, alpha adrenotropic receptors (later called alpha-adrenoceptors) and the receptors for the second set of responses, where isoprenaline was most potent, beta-adrenotropic receptors (beta adrenoceptors). He arranged adrenoceptor functions according to the accompanying table (Table 4.4). Ahlquist's classification of adrenoceptors into alpha and beta types has been repeatedly verified and confirmed and remains a major basis for drug development. It is useful to consider two further ex-amples.

Schild-Black classification of histamine receptors

In 1966, Ash and Schild measured the activities of several histamine analogues on gastric secretion (rat stomach), inhibition of rat uterine muscle contraction, smooth muscle contraction (guinea-pig ileum). The rank orders of potency of the analogues on gastric secretion and inhibition of rat uterus were similar, suggesting that the receptor types for these effects were similar. In contrast, the rank order for smooth muscle contraction was different. Ash and Schild named the receptor mediating smooth muscle contraction, H_1-receptor, and emphasised that this receptor type was different from the receptor type for acid secretion and uterine muscle relaxation. Six years later in 1972, Black and his colleagues confirmed and extended this finding by discovering that 2-methylhistamine was a relatively selective agonist at H_1-receptors while 4-methylhistamine was selective at the non-H_1-receptors which they named H_2-receptors. The Schild-Black classification has been extensively verified and confirmed by the use of antagonists (see later). Other selective agonists for the two types of receptors are now known, e.g. 2-pyridylethylamine (H_1-receptors) and dimaprit (H_2-receptors). Histamine is a non-selective agonist.

Beta₁ and beta₂ adrenoceptors

In 1967, Lands and his colleagues studied the lipolytic, car-diac, bronchodilator and vasodepressor activities of a series of catecholamines in rats, guinea-pigs, dogs and rabbits. A comparison of activity ratios showed that the beta-adrenoceptors mediating lipolysis

Table 4.4   *Functions associated with each of the two adrenotropic receptors*

Alpha adrenoceptor functions	Beta adrenoceptor functions
Vasoconstriction	Vasodilation
Viscera ⎱ vessels Skin ⎰	Skeletal muscle ⎱ Coronary vessels ⎰ vessels Viscera (few)
Nictitating membrane (contraction)	
Uterus (excitatory)	Myocardium (excitation)
Intestine (inhibition)	Uterus (inhibition)
Ureter (contraction)	Bronchodilation
Dilator pupillae (contraction)	Intestine (inhibition).

and cardiac stimulation were similar and could be distinguished from the receptors mediating bronchodilation and vasodepression. They named the beta-adrenoceptor for the first set of responses, beta 1, and the second, beta 2 adrenoceptor. The classification was confirmed when it was discovered that certain sympathomimetic agonists stimulate beta-adrenoceptors in the bronchioles more effectively than those on the heart. For example, isoprenaline is nearly equally effective in stimulating beta-adrenoceptors on cardiac and bronchiolar muscle. Isoprenaline is some 2500 times more potent than salbutamol in stimulating guinea-pig cardiac muscle; but it is only 6 times more potent than salbutamol in relaxing guinea-pig trachea. Isoprenaline has *specific* action at beta-adrenoceptors but it is not *selective* in differentiating between beta 1 and beta 2 adrenoceptors. Salbutamol and many other sympathomimetics used in the treatment of asthma are selective as agonists at the beta 2 adrenoceptor (see Fig. 4.10).

Alpha 1 and alpha 2 adrenoceptors

Alpha adrenoceptors are also of two types, namely, alpha 1 (present at postsynaptic membranes of smooth muscles, cardiac muscles and glands) and alpha 2 adrenoceptors (present in presynaptic nerve cells and some non-nervous tissues such as platelets and uterine muscle). Postsynaptic alpha 1 receptors mediate the vasoconstrictor actions of catecholamines and presynaptic alpha 2 receptors mediate a negative feedback control of noradrenaline release from sympathetic nerves. Noradrenaline and adrenaline stimulate both types of alpha adrenoceptors. Phenylephrine and methoxamine are alpha 1 agonists whereas clonidine and alpha methylnoradrenaline are selective alpha 2 agonists (Fig. 4.11). These drugs can reduce the amount of noradrenaline released from sympathetic nerves without an effect on the postsynaptic effector cell. Clonidine and alpha-methylnoradrenaline (derived from alpha-methyldopa) probably owe their antihypertensive effects to a reduction of noradrenaline release from sympathetic nerves.

Fig. 4.10. Structures for isoprenaline and beta-2 selective agonists salbutamol and terbulaline.

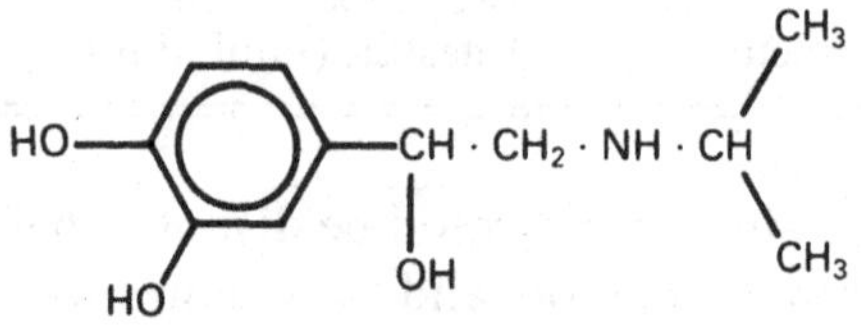

Isoprenaline

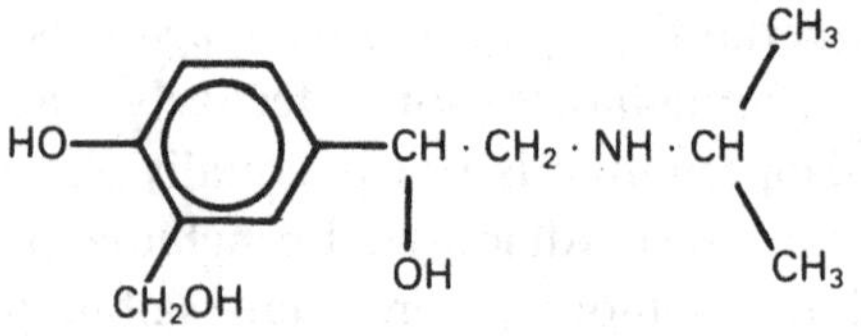

Salbutamol

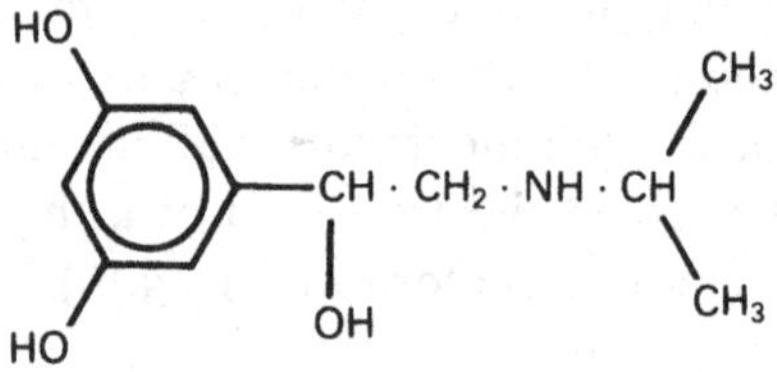

Terbulaline

Fig. 4.11. Alpha-2 adrenoceptor agonists alphamethylnoradrenaline and clonidine.

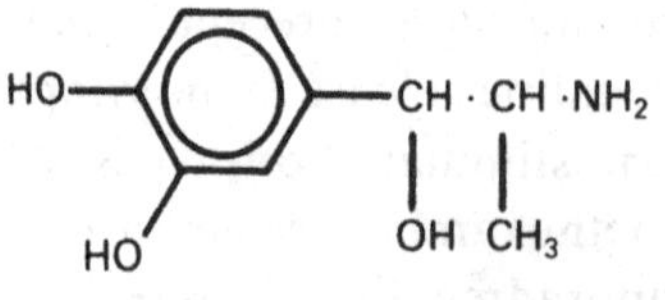

Alpha methylnoradrenaline

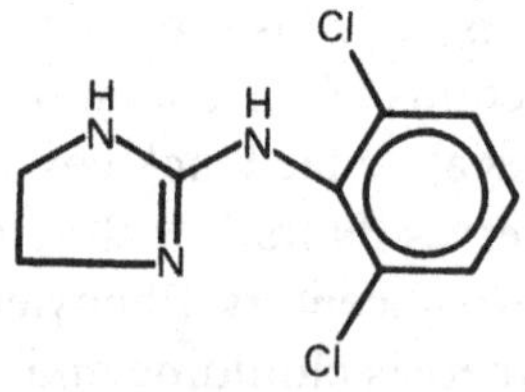

Clonidine

The use of antagonists

A common approach to receptor classification is measurement of the potency of compounds as antagonists at the receptor, the idea being that similar receptors should be antagonised to the same extent by a given antagonist molecule. What is frequently measured is the pA_2 value which in the case of simple competitive antagonism is a measure of antagonist K_B or affinity constant. This method, described on pages 95–96, gives highly reproducible results. It has been successfully applied to characterise receptors and to develop a number of highly selective antagonist drugs. Some examples are given below.

Selective beta₁ antagonists

We have seen that cardiac beta adrenoceptors (beta 1) can be differentiated from, for example, bronchial beta adrenoceptors on the basis of agonist potencies (page 102). This result is confirmed by the finding that practolol is some 100 times more potent in antagonising the effects of isoprenaline in cardiac muscle than in bronchial muscle. Practolol and several other drugs of its type are described as *selective* beta 1 antagonists. Propranolol is equally effective in blocking isoprenaline in both organs. It is said to be *non-selective*, although it is a specific beta adrenoceptor antagonist. The finding that beta 1 and beta 2 adrenoceptors can be differentiated and the subsequent discovery of selective beta 1 antagonists were a significant breakthrough in medicine. The 'cardioselective beta blockers' can be used in the treatment of angina pectoris, hypertension or cardiac arhythmias without the danger of blocking bronchial beta adrenoceptors. When propranolol was used initially for these conditions, the drug precipitated dangerous, sometimes, fatal bronchospasms in asthmatic patients. The mechanism of action of beta blockers in the treatment of cardiovascular disorders, is however, more complex than simple blockade of beta adrenoceptors. The reader should consult a standard text on applied pharmacology for a fuller discussion. Selective beta 2 antagonists have not been developed apparently because there is no obvious clinical indication for such a drug.

Histamine H₂-receptor antagonists

Measurement of antagonist potency has also been used to define histamine H₂-receptors as shown in Table 4.5.

The pA_2 values for burimamide in atrium, rat uterus, rat gastric acid secretion and guinea-pig pulmonary vasodilation are close showing that the receptors are of the same type (H₂) but differ from the type of

Table 4.5   *pA$_2$ values for burimamide tested against histamine and 4-methylhistamine in four mammalian preparations*

Tissue	Agonist	Slope of Schild plot	pA$_2$
Guinea-pig atrium	Histamine	0.98	5.17
Rat uterus	Histamine	0.96	5.11
Rat gastric acid secretion *in vivo*	Histamine	1.07	5.14
Guinea-pig pulmonary vasodilation (in the presence of mepyramine)	4-methyl-histamine	0.95	5.0
Guinea-pig ileum	Histamine	1.32	non-competitive antagonism

receptor mediating histamine contraction of guinea-pig ileum (H$_1$). Other more potent antagonists at the H$_2$-receptor, e.g. cimetidine and ranitidine are used in the treatment of peptic ulcer.

FURTHER READING

Ahlquist, R.P. (1948). A study of adrenotropic receptors. *Am. J. Physiol.* **153**, 586–600.

Arunlakshana, O. & Schild, H.O. (1959). Some uses of drug antagonism. *Brit. J. Pharmacol. Chemotherap.* **14**, 48–58.

Ash, A.S.F. & Schild H.O. (1966). Receptors mediating some actions of histamine. *Brit. J. Pharmacol. Chemotherap.* **27**, 427–39.

Black, J.W., Duncan, W.A.M., Durant, C.J., Ganellin, C.R. & Parsons, E.M. (1972). Definition and antagonism of histamine H$_2$-Receptors. *Nature* **236**, 385–90.

Dale, H.H. (1913). On the action of ergotoxine; with special reference to the existence of sympathetic vasodilators. *J. Physiol.* **46**, 291–300.

Lands, A.M., Arnold, A., McAuliff, J.P., Luduena, F.P. & Brown, T.G. (1967). Differentiation of receptor systems activated by sympathetic amines. *Nature* **214**, 597–8.

Paton, W.D.M. (1961). A theory of drug action based on the rate of drug receptor combination. *Proc. Roy. Soc. B*, **154**, 21–69.

Paton, W.D.M. & Rang, H.P. (1965). The uptake of atropine and related drugs by intestinal smooth muscle of the guinea-pig in relation to acetylcholine receptors. *Proc. Roy. Soc. B*, **163**, 1–44.

Rang, H.P. (1973). Receptor mechanisms. Fourth Gaddum Memorial Lecture, School of Pharmacy, University of London, January 1973. *Br. J. Pharmac.* **48**, 475–95.

Schild, H.O. (1947). *p*A₂, a new scale for the measurement of drug antagonism, *Brit. J. Pharmacol. Chemotherap.* **2**, 189–206.

Schild, H.O. (1968). A pharmacological approach to drug receptors. In *Importance of fundamental principles in drug evaluation*, ed. D.H. Tedeschi & R.E. Tedeschi. Raven Press, New York.

Stephenson, R.P. (1956). A modification of receptor theory. *Br. J. Pharmac.* **2**, 379–93.

Taylor, I.K., Cuthbert, A.W. & Young, M. (1975). Muscarinic receptors in rat intestinal muscle: comparison with the guinea-pig. *European J. Pharmacol.* **31**, 319–26.

PART III
Fundamental Pharmacokinetic Principles
in Drug Disposition

5

Drug administration and factors affecting drug metabolism

5.1   INTRODUCTION

Many adult Nigerian patients prefer an injection to other routes of drug administration. The injection is merely a device by which the drug is delivered into the circulation. So, it should not really matter if the drug is taken by mouth provided absorption is adequate. However, it seems that the needle is perceived by some traditional people as a form of treatment in itself. This brings to mind the point made in chapter 1 that in traditional medicine, the method is as important as the material. The story has frequently been told of the man who suffered intermittent headaches and had been treated by various doctors. On one occasion he insisted on an injection. The doctor dutifully obliged by drawing a few microlitres of sterile distilled water into a syringe in preparation for an intramuscular injection into the buttocks. On being asked to pull down his pants the dignitary had exclaimed indignantly that he had not complained of bottomache but of headache. Again the doctor had obliged by giving the injection subcutaneously in the scalp. We are told that the old man returned later, laden with gifts for the doctor. For the first time in his life, he had had no headaches for months after the doctor's treatment!

This is not a recommendation of the quack's method, for although this particular incident had a happy ending, there are other instances where indiscriminate use of the needle has had disastrous consequences. The point being made is that many traditional patients often wish to be injected. The doctor/pharmacist has a duty to explain carefully that in modern medicine, what is important is that the drug in the preparation enters the circulation and not how it is administered. The dangers of injection especially in the hands of quacks should be borne in mind and explained.

5.2   CHOICE OF ROUTE OF DRUG ADMINISTRATION
Drugs can be administered by various routes after considering such factors as the state of the patient, how critical is the desired time of onset of drug action, the chemical nature of the drug, the duration of action required, how accurate the dose of drug needs to be, available personnel, etc.

State of the patient
If the patient is too ill, the drug has to be given by injection or other route which does not require the patient's active participation. For example, although an asthmatic attack can usually be treated by drugs administered sublingually or by inhalation, in status asthmaticus, intravenous prednisolone or aminophylline may be necessary. Frequent vomiting may make the oral route ineffective, e.g. febrile children who are vomiting may require parenteral chloroquine, but this should be administered with great care as many fatal accidents have happened with chloroquine given in this way.

Onset of action
Inhalation or intravenous (i.v.) injection are the most appropriate routes if a quick onset of action is required. Examples are inhalation of amyl nitrite in angina pectoris, and of salbutamol in asthma. The intravenous route is the most rapid and is used, for example, in the administration of thiopentone in the induction of anaesthesia (great care should be taken not to enter an artery as this can cause necrosis and gangrene of extremities). Drugs with powerful actions on the heart such as isoprenaline must never be administered intravenously. Intramuscular (i.m.) and subcutaneous (s.c.) routes can also be used when a rapid onset is required. The blood supply to skeletal muscle is greater than to cutaneous tissues. Therefore onset of action after the i.m. route is more rapid than after the s.c. route. Another site from which rapid absorption can occur is the sublingual route. Glyceryltrinitrate is administered sublingually for rapid relief of the pain of angina pectoris. Isoprenaline can also be administered in this way to treat bronchial asthma.

Chemical nature of the drug
Some drugs have to be given parenterally; quarternary ammonium compounds such as pentolinium are irregularly absorbed from the gastrointestinal tract. Insulin and penicillin G are destroyed by the high acidity of the stomach, and the enzyme monoamine

oxidase present in the wall of the gut destroys monoamines so that drugs such as adrenaline and noradrenaline are not absorbed from the gut.

Duration of action

When a long duration of action is desired, the drug may be given intramuscularly in the form of a 'depot', e.g. protamine zinc insulin, or implanted subcutaneously in the form of pellets, e.g. deoxycorticosterone acetate (DOCA) implant in the treatment of Addison's disease. The drug is then slowly released into the circulation from the depot over a period of time. Another form of *sustained release* is encountered with drugs such as the long acting sulphonamides, e.g. sulphamethoxypyridazine. These are highly bound to plasma protein from which therapeutic amounts of free drug are slowly released. Renal excretion of the drug is delayed because at any time most of the drug is bound to protein. The action of a drug can also be prolonged by restricting it to its site of action e.g. the use of the vasoconstrictor adrenaline in combination with the local anaesthetic procaine to limit diffusion of the latter after subcutaneous injection.

Control of dose administered

We may wish to adminster a drug continuously until a particular pharmacological effect has been achieved. Inhalation, e.g. of halothane or ether in anaesthesia or intravenous infusion of oxytocin in induction of labour are examples of controlled dose administration.

The first pass effect

Some drugs after absorption from the gastrointestinal tract (GIT) are almost completely inactivated after a single passage through the liver (the first pass effect, see Fig. 5.1). An example is isoprenaline, which is metabolised by catechol-0-methyl transferase and cytochrome P-450 enzymes in the liver. Since all drugs absorbed from the GIT (except those absorbed from the buccal cavity or rectum) must enter the portal circulation, then drugs which undergo extensive first pass metabolism are usually inactive after oral administration. Extensive first pass metabolism is used as an explanation of the relative ineffectiveness of propranolol as an antihypertensive in black people. Note that first pass metabolism can also result in the formation of a more active product (Table 5.1).

For convenience (of patient and doctor) the best route of administration is the oral route. The patient can be instructed to take the drug

Tables 5.1   *Examples of drugs which are activated in the liver*

Drug	Active metabolite	Pharmacological effect of metabolite
Acetylsalicylic acid	salicylic acid	analgesic, antipyretic, anti-inflammatory
Phenacetin	paracetamol	analgesic, antipyretic
Cyclophosphamide	nitrogen mustard	antineoplastic
Azathioprine	6-mercaptopurine	antineoplastic
Prednisone	prednisolone	anti-inflammatory
Proguanil	cycloguanil	anti-malarial

Fig. 5.1. Fate of drugs absorbed from: (a) buccal cavity, (b) gastro-intestinal tract, and (c) rectum. Drugs absorbed from (a) and (c) enter the systemic circulation (e) directly to produce effects at the required sites. Drugs absorbed from (b) must pass through the liver (d) via the portal vein and are subject to first-pass metabolism.

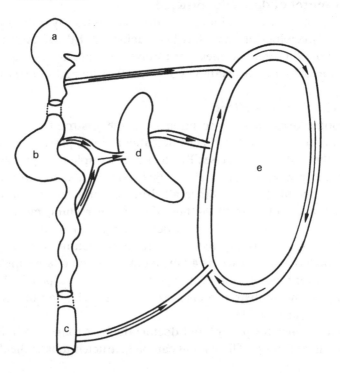

without frequent visits to the hospital which also reduces costs. Unfortunately not all drugs are active after oral administration – some of the reasons for this have already been stated – but the majority are taken by mouth so, much attention is paid to their absorption after oral administration.

5.3 ABSORPTION OF DRUGS FROM THE GASTROINTESTINAL TRACT

Mammalian cell membranes

An important consideration is the absorption of drugs into the general circulation after oral ingestion. Absorption involves passage of the drug across cell membranes. It is therefore useful to describe here the essential features of mammalian cell membranes (Fig. 5.2).

A phospholipid/cholesterol bilayer and a protein layer constitute the framework of the mammalian cell membranes. The hydrophilic (water-attracting) ends of the lipids (complexes of ethanolamine, serine or choline) orientate themselves at both the outer and inner surfaces of a membrane. The hydrophobic (water-repelling) chains of the lipids occupy the centre of the membrane. The integral proteins traverse the entire width of the membrane. Monosaccharide sugars (galactose, mannose), aminosugar derivatives (N-acetylglucosamine) or sialic acids (N-acetylneuraminic acid, NANA) attach to the outer surface of the membrane to form glycoproteins or glycolipids. Also the membrane has the following properties.

(a) Membrane-bound water associated with ionised polar groups such as Ca^{2+}.

(b) Water-filled pores which act as ultrafilters allowing substances

Fig. 5.2. Diagrammatic representation of mammalian cell membrane essential features.

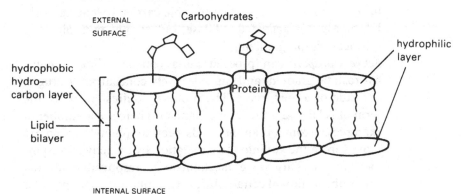

of small molecular weight (up to 100) to diffuse in and out of the cell freely.

(c) Carrier enzyme systems such as Na_+, K_+ – ATPase and other mechanisms for the translocation of cations such as Ca^{2+}, Mg^{2+} across the membrane. Such transport systems can be activated by substances called ionophores, e.g. valinomycin. An additional characteristic is that the charge distribution between the inside and outside of the membrane is uneven giving rise to a potential difference between the two sides. It is therefore possible to electrically excite or inhibit the membrane by interfering with the distribution of charged ions. Most mammalian cell membranes have special components (receptors) which can recognise and bind specific hormones and link extracellular to intracellular events.

Transfer mechanisms at cell membranes

(a) *Diffusion* can take place through water-filled pores. Only substances of limited molecular weight can be transferred in this way, which is called ultrafiltration. Simple diffusion also takes place through the integral protein layer down a concentration gradient, i.e. for the substance to diffuse into the cell, its concentration on the outside of the membrane must be higher than it is on the inside. Another requirement for simple diffusion is lipid solubility. Highly ionised molecules whether they are positively charged, e.g. quaternary ammonium compounds such as $(CH_3)_3$ $N^{(+)}$ – $(CH_2)_6$ –$N^{(+)}$ $(CH_3)_3$ or negatively charged, e.g. acetylsalicylic acid at high pH (see below) attract a shell of water around them. This hinders their passage through the hydrophobic centre of the membrane.

(b) *Facilitated diffusion* takes place at a faster rate than simple diffusion; it involves a specific saturable carrier system e.g. Na^+, K^+ or Mg^{2+} – activated ATPase, but cannot take place *up* a concentration gradient.

(c) *Active transport* can proceed *up* a concentration, osmotic, hydrostatic gradient and can selectively concentrate a drug at one side of a membrane. The process requires energy in the form of ATP and a carrier mechanism. There are a number of examples. Aromatic amino acids such as phenylalanine are moved from the gut into the circulation by an active transport mechanism. This same mechanism is responsible for the active absorption of certain drugs, e.g. alpha-methyldopa, after ingestion. Guanethidine and certain other adrenergic neurone blockers are concentrated in adrenergic nerve terminals by the uptake mechanism which normally repeats uptake of noradrenaline after release.

5.4 IONISATION AND ABSORPTION

An ionised molecule attracts water molecules to itself and has difficulty diffusing through the hydrophobic bilayer of the membrane. Therefore the degree of ionisation of a drug at the site of absorption is an important factor. The tendency of a molecule to ionise is described by its pKa, which *is the pH at which ionised and unionised forms of the drug are present in equal numbers.* At higher or lower pH values, ionised or unionised forms of the drug will predominate depending on whether the drug is acid or base. For an *acid* (e.g. aspirin or barbiturate) more of the drug is in the ionised form as the pH is *increased* (i.e. increased alkalinity), whereas for a *base* more of the drug is in the ionised form as the pH is decreased (i.e. increased acidity). This relationship is usually described by the general Henderson-Hasselbach equation:

$$p^H = p^{Ka} + \log [\text{ionised form}]/[\text{nonionised form}]$$

In general, for a pH change of one unit, there is a 10-fold change in the proportion of ionised or unionised form of the drug. For example indomethacin is an acidic drug with a pKa of 3.5, i.e. at pH 3.5, there are equal numbers of ionised and unionised molecules. At pH 5.5, there are 100 times more ionised molecules than unionised ones, whereas at pH 1.5, there are 100 times more unionised than ionised molecules.

To determine the pKa of a drug, the relative concentrations of ionised and unionised forms of the drug must be known at a particular pH and these are measured by potentiometric titrations, solubility determination or spectrometry.

Ionisation and absorption in the GIT

The way in which ionisation affects absorption in the gastrointestinal tract may be illustrated by considering the absorption of acetylsalicyclic acid (aspirin), a weak acid (pKa, 3.4).

Stomach

In the stomach where the pH is low (about 1.4) there are 100 times more unionised than ionised molecules of aspirin, which should favour rapid absorption. But at such a low pH, solubility is also very low. This limits absorption. Note that the pH of the stomach is not constant, but rises temporarily after a meal and decreases during fasting. This is why it helps the ulcer patient to eat frequent small meals. After traversing the cell membrane, aspirin encounters a higher pH (7.4) in the cytoplasm of the mucosal cell where the drug would now become highly ionised. This form can only pass from the cell into the blood stream with difficulty: The drug is trapped in the cell. Ion-trapping is a process whereby a molecule or ion passes a membrane only to encounter a milieu of a different pH from which it has difficulty in escaping (Fig. 5.3). Ion-trapping gives rise to high concentrations of aspirin in mucosal cells and is thought to account for the gastric irritation and erosion caused by the drug.

Small intestine

In the small intestine where the pH is about 7.4, there are 10000 times more ionised forms of aspirin than nonionised forms. In spite of this apparently unfavourable condition, most of the absorption of aspirin in fact takes place in this part of the gut due to

    (a) higher solubility of the drug at this pH;

    (b) a larger absorptive surface area, and

    (c) the longer transit time in this part of the GIT.

Fig. 5.3. *The phenomenon of ion-trapping.* In the stomach (pH 1.4) aspirin is relatively easily absorbed and inside the mucosal cell cytoplasm (pH 7.4), aspirin is mostly ionised. It then enters the bloodstream with difficulty.

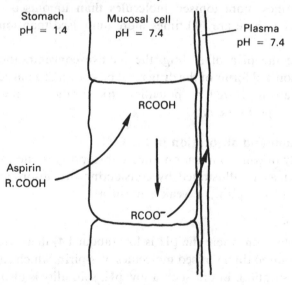

There is no ion-trapping here as the drug enters the bloodstream at the same rate as it traverses the mucosal cell membrane from the intestinal lumen. What this shows is that lipid solubility which facilitates the passage of the molecule through the hydrophobic layer of the membrane as well as sufficient solubility in the vicinity of the absorptive surface are necessary requirements for drug absorption.

Absorption of drugs into the brain

The capillaries in the central nervous system (CNS) differ from those in the peripheral circulation. The former constitute the *anatomical blood–brain barrier*. Only lipid-soluble drugs can traverse the wall of these capillaries. Peripheral capillaries can be traversed by lipid-soluble drugs by simple diffusion, or if poorly lipid soluble, by ultrafiltration whereby substances with molecular weight of up to 30000 pass through pores in the capillary membrane. These pores lie between endothelial cells. Therefore virtually all drugs can pass through peripheral capillaries unless they are bound to plasma protein. In the CNS the capillaries do not have such pores; the endothelial cells are tightly packed. CNS capillaries therefore constitute a barrier to all but lipid-soluble molecules. Hence highly ionised molecules cannot gain access into the neuraxis and cerebrospinal fluid unless the protective membranes have been damaged by infection such as occurs in meningitis.

The clinical uses of a number of drugs are based on these considerations. For example, in the treatment of *myasthenia gravis* or tubocurarine overdose, the anticholinesterase neostigmine is preferred to physostigmine (Fig. 1.3). The former, with a highly ionised quarternary nitrogen, does not penetrate the blood–brain barrier and therefore lacks CNS toxicity. Conversely, physostigmine is preferred to neostigmine for topical use, e.g. in the treatment of narrow-angle glaucoma. Physostigmine is better absorbed through mucous membranes than neostigmine.

Another barrier to the free entry of substances into the brain from the general circulation is the presence of inactivating enzymes in the endothelium of CNS capillaries. For instance, the enzyme L-amino acid decarboxylase (dopa decarboxylase) present in CNS endothelial cells restricts the entry of certain amino acids, e.g. L-dopa, 5-hydroxytryptophan, into the brain. This is why, in the clinical use of L-dopa to treat Parkinsonism, another compound, carbidopa, which does not penetrate the CNS, is combined with L-dopa. Carbidopa inhibits peripheral L-amino acid decarboxylase. Other components of this *enzymatic barrier* are monoamine oxidase (restricts the entry of tyramine, noradrenaline, adrenaline, 5-hydroxytryptamine) and esterases which inactivate esters such as acetylcholine.

Drugs in breast milk

Many drugs taken by a nursing mother subsequently appear in the breast milk. The nursing infant thus stands the risk of being poisoned. The mechanism of transfer is not fully understood. The concentration of some drugs in breast milk is higher than in the mother's plasma (e.g. propylthiouracil). This may mean, therefore, that in some cases, active secretion is involved. The matter of drugs in breast milk is one which should command the attention of drug experts in the tropics since mothers in traditional societies may both misuse drugs and breast feed. Most drugs are transferred, but the concentration of many in breast milk is low. In the tropics even low concentrations may be toxic to the infant who may be undernourished. It is worth bearing in mind that even well fed infants have under-developed drug-metabolising enzyme systems.

The following drugs have been shown to have increased half lives in neonates: ampicillin, furosemilde, and indomethacin. The under-nourished infant is at even greater risk. The following are examples of drugs which have been detected in breast milk.

Corticosteroids

These are transferred to milk and if the mother is taking large doses, sufficient may be taken to depress the infant's growth or exert other unwanted steroid effects.

Antithyroid drugs

E.g. propylthiouracil, appear in breast milk in sufficient amounts to affect the baby's thyroid. Radioactive iodine is similarly secreted in milk.

Penicillin

May induce hypersensitivity reactions in the infant. Nalidixic acid and sulphonamides are secreted in breast milk and have been reported to produce haemolytic anaemia in the baby. This would be severe if the infant has G6-PD deficient red blood cells (page 186).

Anticoagulants

Maternal use of orally active anticoagulants can result in impaired coagulation and haemorrhage in the breast fed infant. The use of large doses of aspirin by the mother can have the same effects. These risks are greater if there is vitamin K deficiency.

Antipsychotic drugs
Reserpine taken by the mother has been observed to produce lethargy and other signs of reserpine intoxication in breast fed infants.

Membrane-crossing mechanisms in the kidney
Drugs cross membranes at three major sites in the kidney (Fig. 5.4).

(1) Glomerulus
The pores in the membranes of the glomerular capillaries are larger than capillary pores elsewhere. Therefore only very large macro-

Fig. 5.4. Membrane-crossing mechanisms in the kidney. (1) Ultrafiltration at the glomerulus; (2) Reabsorption into the bloodstream by the kidney tubules; (3) Active secretion from the blood into the tubules.

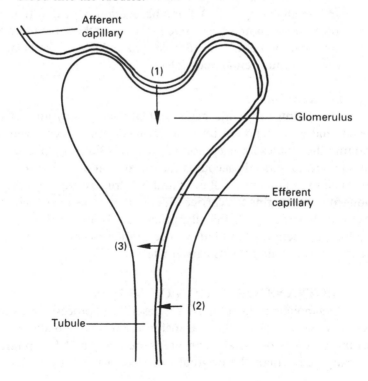

molecules or drugs bound to plasma proteins are excluded from the ultrafiltrate.

(2) Kidney tubules

Lipid-soluble substances filtered by the glomerulus can be reabsorbed by the kidney tubules into the bloodstream. This has a number of consequences.

(a) Highly lipid-soluble substances which are not metabolised are retained in the body by this mechanism of filtration and reabsorption. Examples are DFP, alcohol and DDT.

(b) Metabolic transformation of drugs decreases their lipid solubility and this increases their renal excretion.

(c) In poisoning, the principle employed for treatment is to accelerate the renal excretion of certain drugs. For example aspirin with a pKa of 3.4 is ionised in the tubular fluid (pH 6.0), but its ionisation is increased and hence renal excretion is accelerated by increasing the pH of tubular fluid with sodium bicarbonate or potassium citrate to treat aspirin poisoning. Other acidic drugs whose renal excretion can be accelerated by making the urine alkaline are barbiturates (pKa 7.25 - 7.9), and indomethacin (pKa 3.5). For a base, that is a drug with a high pKa, elimination is accelerated by making the urine more acid by giving ammonium chloride. Examples are amphetamine (pKa 9.4), and gentamicin (20.5).

(3) Secretion

Many drugs (organic acids and organic bases) are actively secreted, that is, transported by a carrier-mediated process, from the blood into the tubules for excretion in the urine. For example penicillin is so secreted and this accounts for its rapid elimination from the body. Such excretion can be slowed and the drug's duration of action prolonged by presenting the carrier with another molecule which competes for its binding site. Clinically, probenicid is used with penicillin to prolong the action of the latter since probenicid blocks penicillin secretion by competing for its carrier site.

5.5   BIOTRANSFORMATION OF DRUGS

Metabolism is the term used to describe all processes by which drugs undergo enzyme-catalysed transformations in the body. In most cases the products of metabolism are more polar and less pharmacologically active than the original drug (see Table 10.1, p. 226, for examples of exceptions). Consequently, metabolites are in general, both less toxic and more easily excreted from the body. Reference has already been made to drugs such as DDT which are highly lipid-soluble, undergo little biotransformation and therefore accumulate in fatty tissues. There are also drugs such as hexamethonium which are not metabolised but are lipid-insoluble and are therefore rapidly excreted. In some cases the toxicity of a drug is due to its metabolite. For example, the phenacetin - induced methaemoglobinaemia is due to its metabolite, para-phenetidin (see Fig. 5.5). The hepatotoxicity of paracetamol is also attributed to a metabolite, possibly N-acetyl-*p*benzoquinone. Many enzymes concerned with biotransformation are located in the hepatic smooth endoplasmic reticulum (SER). When liver cells are homogenised and the suspension is subjected to differential centrifugation, SER occurs in the fraction of the homogenate known as microsomes. SER contains oxidative enzymes called mixed function oxidases (MFO) or monooxygenases which, to act, require reduced nicotinamide adenine dinucleotide phosphate (NADPH) and molecular oxygen.

Drugs undergo two main types of biotransformation. These are nonsynthetic (phase I metabolism), and synthetic or conjugation biotransformation (phase II metabolism). Phase I and II description may suggest that one form of transformation is preceded by the other. In fact, nonsynthetic and synthetic metabolism can occur concurrently or consecutively.

Nonsynthetic

In nonsynthetic biotransformation, the drug is degraded. Examples of such reactions are oxidation, hydrolysis, and reduction. The student should always note the structure of drug molecules and attempt to deduce from first principles, the possible mode of biotransformation. Some examples are given below as a guide.

Oxidation

Most oxidative biotransformations are catalysed by MFO but some are also catalysed by nonmicrosomal enzymes. MFO oxidation of primary alcohols is described on page 182. Other oxidative reactions are: O-dealkylation of phenacetin (see Fig. 5.5); N-dealkylation of imipramine, deamination of primary and secondary amines (see Fig. 5.6), and hydroxylation of propranolol and debrisoquine (see page 183).

Fig. 5.5. Biotransformation of phenacetin.

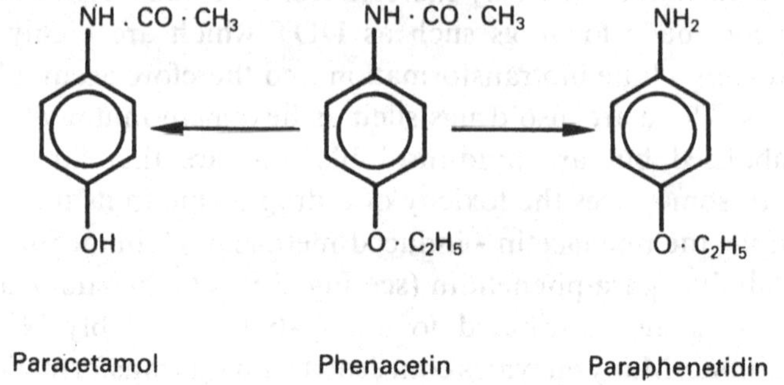

Paracetamol   Phenacetin   Paraphenetidin

Fig. 5.6. N-dealkylation of imipramine and deamination of adrenaline.

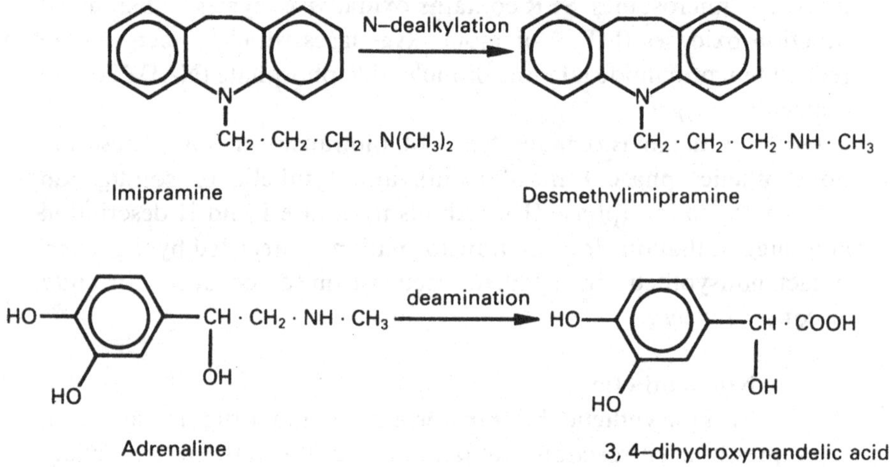

Imipramine   Desmethylimipramine

Adrenaline   3, 4–dihydroxymandelic acid

Hydrolysis of esters and amides

Good examples to remember are hydrolysis of the muscle relaxant succinylcholine by plasma cholinesterase (page 390), acetylsalicylic acid, lignocaine, and procaine (see Table 5.2).

Reduction

An important example of a reduction biotransformation is the hypnotic prodrug chloral hydrate which is rapidly reduced to the active metabolite, trichloroethanol under the influence of alcohol dehydrogenase:

Table 5.2 *Biotransformation of drugs*

Type of transformation	Drug type	Enzyme(a)	Product	Therapeutically active or inactive
Oxidation				
O-dealkylation	phenacetin	MFO	paracetamol	active
N-dealkylation	imipramine	MFO	desmethylimipramine	active
	pethidine	MFO	norpethidine	inactive
	diazepam	MFO	desmethyldiazepam	active
Primary alcohol	ethanol	MFO	acetic acid	inactive
Deamination	adrenaline	NM	3, 4-dihydroxymandelic acid	inactive
Hydroxylation	propranolol	MFO	4-hydroxypropranolol	active (short duration)
	debrisoquine	MFO	4-hydroxydebrisoquine	inactive
Hydrolysis				
Amide	lignocaine	NM + MFO	xylidine	inactive
Ester	procaine	NM + MFO	diethylaminoethanol + PABA	inactive
	acetylsalicylic acid	NM + MFO	salicylic acid	active
Reduction				
Aldehyde to alcohol	chloral hydrate	NM	trichloroethanol	active
Ketone to alcohol	cortisone	MFO + NM	hydrocortisone	active
	prednisone	MFO + NM	prednisolone	active
Synthetic (conjugation)				
Glucuronylation	salicylic acid	MFO + NM	glucuronide	inactive
	paracetamol	MFO + NM	glucuronide	inactive
Sulphonation	morphine	MFO + NM	morphine sulphonate	inactive
N-acetylation	isoniazid	MFO	acetylisoniazid	inactive
	sulphonamide	MFO	acetyl derivative	inactive
O-methylation	isoprenaline	NM	3-methoxyisoprenaline	inactive (B₂-receptor blocker

(a)NM = non-microsomal enzyme; MFO = microsomal mixed function oxidase.

C.(Cl)$_3$. CHO ⇌ C.(Cl$_3$).CH$_2$ OH
chloral   trichloroethanol
                                           (inhibits alcohol
                                           dehydrogenase)

Synthetic (conjugation reactions)
Examples of conjugation reactions are given below.

(a)   Combination of the drug or its metabolite with glucuronic acid (glucuronylation). This reaction occurs with molecules containing free phenolic/alcoholic -OH or free COOH groups. A large number of drugs are glucuronated either before or after nonsynthetic bio-transformation (see Table 5.2). The hepatic microsomal enzyme which catalyses this reaction is *glucuronyl transferase*. Its deficiency can result in the 'grey baby' syndrome in infants treated with chloramphenicol or in a condition known as *kernicterus* (failure in the conjugation of bile pigments). Urinary D-gluconic acid is a reliable measure of liver microsomal glucuronylation activity.

(b)   N-acetylation of, e.g. noradrenaline, isoniazid, and hydrallazine (page 180).

(c)   O-methylation of isoprenaline is another important example of a conjugation reaction (see summary Table 5.2).

Microsomal enzymes can be activated (induced) by drugs and environmental xenobiotics. The induced enzyme can usually remain active for several weeks after the inducer drug has been removed. Barbiturates are powerful inducers of MFO. Inducer drugs can profoundly influence the action of other drugs administered concurrently, e.g. phenobarbitone accelerates the metabolism of warfarin by enzyme induction. The enzymes are impaired by liver disease and chronic alcoholism and by some drugs, e.g. allopurinol and cimetidine.

5.6   PROTEIN BINDING

This is discussed in detail in relation to protein energy malnutrition (Chapter 7). It is essential to note here that drug binding to plasma protein has important consequences on the pharmacokinetics of the drug concerned. In general, acidic drugs, e.g. nonsteroidal antiinflammatory drugs, oral anticoagulants, and sulphonamides are bound to plasma albumin whereas basic drugs such as propranolol, chloroquine, and imipramine are bound to alpha$_1$-acid glycoprotein. The concentration of these proteins is affected by disease. For example plasma albumin concentration is drastically reduced in kwashiorkor and liver disease. Whereas that of alpha₁-acid glycoprotein is known to increase in diseases such as rheumatoid arthritis. Up to 95% of the total concentration of certain drugs in the plasma is in the bound form (see Table 6.2, page 152). It is the free form of the drug that exerts pharmacological action. For heavily bound drugs, the free concentration of drug in plasma can be severely affected by disease (see above) or by other drugs which can displace them from binding sites. To take an example, acetylsalicylic acid and warfarin appear to bind to a common site on human serum albumin. After a therapeutic dose of warfarin, 99% of the drug is bound to plasma albumin. The clinical effect is thus due to 1% of the given dose. If sufficient aspirin is co-administered to displace 1% of the bound warfarin, the dose of the latter is effectively doubled. This can lead to toxic manifestations of warfarin such as haemorrhage. Drugs that are highly bound to plasma proteins tend to have low apparent volumes of distribution, long half lives (because renal clearance is low as the bound drug is not filtered by the glomerulus nor is it available for metabolism by the liver enzymes (however see section 7.3).

5.7 FACTORS AFFECTING DRUG ABSORPTION AND METABOLISM
Liver diseases

These affect the organ's capacity to synthesise plasma protein and the enzymes responsible for the metabolism of drugs and can have profound effects on drug disposition and metabolism. For example, liver synthesises plasma albumin at the rate of about 10 g per day. Most of the globulins are also synthesised in the liver. These functions of the liver are adversely affected by diseases such as cirrhosis. This is a disorder of the liver characterised by loss of hepatocytes and their replacement by fibrous connective tissue. The causes of cirrhosis include viral hepatitis, malnutrition, congestive heart failure and hepatotoxic agents, e.g. alcohol. Excessive and prolonged intake of alcohol is a major cause of cirrhosis: 10% of heavy drinkers have cirrhosis and 50% of patients with cirrhosis have a history of alcoholism. In moderate to severe cirrhosis, plasma albumin is low (hypoalbuminaemia) and there is a reduction in activity of a whole range of metabolising enzymes normally synthesised by the liver. Drugs therefore tend to produce prolonged effects. Occurrence of severe toxicities has been observed with amylobarbitone, chloramphenicol, phenylbutazone, rifampicin and tolbutamide. Half lives of the following drugs are increased in cirrhotic patients: ampicillin, carbenicillin, chloramphenicol, chlordiazepoxide, diazepam, phenobarbitone, rifampicin, quinidine, and valproic acid. No doubt, the risk of toxicity also exists for other drugs which are bound to albumin and similarly metabolised by the liver. Reduced plasma binding in liver disease is due to hypoalbuminaemia as well as to drug displacement from protein-binding sites by bilirubin whose plasma concentration is greatly raised in cirrhosis.

Protein energy malnutrition (PEM)

This is a disease condition which may be encounterd frequently in the tropics and which has profound effects on drug action. A detailed discussion of the ways in which this disease can affect drug absorption, drug distribution and metabolism can be found in Chapter 7. Briefly, absorption is impaired in PEM because of (i) atrophied jejunal mucosa, (ii) diarrhoea, and (iii) altered pH of the stomach and intestinal contents; drug distribution is altered due to hypoalbuminaemia and possibly changes in the concentration of other plasma proteins; there is reduction in the activities of mixed function oxidases leading to reduced metabolism of a wide range of drugs. Some of the evidence derived from animal and human experiments and the drugs most affected are described in Chapter 7.

Food substances

Studies suggest that in the tropics, chronic intake of certain foods can cause harmful effects. Two food-derived intoxicants which have been widely studied are hydrocyanic acid (HCN) which is said to be responsible for ataxic neuropathy among populations whose main source of carbohydrate is cassava, and mycotoxins (e.g. aflatoxins) produced by fungi which commonly contaminate tropical food products. These are discussed in detail in Chapter 6.

There have been no studies specifically relating drug metabolism to chronic intake of these toxins. It is nevertheless important to note the likelihood that these substances may adversely affect the metabolism of drugs.

Aflatoxin B1 (see Fig. 7.2)

Is both an inhibitor of protein synthesis and paradoxically a powerful inducer of microsomal hydroxylating enzymes. These actions could have complex effects on the metabolism of a whole range of drugs in people exposed to mycotoxin intoxication. Aflatoxins are coumarin derivatives and as such they possess anticoagulant properties. Aflatoxin B1 has been shown to be a powerful anticoagulant in several animal species and is active at concentrations expected to be achieved in plasma by people eating contaminated foods. The toxin competes with vitamin K for an enzyme site in the synthesis of prothrombin in the liver. Also, aflatoxins bind strongly to plasma albumin. There is therefore the likelihood, although this has not been demonstrated, that in people of the tropics who are exposed to mycotoxins on a continuous basis, their effects may increase the toxicity of warfarin or similar drugs used as anticoagulants.

Hydrocyanic acid

It is known that HCN is a potent inhibitor of cytochrome P-450 microsomal drug metabolising enzymes. Conceivably, therefore, in chronic cyanide intoxication such as manifests in ataxic neuropathy, there could be sufficient effect on liver enzymes to cause abnormal metabolism of a variety of drugs. This would seem to be an important area for further research.

6

Pharmacokinetic principles

6.1 INTRODUCTION

Pharmacokinetics is the study of rates of drug absorption, metabolism and excretion. Since the sites of absorption, metabolism and excretion are not accessible to direct study, pharmacokinetic investigations usually involve mathematical analyses of model systems based on plasma concentrations of drug determined at different times after administration. This branch of study has gained prominence in the last two decades for the following reasons:

(a) Individuals or groups of individuals may absorb, metabolise and excrete a given drug to different extents after being given the same dose (due to genetic and other factors referred to elsewhere in this book). That being the case, the plasma concentration of a drug is a better indicator of its pharmacological activity than the dose administered. Pharmacokinetic methods are used to achieve refined dose regimens relevant to the required plasma concentration.

(b) During the formulation of a new drug into dosage forms, pharmacokinetic studies provide data from which (i) bioavailability can be assessed, and (ii) dosage frequencies can be determined.

(c) It is sometimes necessary, especially for a drug with low therapeutic index, e.g. antitumour drugs, to adjust the dosage for individual patients, so as to maintain critically effective but nontoxic plasma concentrations. Pharmacokinetic measurements can help to achieve this purpose.

A detailed treatment of pharmacokinetics requires a good knowledge of calculus since the subject is concerned with rates of change.

But the essential principles can be understood without a great deal of mathematics. The aim in this chapter is to explain, without the burden of the calculus, the basic principles of the subject and the meaning and significance of pharmacokinetic data for various drugs. The reader interested in a more detailed treatment of the subject should consult specialised texts on pharmacokinetics. Some are listed at the end of this chapter.

6.2   METHODS IN PHARMACOKINETICS

The usual approach in pharmacokinetics is to determine drug concentrations in plasma or urine at different times after administration. Suitable data are then derived from the graph relating changes in plasma concentration to time. Recent advances in analytical chemistry techniques have greatly contributed to the ease and accuracy with which low concentrations of most drugs can be determined. Examples of such techniques are spectrofluorometry, gas chromatography – mass spectrometry (GC – MS), saturation analysis, radioimmunoassay, and the use of isotope-labelled drugs.

6.3   FIRST-ORDER OR LINEAR PHARMACOKINETICS

In general, changes in plasma concentration of drug with time result from decay processes (absorption, metabolism and excretion); the amount of drug at the absorption site after administration decreases with time as the drug is absorbed into the systemic circulation and distributed throughout the tissues. The amount of drug in the systemic circulation is also not constant; it is continuously subjected to metabolism and elimination processes. In general, drug handling by the body (absorption, metabolism and elimination) obey *first–order* or linear kinetics, that is, the rate of a given process is proportional to the concentration of drug being handled. A first-order reaction has the following characteristics:

(i) A graph of concentration versus time gives an exponential curve described by the general equation:

$$Cp_t = Cp_0 \exp(-kt) \tag{6.1}$$

Where Cp_t = concentration of drug at time t, Cp_0 = concentration of drug at time $t = 0$ = initial concentration of drug, and k = rate constant for the decay process.

The graph of log concentration versus time gives a straight line (Fig. 6.1). A straight line also results if the data are plotted on semi-logarithmic paper.

The rate constant is characteristic of the particular drug. A drug, with for example, a high absorption rate constant would appear very rapidly in the systemic circulation after oral administration; its plasma concentration at any given time would depend on its rate constants of elimination and metabolism.

(ii) An important relationship in first-order decay kinetics is that the concentration of drug declines by *a fixed amount in a given time and by 50% in a fixed time*. The time for 50% of the drug to be eliminated from the plasma is called the $t_{1/2}$ and is characteristic of a given drug in a defined system. The $t_{1/2}$ can be estimated from the graph of concentration versus time between any two time points. Note that in zero-order and second-order reactions, $t_{1/2}$ is a function of concentration and is therefore not constant. The $t_{1/2}$ in first-order kinetics is related to the elimination rate constant, k_{el} (that is a rate constant for metabolism and excretion, see page 139) as follows:

$$t_{1/2} = \frac{0.693}{k_{el}} \tag{6.2}$$

Knowledge of $t_{1/2}$ and k_{el} for a drug is very important because they give some idea of how long the drug persists in the body. You have to bear in mind, though, that a $t_{1/2}$ does not tell the whole story about the duration of action of a drug. If a drug is bound to tissue sites to a negligible extent or if the binding is reversible, then the $t_{1/2}$ is a good estimate of its duration of action: for example, the $t_{1/2}$ of hexamethonium which is not bound to body tissues to any appreciable extent and is excreted

Fig. 6.1. Graph of plasma concentration (a), and log plasma concentration (b), of drug versus time t.

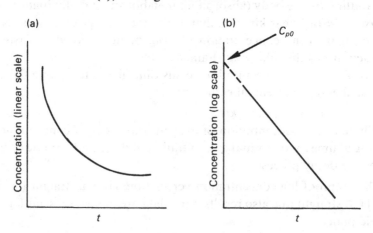

unchanged, gives an estimate of its duration of action. On the other hand for a drug such as guanethidine which is selectively concentrated in adrenergic neurones where it interferes with sympathetic nerve function, the pharmacological effect of the drug can be apparent even when it is no longer detectable in plasma. In this case the $t_{1/2}$ has little value in predicting the duration of drug action. This kind of drug is sometimes described as 'hit and run'. Also, if a metabolite of the drug is pharmacologically active, $t_{1/2}$ of the drug itself is not useful in estimating how long the drug would act.

(iii) Another important characteristic of first-order kinetics in drug therapy, is that the mean steady state plasma level during multiple dosing is directly proportional to dose and $t_{1/2}$. If the same dose is given at regular and equal intervals, the number of doses necessary to reach a given percentage of the steady state level depends on the dose interval and the $t_{1/2}$. This point is further discussed under the *Plateau principle* on page 147.

(iv) In first-order kinetics, the area under the plasma concentration time curve (AUC) is directly proportional to dose. AUC is discussed later but it can immediately be seen that the shape of this curve (Fig. 6.2) provides a measure of how much drug is available in plasma over a period of time ($t_1 - t_2$) and hence the duration of action of the drug.

Fig. 6.2. Area under the plasma concentration versus time curve (AUC) after oral administration of drug. The broken line indicates the minimum effective concentration (MEC).

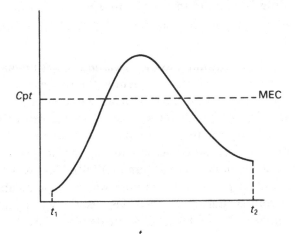

6.4   NON-LINEAR PHARMACOKINETICS

The pharmacokinetic behaviour of some drugs does not follow first-order linear kinetics with fixed rate constants. Rather, their rates of absorption and elimination depend on the concentration of the drug. Ethanol, aspirin and phenytoin are examples of drugs that exhibit dose-dependent elimination or non-linear pharmacokinetics. Ethanol distributes readily between water and lipid. It is rapidly filtered by the glomerulus, but it is also rapidly reabsorbed in the tubules. Both glomerular filtration and tubular reabsorption are first-order processes. Therefore elimination from the body depends largely on the liver. However the amount of alcohol dehydrogenase in the liver and elsewhere is small and easily saturated, after which an increase in ethanol concentration does not lead to an increase in the rate of elimination. From then on, ethanol metabolism follows *zero-order kinetics*. With drugs showing this sort of kinetics, the first-order fixed rate constant obtains only over a narrow range of low doses. Once the elimination process is saturated elimination half times and drug effects increase disproportionately with increase in dose with unpleasant consequences if care is not taken. In the case of ethanol, for example, the drug is eliminated from the body at the rate of about 10 ml h^{-1}. If you take three pints of beer at lunch time and another three in the evening, by mid-day the following day, you might still have enough ethanol in your blood to make you a dangerous driver.

Another instance in which a zero-order phenomenon is encountered is when a drug is given by continuous infusion. The concentration of the drug in plasma is virtually unchanged with time during the infusion after attainment of steady state when the rate of removal of the drug is equal to the rate of infusion. The steady state concentration of drug, C_{ss}, is given as

$$C_{ss} = k/Cl \qquad (6.3)$$

where k = infusion rate constant and Cl = *clearance*. C_{ss} is unchanged because, $k = Cl$, at steady state. Consequently, the rate at which the drug is removed from circulation is constant since its concentration in plasma is constant. Zero-order release is achieved for a variety of drugs by slow intravenous infusion, in for example, dextrose saline by constant infusion pumps. Constant release can also be achieved by a device called the elementary osmotic pump (EOP). This is a tablet specially coated with a polymer membrane which is permeable to water. In the gastrointestinal tract, the tablet absorbs water and the drug in its core dissolves. The internal pressure developed by the entry of water forces the drug solution through an orifice in the polymer membrane. EOPs can be designed so that constant rate release is achieved for prolonged periods.

6.5   COMPARTMENT MODELS

For a first-order elimination process, the graph of log Cp_t versus time should give a straight line with a slope characterised by the elimination rate constant. This is the case if the drug is distributed only in the plasma compartment. In practice, for most drugs, the decay curve is characterised by two or more elimination rate constants (e.g. α and β in Fig. 6.3). This is a graph of log Cp_t versus time after intravenous injection of a drug that is distributed in two compartments. The graph shows two phases: a phase of rapid decline and one of slower decline. Such a curve is described as a double exponential decay curve and the equation is:

$$Cp_t = A \exp(-\alpha t) + B\exp(-\beta t) \tag{6.4}$$

where Cp_t = plasma concentration at time t, A = initial concentration in central compartment, B = steady state concentration in central compartment. α = initial elimination rate constant from central compartment, and β = elimination rate constant from central compartment at steady state.

Fig. 6.3. Determination of A, B, α and β from experimental data (●) by the method of residuals. A line of best fit is constructed through the terminal slow mono-exponential phase (β). Subtraction of this line from the remaining data yields a second series of points (○) through which the residual line is fitted to yield A and α (see text).

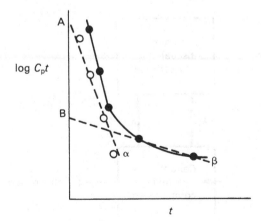

A double decay curve indicates that the drug is transferred through a two-compartment open system which may be represented as in Fig. 6.4. Two exponential components suggest two straight lines with different decay constants, α and β and the intercepts A and B on the concentration axis represent the initial concentrations in the two compartments. The two lines can be separated by the method of residuals (see Fig. 6.3).

Fig. 6.4. Diagrammatic representation of (A) one- and (B) two-compartment models.

$k_a =$ rate constant of absorption after oral or other non-intravenous route of administration.

$k_{12} =$ rate constant for transfer of drug into peripheral compartment.

$k_{21} =$ rate constant for transfer of drug from peripheral to cenral compartment.

$k_{el} =$ rate constant of elimination by all processes from a single compartment.

$k_{10} =$ rate constant of elimination from a multicompartment system.

(A)

Drug after i.v. injection or absorption from site of administration

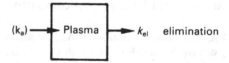

$(k_a) \longrightarrow$ Plasma $\longrightarrow k_{el}$ elimination

(B)

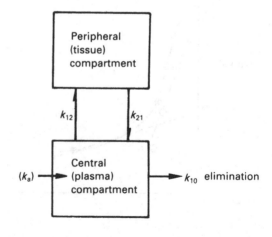

Peripheral (tissue) compartment

k_{12} k_{21}

$(k_a) \longrightarrow$ Central (plasma) compartment $\longrightarrow k_{10}$ elimination

When the drug reaches the plasma, it is rapidly distributed in the compartment made up of the plasma and highly vascular organs. This is called the *central compartment* from which sampling is usually done. The rapid phase of decline in plasma concentration therefore represents distribution between the central compartment and the *peripheral compartment* which may be viewed as consisting of less well-perfused organs. Since the peripheral compartment is initially empty of drug, the rate of entry of drug into it (k_{12}) is at first high, hence a rapid phase of decline in plasma concentration. As the amount of drug in the peripheral compartment approaches equilibrium concentration, that is as k_{21} approaches k_{12}, the rate of net transfer of drug into it from the central compartment diminishes, giving rise to the phase of slower decline (Fig. 6.3). The slope of the curve declines until the line becomes virtually straight. Both central and peripheral compartments are now at equilibrium and the rate constant of elimination (k_{10}) measured from the slope of the log linear phase represents the rate constant of elimination for all compartments just as k_{el} is rate constant of elimination for a single compartment model. k_{10} is derived from several rate constants, but overall it is responsible for the biological half life of the drug.

The idea of compartments is helpful in accounting for the complex ways in which drugs are distributed in the body. It is obvious that a drug would reach equilibrium concentration faster in highly vascular tissues such as heart and lung than it would in less vascular tissues such as muscle and fat. A drug compartment may therefore be regarded as a group of tissues in which the drug achieves equilibrium concentration simultaneously. The rate at which a drug attains equilibrium concentration would depend on its physicochemical properties, such as its lipid solubility.

In theory, the number of compartments should be very large. In practice however, drugs are distributed in (a) plasma, (b) a compartment of highly vascular, highly perfused tissues – liver, kidney, spleen, lungs, heart and brain (for drugs which cross the blood–brain barrier), and (c) a compartment of poorly perfused tissues – fat depots, skeletal muscle and brain (for molecules which do not cross the blood–brain barrier easily). Plasma and the compartment of highly perfused tissues are practically indistinguishable and are roughly referred to as the central compartment; but the compartment of poorly perfused tissues (peripheral compartment) can often be separated into sub-groups, e.g. lean tissue (muscle) and adipose tissue compartments.

Consider the anaesthetic thiopentone; this drug has a very short duration of action producting surgical anaesthesia lasting only a few minutes after intravenous injection. The short duration of action is not due to rapid metabolism but instead it is due to rapid redistribution in different compartments. The Cp_t versus t curve for thiopentone is a triple exponential, meaning that the pharmacokinetics of thiopentone can be described by a three-compartment model. Rapid return of consciousness after intravenous thiopentone is due to restribution of the drug from the central compartment to the lean tissue compartment. Later the drug finds its way into the adipose tissue compartment. Thence it slowly returns to the central compartment where, over several hours or days, it is metabolised in the liver to phenobarbitone.

Determination of drug compartments

The number of compartments in which a drug is distributed can be determined in two ways. The semilogarithmic plot of plasma concentration versus time is analysed. The number of exponentials in the graph corresponds to the number of compartments. The drug penetrates each compartment at a different rate, so that equilibrium is achieved in a time characteristic of the drug and the compartment. Thus the pattern of decline in plasma concentration reflects the different compartments into which the drug is distributed (see Fig. 6.3). This method involves complex mathematical treatments of concentration- time curves.

A more direct way of determining the number of compartments is to measure the drug concentration in plasma and in different tissues after intravenous injection. Plasma concentrations will show decline while tissue concentrations may show rise and fall with time. In any given tissue, peak drug concentration will indicate the time when equilibrium concentration was reached in that tissue. A group of tissues having peak drug concentration at the same time constitute a compartment. This method is applicable in experimental animals and has been used by Adelusi & Salako (1982) to determine the distribution of chloroquine in rats (Fig. 6.5). Following 10 mg kg^{-1} chloroquine, i.p., peak plasma concentration is reached within one hour. The plasma concentration then declines steadily over the next 170 h. On the other hand, the concentrations in liver, spleen, lung, kidney, heart, brain, eye, skeletal muscle, and skin show rises and then falls. These measurements show that in the rat chloroquine is distributed in at least three compartments.

Drug distribution in a single compartment after intravenous injection

Some basic ideas in pharmacokinetics can be appreciated by considering the decline in the plasma concentration of a drug following intravenous injection in the simplest case, where the drug is distributed in the plasma compartment only. The drug will be thoroughly mixed in the compartment and will attain peak concentration instantaneously. This phase will be followed by an exponential first-order decline in plasma concentration. The rates of metabolism and excretion are proportional to the amount of drug to be metabolised or excreted, so that

$$\text{Rate of metabolism} = Q_d/dt = k_m Q_d \qquad (6.5)$$
$$\text{and Rate of excretion} = Q_d/dt = k_e Q_d \qquad (6.6)$$

where k_m and k_e are the rate constants for metabolism and excretion respectively; Q_d is the amount of drug remaining at time t.

Now, metabolism and excretion are elimination processes. Therefore k_m and k_e can be combined as k_{el}, the rate constant of elimination, and (6.5) and (6.6) above can be combined as

Fig. 6.5. Distribution of chloroquine in different tissues of rat following the intraperitoneal administration of 10 mg kg^{-1}. (a) plasma, (b) skeletal muscle, (c) heart, (d) liver. (Redrawn from Adelusi & Salako, 1982.)

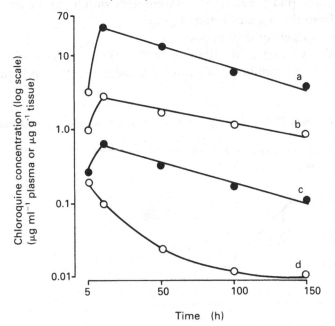

Rate of elimination, $Q_d/dt = k_{el} Q_d$ (6.7)

The equation for the time course of elimination is therefore

$$Q_{dt} = Q_{do} \exp(-k_{el}t)   (6.8)$$

where Q_{do} = initial quantity of drug injected. This is equivalent to the dose injected at the time 0, assuming that mixing with plasma is instantaneous and distribution is strictly in the vascular compartment.

What we measure is not the total quantity of drug in the body, but the concentration in plasma. Hence equation (6.8) can be rewritten as

$$Cp_t = Cp_0 \exp(-k_{el}t)   (6.9)$$

where Cp_t = concentration in plasma at the time t, and Cp_0 = concentration at time $t = 0$. The negative sign indicates that the quantity is declining. Taking logarithms to base e, then

$$\ln Cp_t = \ln Cp_0 - k_{el}t   (6.10)$$

and since $\ln x = 2.303 \log_{10}x$, then

$$2.303 \log_{10}Cp_t = 2.303 \log_{10}Cp_0 - k_{el}t   (6.11)$$

A plot of log Cp_t *versus* t gives a straight line with log Cp_0 as intercept on the y (concentration) axis. The slope of the line is $- k_{el}/2.303$ (Fig. 6.6). Therefore the elimination rate constant can be determined from the slope of the log concentration–time curve. *Never use log t for this plot.*

Some pharmacokinetic parameters which can be derived from the log Cp_t versus t graph
(i) Volume of distribution, V_d
The volume of distribution is the volume of body fluid in which the drug is uniformly distributed at the concentration found in

Fig. 6.6. Plot of log Cp_t versus t in a one-compartment system.

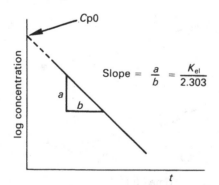

the plasma. It is the fluid volume which would be required to account for all the drug in the body, and is given by

$$V_d = D/Cp_0 \qquad (6.12)$$

where D = dose administered.

The volume of distribution in a two-compartment system is calculated from

$$V_d \text{ (or } V_{dss}) = D/B \qquad (6.13)$$

The concentration B is used because it represents the plasma concentration at a time when concentrations in the two compartments have reached steady states. Hence the volume of distribution calculated as above is usually referred to as steady state volume of distribution V_{dss}. V_d has units of volume or volume per mass (L or L kg^{-1}). Cp_0 is obtained from the Cp_t versus t plot by extrapolation to the concentration axis.

For example, if the dose, D, given to a 70-kg man is 10 mg (10 000 μg) and $Cp_0 = 1$ μg/ml, i.e. 1000 μg/L, then

$$V_d = \frac{10\ 000\ \text{L}}{1000} = 10\ \text{L or } 0.14\ \text{L/kg}.$$

The volume of distribution denotes the volume of body water in which a drug is distributed, assuming that the drug is distributed evenly throughout the body water, and not bound to plasma protein or other tissue structures. A substance distributed uniformly throughout the body water should have a volume of distribution equivalent to total body water which in a 70-kg man is about 42 L (or 0.60 L kg^{-1}); many drugs have V_d values in excess of 42 L. This is due to binding of drug to tissues. Drugs can also have V_d values which are less than the total body water. This is due to plasma protein binding. The V_d derived as above is therefore referred to as the *apparent volume of distribution*.

In the equation (6.12) for V_d, Cp_0 is the denominator in the right-hand term. Therefore a drug that is highly localised in tissues, and so has low plasma concentration at a time when tissue concentrations are high, will have a high V_d. Some examples of drugs which are highly bound to different tissues are shown in Table 6.1. Chloroquine after an intravenous dose of 150 mg has a volume of distribution of over 5600 L in a 70-kg man, more than 100 times the total body water. This is due to extensive tissue binding. Drugs which are restricted to the plasma compartment, for example by extensive binding to plasma protein, have high plasma concentrations. Such drugs have relatively low volumes. Examples are aspirin and warfarin with volumes of about 10

Table 6.1   *Average volumes of distribution of some drugs*

Drug	V_d (L kg^{-1})
Aspirin	0.14
Bethanidine	7.0
Chloroquine	80.0
Desipramine	35.0
Digoxin	10.0
Imipramine	14.0
Propranolol	4.0
Warfarin	0.10

and 7 L respectively in a 70-kg man, less than a quarter of total body water. On the other hand, bethanidine which is highly concentrated in adrenergic neurones has a volume of 490 L. However, some drugs such as desipramine, imipramine and propranolol which are extensively bound to the plasma protein, alpha$_1$-acid glycoprotein, have high volumes of distribution which indicates that they are also extensively bound to tissue protein and fat.

The volume of distribution thus provides an estimate of the extent of binding of a drug to tissue structures or plasma proteins.

(ii) The $t_{1/2}$ of a drug

The $t_{1/2}$ is the time taken for the concentration of the drug in plasma to decline to half the starting concentration. It is sometimes called 'half-life', 'biological half-life' or 'elimination half-life'. Removal of drug from the plasma proceeds according to first-order kinetics. The $t_{1/2}$ can therefore be obtained from the Cp_t versus t graph:

$t_{1/2} = \ln2/k_{el}$ and since $\ln2 = 0.693$

$t_{1/2} = 0.693/k_{el}$ $\hspace{4cm}$ (6.14)

$t_{1/2}$ measures how much drug is disappearing from plasma but does not distinguish between distribution of the drug into tissue compartments and elimination processes such as catabolism and excretion; $t_{1/2}$ is useful in:

Providing some indication of the time to reach steady state concentration in plasma during intermittent dosing. In general 97% of steady state will be reached in 5 half-lives (see page 148).

Estimating the time for the drug to be removed from the body.

Estimating appropriate dosage intervals, including estimate of the loading dose and maintenance dose (see page 148).

(iii) Area under the concentration–time curve or area under the curve (AUC)

For a drug administered intravenously, the area under the Cp_t versus t curve is given by

$$AUC = D/(V_d k_{el}) \qquad (6.15)$$

If the drug is administered by another route, say orally, then

$$AUC = \text{amount absorbed}/(V_d k_{el}) \qquad (6.16)$$

The amount absorbed after oral administration is often less than the total dose administered. The extent of absorption is affected by factors such as the physiochemical properties of the drug, the dosage form and disease. Since for a given dose, V_d and k_{el} are constant for the drug, any difference in AUC after intravenous and oral administration, or after oral administration of different dosage forms of the same drug, can only be due to how much drug is absorbed. Thus the fraction, F of oral dose absorbed can be estimated from

$$F = (AUC_{oral})/(AUC_{intravenous}) \qquad (6.17)$$

The relative extents of absorption after oral dosing with different forms of the same drug can also be determined by comparison of areas. Thus the area under the curve is used to measure the fraction of the drug absorbed or the relative extent of absorption after oral dosing with different dosage forms. AUC has the units of concentration–time i.e. mg ml^{-1}h^{-1}.

If a drug is excreted unchanged in urine in amounts that can be estimated accurately, the relative extent of absorption from different dosage forms after oral administration can also be determined from

$$F = (A_u \text{ dosage form 1})/(A_u \text{ dosage form 2}) \qquad (6.18)$$

where A_u is the amount of drug excreted in urine during a fixed time interval after administration of the drug in two dosage forms.

Determination of AUC

AUC values can be estimated from the plasma concentration–time curve by (i) a planimeter which is an instrument for mechanically measuring the area of plane figures, or (ii) the cut and weigh method in which the area under the curve is cut out and weighed; that weight divided by the weight of a unit area, e.g. 1 µg/ml by 1 h on the same paper, gives the area under the curve, or (iii) the use of the trapezoid rule which is that the plasma concentration–time curve can be described by a series of trapezoids; the area of a trapezoid being equal to

$$\tfrac{1}{2}(C_1 + C_2)(t_2 - t_1) \tag{6.19}$$

Where C_1 and C_2 denote drug concentrations corresponding to sampling times t_1 and t_2 (see Gibaldi, 1984, appendix 1).

Pharmacokinetic studies are not usually carried out to the point where the drug has become undetectable in plasma. Therefore the entire curve from time = 0 to time = ∞ is not available for estimating the AUC. What is done is to carry on the measurement of plasma levels long enough for absorption to be complete and to estimate the area beyond the last concentration (C_1) and last time (t_1) from the equation:

$$\text{Area from } t_1 \text{ to } t_\infty = C_1/k_{el} \tag{6.20}$$

where k_{el} is the first-order elimination rate constant. This area must be added to the area up to time t_1 to obtain the total AUC.

(iv) Bioavailability

The bioavailability of a drug is its rate and extent of absorption after oral administration and is found by measurement of absorption and by comparing AUC values (see page 143). For a given drug the plasma concentration will vary for the same dose given orally or intravenously and the fraction F of drug absorbed can be estimated from the ratio of AUC values (equation (6.18)).

It is not enough that a drug be completely absorbed after oral administration. Its rate of absorption must be adequate. If, for example, the rate of absorption is slow compared to the rates of metabolism and elimination, then a therapeutically effective concentration may not be reached, even if the drug is eventually completely absorbed (see Fig. 6.7). In some instances a rapid rate of absorption is particularly important, for example, when pain relief or sedation is required. The absorption of certain drugs is incomplete for various reasons:

low permeability through cell membranes e.g. neomycin, riboflavin;

low water solubility e.g. phenytoin, griseofulvin;

chemical degradation in the stomach e.g. penicillin G;

preabosorptive metabolism by enzymes in the proximal small intestine and colon (digoxin); and

presystemic metabolism by enzymes in the liver–first pass effect (isoprenaline and propranolol).

Even if the absorption of the drug is not affected by any of the above, the way the tablet or capsule containing the drug is made (formulation) can affect its absorption, and a given drug can be absorbed to different extents depending on the quality of its formulation.

Measurements of absorption and bioavailability are therefore extremely important in determining the quality of a drug. Such measurements are imperative in third world countries where most drugs are imported from industrialised temperate countries (see Chapter 2).

(v) Clearance, Cl

Clearance is defined as the volume of plasma from which the drug is totally eliminated in a unit time. It is expressed as ml min⁻¹ or L h⁻¹. Consider a situation in which blood containing a certain amount of drug flows through an organ, and the drug can be removed by excretion or metabolism. Then the amount of drug entering the organ in a given time depends on the arterial blood flow and the concentration of the drug. The amount of drug leaving the organ can be determined from the venous blood flow and the concentration of the drug in the

Fig. 6.7. Absorption rates of different dosage forms of a drug as measured by its concentration in plasma. The drug is absorbed most rapidly from the dosage form A and the concentration in plasma exceeds the minimum effective concentration (MEC) for the time period t_A. Absorption from the dosage form B is slower and even though the drug concentration in plasma eventually reaches the MEC, the time taken for this to happen is long and the time of exposure to MEC t_B is short compared to t_A. Absorption from dosage form C is both slow and incomplete so that MEC is never reached. Bioavailability of the drug from dosage form A is good. Dosage forms B and C are unsatisfactory.

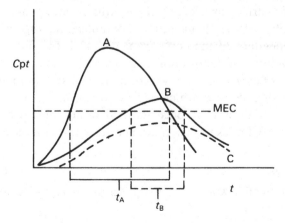

plasma leaving the organ. If the organ eliminates the drug very efficiently, the concentration of drug in the effluent plasma will be low compared to its concentration in the arterial plasma. This difference is known as the *extraction ratio* (ER) and is a measure of the elimination capacity of the organ for the particular drug. ER is defined as

$$ER = \frac{C_{AB} - C_{VB}}{C_{AB}} \tag{6.21}$$

where C_{AB} = drug concentration is arterial blood and C_{VB} = drug concentration in venous blood.

ER is zero if $C_{AB} = C_{VB}$, that is, no drug is eliminated at all, and is unity if $C_{VB} = 0$, that is all the drug is eliminated by the organ. Thus organ clearance (hepatic, biliary or renal) is the volume of blood cleared of the drug by the organ in unit time. This concept which was originally developed for a single organ, e.g. the kidney, is here applied to the elimination of a drug from the whole body. So clearance describes removal of drug by all processes and all organs. Renal clearance is often a major fraction of total body clearance. For drugs that are excreted exclusively in the urine unchanged, renal clearance equals total body clearance, e.g. inulin, creatinine. Total body clearance can be estimated from the Cp_t versus time graph after intravenous drug administration from the relationship:

$$Cl = D/AUC \tag{6.22}$$

Clearance can only be meaningfully estimated after intravenous administration since after administration by other routes, the amount of drug reaching the systemic circulation is variable.

Clearance is a more accurate measure of the efficiency with which the eliminating organs remove a drug since it is defined as the fraction of the volume of distribution cleared of the drug in unit time by all processes. It is a physiologically meaningful parameter having units of flow and is independent of the compartment model. In contrast, $t_{1/2}$ depends on the volume of distribution and clearance.

The calculation of clearance in a two compartment system involves consideration of all processes which are occurring at a time when steady state concentrations have been reached in all compartments. Hence, from Fig. 6.3 for example, clearance in a two-compartment model is given by

$$Cl = V_{dss}/B \tag{6.23}$$

It gets more complicated when an absorption factor is added to the equation of Cp_t versus t.

6.6 PLATEAU PRINCIPLE

So far we have considered what happens to the drug after its administration in a single dose. In therapeutics the patient rarely takes just a single dose. More usually, a given dose is taken repeatedly, the dosing interval being such that an effective therapeutic concentration is maintained in plasma throughout the period of treatment. This objective would also be achieved by infusing the drug at a constant rate, so that at a steady state, the amount of drug entering the body is equal to the amount removed by all processes of elimination. Constant rate infusion (CRI) is easier to visualise than multiple intermittent dosing. So, let us consider CRI first. The maintenance of a therapeutic level of drug in plasma through CRI is achieved by application of the *plateau principle* and is a problem analogous to trying to fill a bucket to a certain level from a tap flowing at a constant rate, but with a hole in the bucket! If you ran the tap at a rate at which the amount of water entering the bucket is the same as the amount leaving it, the bucket would never fill up to the required level. In the case of a drug infused into plasma however, the kinetics of elimination are of first-order, that is the rate of elimination is directly proportional to the concentration of drug. Hence at the onset, the rate at which drug is admitted into the body is greater than the rate at which it is removed. Therefore, drug concentration increases gradually but at a diminishing rate (Fig. 6.8). If infusion is continued long enough, drug concentration eventually

Fig. 6.8. Drug concentration in plasma during constant-rate infusion. At the start of infusion, the rate of drug elimination is low compared to the rate of infusion. There is therefore drug accumulation and the concentration increases steadily until the steady state concentration (C_{ss}) is reached when the rate of infusion equals the rate of elimination. On ceasing infusion plasma concentration declines.

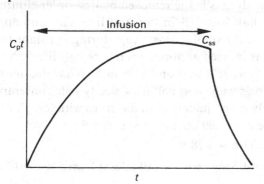

reaches a plateau or steady state at which the amount of drug in plasma is such that its rate of elimination is equal to the infusion rate.

Steady state concentration

For clinical purposes, we are interested in the actual steady state concentration because this must be high enough to be pharmacologically effective, but not so high as to be in the toxic range. We must also know how long it takes for the steady state concentration to be reached. Drug concentration at steady state (C_{ss}) is given by:

$$C_{ss} = k_o/k_{el} V_d \qquad (6.24)$$

where k_o = infusion rate.

In a two-compartment system

$$C_{ss} = k_o/\beta V_{dss} \qquad (6.25)$$

and $\quad k_o = \beta V_{dss} C_{ss}$

where β = steady state elimination rate constant for the drug and V_{dss} = its volume of distribution at steady state. Suppose in a clinical situation we wished to achieve a steady plasma concentration of 2 mg L^{-1} of drug, e.g. lignocaine in a 70-kg man given that for lignocaine V_{dss} = 1.7 L kg^{-1} and β = 0.39 h^{-1}. The infusion rate (k_o) to achieve the required steady state concentration is

$$k_o = 2 \times 1.7 \times 70 \times 0.39 = 92.8 \text{ mg h}^{-1} \text{ or } 1.5 \text{ mg min}^{-1}$$

Loading dose and maintenance dose

Next, we must know how long it takes to achieve the steady state concentration since this is important for the clinical goal we wish to achieve. The time it takes to reach C_{ss} is independent of dose or volume of distribution, but is dependent on the $t_{1/2}$. In general, the steady state concentration is reached during constant rate infusion in approximately 5 half lives ($5 \times t_{1/2}$). The easiest way to understand this is to remember that the drug is being removed by first-order elimination processes, 50% in 1 half life, 75% in two half lives etc., and approximately 97% in $5 \times t_{1/2}$. By similar reasoning, during constant rate infusion, 50% of what is infused accumulates in one half life, 75% in two half lives, 87.5% in 3, 93.75% in 4 and 97% in 5. What this means in practice is that for drugs with short half lives, steady state concentrations are reached relatively more quickly than for drugs with long half lives. Since for lignocaine $t_{1/2} = 0.693/\beta$, and $\beta = 0.39$ h^{-1},

$$t_{1/2} = 0.693/0.39 \text{ h} = 1.78 \text{ h}$$

At an infusion rate of 1.5 mg min^{-1}, it will take at least 5×1.78 (8.7) h to reach the required steady state concentration of 2 mg L^{-1}. This is too long for practical purposes and this problem brings us to the idea of the loading dose.

The loading dose is simply the amount of drug one has to administer in order that the steady state concentration is reached soon after the start of constant rate infusion. The amount infused subsequently represents the *maintenance dose*. The meaning of the maintenance dose is clearer if we return to our leaking bucket analogy where we saw that there could be no accumulation of water if the tap delivered the same amount of water into the bucket as leaked out through a hole in a given time. If we kept the input and output rates constant, we can keep a certain level of water in the bucket only by pouring in an appropriate amount of water from another bucket to start with or by increasing the input rate so that initially the amount of water entering the bucket is much greater than the amount leaking out.

In practice the loading dose is given by a single bolus injection or it may be administered orally It is obtained from the relationship:

$$\text{Loading dose} = C_{ss} V_{dss} \qquad (6.26)$$

In the lignocaine example, the loading dose

$$= 2 \times 1.7 \times 70 \text{ mg} = 238 \text{ mg}.$$

Also, since

$$k_o = C_{ss} V_{dss} \beta \qquad (6.27)$$

then $\quad C_{ss} V_{dss} = k_o/\beta$

$$= 92.8/0.39 \text{ mg} = 238 \text{ mg}.$$

The idea of a loading dose applies whether the drug is to be given by continuous infusion or by oral repetitive administration (see next section). There are many examples of drug therapy in which a maintenance dose is preceded by a loading dose administered singly or in divided doses. With digoxin therapy, loading or digitalisation is always carried out with 3 or 4 divided doses over the first one or two days. Guanethidine is another example. The drug has a $t_{1/2}$ of about 5 days. Therefore with normal dosage, it would take 3 – 4 weeks to establish a full therapeutic effect. The dosage regimen therefore usually involves the administration of a loading dose.

Doses administered at regular intervals

Let us now consider the situation we started with in which the same dose of drug is administered at regular intervals usually by the oral route. In principle the difference between repeated dosage and constant rate infusion is that in the former case, there is a time interval between the doses. Just before a dose, the concentration of the drug in plasma is at a minimum level and the concentration rises to a maximum soon after the dose is administered. The aim in therapy is to ensure that the minimum concentration is within the effective therapeutic range and the maximum concentration is not in the toxic range (see Fig. 6.9).

Calculation of the steady state concentration during repetitive dosing

Calculation of the steady state concentration after repetitive dosing is a complicated process since it must take into account: the dose to be administered; the interval between doses; fraction of the drug absorbed after oral, intramuscular or other route of administration; elimination rate constants and volumes of distribution. Such complicated methods involving rigorous application of the plateau principle are available in specialised texts. A simple method of calculation is based on the idea of *average drug concentration at steady state* (C_{ss}) which is the mean between the maximum and minimum concentrations during fluctuations occurring at steady state (see Fig. 6.9). C_{ss} is analogous to C_{ss} during constant rate infusion. We can also view drug administration at regular intervals in terms of an *average dosing rate (DR)*. Thus if a drug is given at 600 mg every 6 h, the average dosing rate is 100 mg h^{-1}. *DR* thus becomes analogous to infusion rate constant (k_o) in equation (6.24), which can now be applied to the cal-

Fig. 6.9. Plasma concentration of a drug during repetitive dosing at regular intervals. At steady state the plasma concentration fluctuates between maximum (C_{max}) and minimum (C_{min}), but the average drug concentration ( ) is within the therapeutic range for the drug.

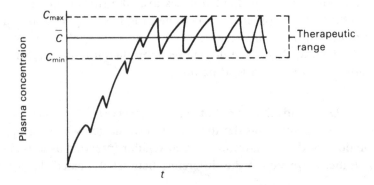

culation of C_{ss} during repeated application of a dose at regular intervals.

$$C_{ss} = \frac{F(DR)}{V_{dss}\,\beta} \qquad (6.28)$$

Where F is the fraction of the dose that actually reaches the blood stream. Another way of estimating C_{ss} is to think of each dose as giving rise to an average concentration that is the equivalent of the height of a rectangle whose base is the dose interval (di) (see Fig. 6.10). The area of the rectangle is $C_{ss} \times di$, and is equal to the area under the plasma concentration versus time curve (AUC) for a single dose and a stated time interval. Then, approximately,

$$C_{ss} = \text{AUC}/di \qquad (6.29)$$

where AUC is from time $t = 0$ to $t = \infty$ after a single dose administered in the same way as the drug would be during repetitive dosing, and di is the dosing interval. Thus, by knowing the AUC for a given dose of drug and the dosing interval, the average plasma concentration at steady state can be estimated.

6.7   GENERAL CONCLUSION

In this simplified introduction to pharmacokinetics, some basic principles are introduced and explained. It can be seen that from plasma concentration versus time curves, several useful parameters which describe the behaviour of drug in the body can be measured. It is possible to estimate fairly accurately what dose to give, and how frequently to give it in order to achieve the desired pharmacological effect without approaching toxic levels. Determination of dosage regimen is

Fig. 6.10. Estimating the average drug concentration at steady state (C_{ss}) during repeated dosing at regular intervals (di).

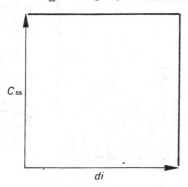

Table 6.2 *Pharmacokinetic data for some orally active drugs*

Drug	Pharmacokinetic Data					
	Bioavailability (%)	Plasma binding (%)	Clearance (ml min^{-1} kg^{-1})	Volume of distribution (L kg^{-1})	Half-life (h)	Urinary excretion (%)
Acetylsalicylic Acid	68	49	9.3	0.15	0.25	1.4
Amoxicillin	93	18	5.3	0.41	1	52
Ampicillin	29–62	18	3.9	0.28	1.3	90
Cephalexin	90	14	4.3	0.26	0.9	96
Chloramphenicol	75–90	53	3.6	0.92	2.7	5
Clindamycin	87	93	3.5	0.66	2.7	9–14
Ethambutol	77	20–30	8.8	1.6	3.1	79
Methotrexate	65	45	1.5	0.4	8.4	94
Sulphamethoxazole	100	62	0.32	0.21	8.6	30
Trimethoprim	100	70	2.2	1.8	11	53
Tetracycline	77	65	1.9	1.3	9.9	48
Warfarin	100	99	0.045	0.11	37	0

The data have been extracted from Appendix II of Goodman & Gilman's *The Pharmacological Basis of Therapeutics*, 6th edn (1980), which should be consulted for references to original papers. The data are approximate and are reproduced here to aid understanding of pharmacokinetic principles, not as a guide to the clinical uses of the drugs listed.

therefore no longer empirical but based on the knowledge of the physicochemical properties of the drug and its pharmacokinetic profile. This means that dosage requirements can be worked out for each individual especially where the drug is toxic as in cancer chemotherapy. Pharmacokinetic data for some drugs are given in Table 6.2.

FURTHER READING

Adelusi, S.A. & Salako, L.A. (1982). Kinetics of the distribution and elimination of chloroquine in the rat. *Gen Pharmac.* 13, 433–437.

Benet, L.Z., Massoud, N. & Gambertoglio, O. (1980), eds. *Pharmacokinetic Basis for Drug Treatment*. Raven Press, New York.

Curry, S.H. (1980). *Drug Disposition and Pharmacokinetics. With a consideration of Pharmacological and Clinical Relationships*, 3rd edn. Blackwell Scientific Publications, Oxford.

Curry, S.H. & Whelpton, R. (1983). *Manual of Laboratory Pharmacokinetics*. John Wiley and Sons Ltd., Chichester, New York.

Gibaldi, M. (1984). *Biopharmaceutics and Clinical Pharmacokinetics*, 3rd edn. Lea and Febiger, Philadelphia.

Rogers, H.J., Spector, R.G. & Trounce, J.R. (1981). *A Textbook of Clinical Pharmacology*, Hodder and Stoughton, London.

PART IV

Factors Affecting Drug Metabolism

7

The influence of malnutrition and food-derived intoxicants

7.1   INTRODUCTION

The term malnutrition refers to a range of disease conditions caused by long-term intake of a diet lacking in essential nutrients, or if the diet contains essential nutrients, the quantities consumed are inadequate to sustain normal growth and body functions. The diet may be deficient in macronutrients (carbohydrates, proteins or lipids) and/or micronutrients (vitamins and minerals). Overt clinical symptoms of malnutrition can arise from deficiencies in micro- or macronutrients.

The term used to refer to the various disease conditions due to carbohydrate and protein deficiency (see Table 7.1) is protein energy malnutrition (PEM) which is defined by the WHO as

> a range of pathological conditions arising from co-incident lack, in varying proportions of protein and calories, occurring most frequently in infants and young children and commonly associated with infection.

Primary PEM associated with inadequate food intake is encountered widely in countries of the third world. Secondary malnutrition such as may arise from cirrhosis, malabsorption, carcinomatosis, and anorexia is also seen in richer developed societies. Malnourished children also frequently suffer from bacterial and parasitic infections, and since PEM can influence drug action in various ways, the nutritional state of the patient must be considered carefully during drug therapy. The discussion in this chapter is limited to the influence of malnutrition on drug action. There is no attempt to cover all of the extensive field of drug–food interactions. Good reviews by Campbell & Hayes (1974) and Roe (1984) of the broad field are recommended further reading.

Table 7.1   *Classification of PEM*

PEM	Body weight (% of standard)	Oedema
Underweight child	80–60	None
Marasmus	60 or less	None
Kwashiorkor	80–60	Yes
Marasmic kwashiorkor	60 or less	Yes

7.2   SOME FEATURES OF PEM

PEM is a complex condition giving rise to a wide range of dysfunctions in the body. The following are some of the pathophysiological changes brought about by PEM that can alter drug pharmacokinetic profiles and metabolic processes.

Hypoproteinaemia

Low serum albumin (hypoalbuminaemia) is characteristic of kwashiorkor and marasmic kwashiorkor but not of marasmus. The low plasma albumin is caused by a progressive fall in the rate of albumin synthesis due to inadequate supply of the right type of aminoacid(s) in the diet. It is not due to increased clearance of albumin or diminished ability of the liver to synthesise the protein. Diminished albumin concentration is associated with the oedema seen in kwashiorkor. Total body water is increased and there can be up to 40% loss in total body potassium. In kwashiorkor and marasmic kwashiorkor there is an overall reduction in the total concentration of serum proteins (hypoproteinaemia): at the same time different plasma proteins are affected to different extents. Because albumin is reduced more than globulin, the ratio of albumin to globulin (A/G ratio) is characteristically low.

In considering such changes, it is important to note that the normal concentration of plasma gammaglobulin is higher in black Africans than in Caucasians. Table 7.2 shows mean values of serum proteins in Europeans and Nigerians living in Ibadan, Nigeria. Since the albumin concentrations are not greatly different in the two ethnic populations, the A/G ratio is characteristically lower for Nigerians than for Europeans.

Possibly, the hypergammaglobulinaemia in the African has developed in response to the frequent exposure to malaria and other endemic parasitic infections. In one study the gammaglobulin

Table 7.2   *Serum proteins of normal adult Nigerians and Europeans living in Ibadan*

Proteins	Nigerians		Europeans	
	g/100 ml	% total	g/100 ml	% total
Total proteins	6.8	100	6.9	100
Albumin	3.35	49.5	4.05	58.5
Alpha₁ globulin	0.20	2.9	0.31	4.5
Alpha₂ globulin	0.51	7.5	0.52	7.5
Beta₁ globulin	0.64	9.4	0.82	11.9
Gammaglobulin	2.10	31.3	1.20	17.6
Total globulin	3.45	50.5	2.85	41.5
A/G ratio	0.97		1.42	

The 25 Europeans studied had lived in Ibadan for between 3 months and 15 years. Data taken from Edozien (1957), with permission.

concentration in the plasma of children protected from malaria with weekly pyrimethamine was found to be lower than that in unprotected children living in the same hyperendemic area. However, the gammaglobulin values of protected children were still higher than the values for European children similarly protected.

Other data show that the high gammaglobulin concentration seen in blacks is not always associated with continuing exposure to parasitic infections. In Venezuela where malaria was once endemic, but is no longer so, blacks still have an excess of gammaglobulin. American blacks have a higher concentration of this protein in their plasma than healthy whites of comparable socioeconomic status. West African blacks resident in London have higher gammaglobulin concentrations than their European counterparts even after several years of continuous residence in the United Kingdom. Edozien (1957) has proposed that the ability to maintain high plasma concentration of gammaglobulin is an inherited characteristic which has been selected for the protection it offers against malaria and other endemic parasitic infections. The excess gammaglobulin represents a component of immunity against infection. The hypergammaglobulinaemia gene also permits the system to switch on the production of additional gammaglobulin in the event of an infection. Thus Africans living in hyperendemic areas of parasitic infection have higher gammaglobulin values than those living in non-endemic areas, while the latter have higher values than Caucasians. It must be added that the genetic basis of hypergammaglobulinaemia has not been established.

In kwashiorkor, the protein fraction most dramatically affected is albumin. The data in Table 7.3 show that there is also a significant fall in the mean absolute concentration of total proteins, alpha2-globulin and beta-globulin. Gammaglobulin shows a tendency to increase in both kwashiorkor and recovered children. From the point of view of drug binding, the changes in serum albumin are the most relevant. The marked fall in serum albumin (the value in kwashiorkor is only 42% of normal) can be due to a reduced capacity of liver to synthesize albumin, increased catabolism of albumin, or lack of the essential aminoacids for synthesis of the protein. When kwashiorkor patients are fed with adequate supply of proteins, the serum albumin concentration rises to normal values very rapidly. Also the $t_{1/2}$ of albumin in kwashiorkor is no different from that after re-covery. Thus hypoalbuminaemia in kwashiorkor is not due to a reduced synthetic capacity of the liver or to increased breakdown of this protein, but to inadequate supply of the right type of aminoacids in the diet. There are more sulphur-containing aminoacids (cystine, cysteine, methionine) in albumin and beta-globulin than in alpha- and gammaglobulin. The major source of sulphur-containing amino- acids in diet is animal proteins (milk and meat), the deficiency of which leads to kwashiorkor. Albumin and beta-globulin are thus the most affected protein fractions.

Endocrine changes

Growth hormone secretion is normal or even above normal in kwashiorkor and marasmus. Hence there is usually intense anabolism and growth activity once the protein deficiencies are corrected. Because plasma albumin concentration is low, there is more free cortisol than normal. Signs of cortisol toxicity such as moon face and abnormal glucose tolerance characteristic of kwashiorkor are explained on this basis. Catecholamine excretion is low in these children, suggesting a decreased synthesis of these amines.

7.3   PEM AND DRUG ACTION

The physiological and biochemical changes in PEM are complex and may alter kinetics and metabolism. However, studies carried out so far have not yielded results from which firm generalisations can be made. One reason for this is that most of the detailed studies have been conducted in animal models. In view of the complexity of mal-

Table 7.3 *Mean values for total serum protein and protein fractions in healthy and kwashiorkor children 1½ to 2½ years of age*

Protein	Control group (96 children)		Kwashiorkor group (39 children)		Recovered (12 children)	
	g/100 ml	% total	g/100 ml	% total	g/100 ml	% total
Total proteins	6.70	100	4.11*	100	6.80	100
Albumin	3.00	44.8	1.27*	31.0	2.77	40.7
Alpha₁ globulin	0.37	5.5	0.26*	6.3	0.40	5.8
Alpha₂ globulin	0.91	13.5	0.53*	12.8	0.82	12.1
Beta globulin	0.87	13.0	0.41*	10.0	0.86	12.6
Gammaglobulin	1.55	23.1	1.64	39.9	1.95	28.6
Total globulin	3.70	55.2	2.84	69.1	4.03	59.3
A/G ratio	0.81		0.45		0.69	

* Significantly lower than control and recovered values

Data modified from Edozien (1960), with permission.

nutrition, extrapolation of data obtained from animal studies to man is not entirely justifiable. Most effects are both animal- and drug-specific and dependent on the duration and degree of malnourishment. On the other hand, studies on human subjects are usually limited to small samples and often complicated by other diseases which may be present at the same time. Furthermore, malnutrition may alter the physiology and biochemistry of the system in a complex way so that opposing kinetic and metabolic effects are exerted on a given drug. Thus, what is known so far about the effects of malnutrition on drug action illustrates the magnitude of the problem rather than serving as a guide to drug therapy in malnutrition.

Drug absorption

In general, absorption of drugs after oral administration is decreased because transit time is short due to diarrhoea, which is a common feature of PEM, and absorption may be impaired due to atrophy of the jejunal mucosa. Malnutrition can also affect absorption indirectly by altering the pH of gastric and intestinal contents.

In malnourished children, the rates of absorption of tetracycline and chloramphenicol are reduced compared to control, well fed children; so is the absorption of iron. This is almost certainly due to absence of carrier proteins. The peak plasma level of rifampicin in malnourished children is lower that it is in well fed controls and this is attributed to impaired absorption.

Drug binding to plasma proteins

One of the most important ways in which PEM can alter drug action is protein binding. The protein most generally involved in the binding of acidic drugs is albumin; globulins play a minor role. Primary binding takes place between anionic groups of acidic drugs and cationic nitrogen groups on the protein. The latter are more available in albumin than in any other plasma protein. Binding of drugs to plasma proteins has the following consequences:

(a) The protein-bound drug does not cross lipid boundaries easily. Important boundaries are the blood–brain barrier, the placenta, the glomerulus and renal tubular epithelium. By reducing the rate of glomerular filtration, protein binding may reduce the rate of renal excretion of drugs, but does not affect tubular secretion.

(b) The protein-bound drug is not available for metabolism. Thus, protein binding may reduce the rate of drug inactivation and alter plasma $t_{1/2}$. However, since drug–protein interactions are reversible processes, with fast rates of dissociation, protein binding does not always prevent availability of drug for metabolism (see (e) below).

(c) Only the unbound fraction of the drug is pharmacologically active. Consequently, reduction in binding, which can occur as a result of displacement from binding sites by other drugs or in hypoalbuminaemia as in PEM, can increase both therapeutic actions and toxicity of normally bound drugs. Also if two drugs bind to the same site on a plasma protein, the drug with the higher affinity can displace the other and so cause an increase in the plasma concentration of unbound drug. This is the basis of the adverse drug interaction between, for example, salicylates and dicoumarol (section 5.6 page 126).

(d) Plasma binding can in theory increase the rate of absorption of a drug from the gastrointestinal tract, because, by binding it, plasma proteins remove the drug from free solution on the side to which the drug is diffusing, thereby increasing the concentration gradient.

(e) Drugs such as penicillin, sulphonamides and salicylates or their metabolites with high affinities for plasma protein may induce hypersensitivity reactions by acting as haptens.

If the bound drug is not available for metabolism, then for a highly bound drug, metabolism and elimination must depend on the relative rates of disassociation of the drug–protein complex and of metabolism. Kinetic consideration of drug–protein interactions suggest that protein binding *per se* may not have significant effects on drug metabolism.

The interaction of a drug, D, with the binding site of a protein, P, is considered a reversible reaction obeying the law of mass action, so that

$$D + P \underset{k_2}{\overset{k_1}{\rightleftharpoons}} DP \qquad (7.1)$$

Where k_1 and k_2 are the rate constants for forward and reverse interactions. At equilibrium

$$B = \frac{1}{1 + 1/K_A nP + D/nP} \qquad (7.2)$$

Where B = fraction of drug bound to protein, K_A = association constant (ratio k_1/k_2), n = number of binding sites per protein molecule, P = concentration of protein, and D = concentration of unbound drug.

Estimates of K_A for interactions of acidic drugs with bovine serum albumin suggest that protein–drug complexes dissociate at very fast rates with half-times in the order of milliseconds. On the other hand, rates of metabolism and elimination are much lower. Thus in the sequence

$$\text{drug–protein complex} \xrightarrow{k_d} \text{drug + protein} \xrightarrow{k_e} \text{drug inactivated or eliminated}$$

where k_d = dissociation rate constant and k_e = elimination or metabolism rate constant for the drug, $k_d > k_e$.

Therefore, dissociation of drug from protein is not the rate-limiting step in the metabolism of drug bound to protein. At any given time there would be dissociated molecules of drug. It is therefore not the case that a proportion of the drug is irreversibly bound to plasma protein and permanently unavailable for metabolism.

The notion that protein binding might reduce drug metabolism has come from observations that many long-acting drugs such as sulphamethoxypridazine are also highly bound to plasma. However, other drugs such as the salicylates and penicillins which are also highly bound are excreted relatively rapidly, probably because they are also actively secreted.

Drug-binding to plasma proteins in PEM

From equation (7.2) above, it can be seen that the fraction of a given drug bound to plasma is directly related to P, the concentration of plasma protein, as well as to the affinity of the drug (K_A) and number of binding sites (n) on the binding protein. In kwashiorkor and marasmic kwashiorkor, the albumin content of the plasma is less than 50% of normal values. Since albumin is quantitatively a very important protein in drug binding, it is no surprise that in malnourished adults and children, reduced plasma binding of acidic drugs (sulphonamides, antimicrobial and antiinflammatory agents) has been observed. Furthermore, the majority of drug–protein interactions involve no more than two primary binding sites and generally only one. The point of a single binding site is that the drug capacity of plasma proteins is limited. The binding sites can be saturated. This can occur with relatively low concentration of drug when plasma albumin is low as in kwashiorkor. After a given therapeutic dose of a plasma-bound drug, the concentration of free drug will be higher in a kwashiorkor patient than in normal subjects.

However, the extent of reduction in binding seen in PEM is not as great as would be expected from the lowered plasma albumin. One explanation for such a discrepancy is that with low albumin levels, binding to other plasma proteins might become significant. It is known that a number of basic drugs such as quinine, quinidine, chloroquine, and other antimalarial quinolines bind to the plasma protein, alpha$_1$-acid glycoprotein more than to albumin. There is no information about concentrations of alpha$_1$-acid glycoprotein in PEM; but it is known that the concentration of this protein is increased in several disease states including rheumatoid arthritis, myocardial infarction and malignancy. If the concentration of this protein is also increased in malnutrition, binding of basic drugs to this protein would increase in that condition and complicate the overall pharmacokinetic picture. Most studies have been concerned with acidic drugs which bind to albumin. Drug binding to oromucoids and globulin and the binding of basic drugs have been little studied in malnutrition.

Renal excretion

Renal excretion of drugs may be affected in PEM due to a combination of reduced cardiac output, reduced glomerular filtration, reduced renal blood flow and inadequate tubular function. However, studies of drug elimination in PEM have not yielded uniform results. This is probably because the extent of alterations in renal physiology depends on the severity of PEM. In undernourished and malnourished adults total body clearance of antibiotics (tetracyclines and rifampicin) is enhanced due to increased renal elimination. This is attributed to decreased plasma binding. On the other hand Buchanan *et al* (1980) found that antipyrine clearance in rehabilitated kwashiorkor children was only 50% of the value in the same children before treatment. The mean serum albumin concentration in rehabilitated children was double its concentration on admission to hospital. This suggests that protein binding had minimal effect on antipyrine elimination.

Drug metabolism

The major site of metabolism of administered drugs is the liver. Metabolism usually occurs in two phases. Phase 1 is oxidation, re-duction or hydrolysis of the drug followed by phase II which is a synthetic reaction such as conjugation (see page 124). The two reactions result in the formation of products with increased polarity, reduced penetrability of cell membranes and greater ease of excretion by the kidney. Probably the most important effects of PEM on drug action are exerted on the drug-metabolising enzymes located in the endoplasmic reticulum of liver cells. The enzyme complex consists of a carbon monoxide sensitive haemoprotein called cytochrome P-450, and a flavoprotein reductase. The enzymes require NADPH (or NADH) and oxygen and can metabolise a wide variety of drugs and chemicals. The complex is therefore termed a mixed function oxidase (MFO) or monoxygenase(s). This enzyme system can be induced by a variety of environmental pollutants and drugs such as phenobarbitone, and can be inhibited by others such as SKF 525-A. Induction implies stimulation of new enzyme synthesis as well as modification or activation of existing enzymes. In the malnourished state, the activity of MFO is greatly reduced.

Laboratory animal studies

In malnourished rats, hepatic microsomal drug metabolism is depressed. Hexobarbitone sleeping time is prolonged. Phenobarbitone, 4-methylcoumarin and carbon tetrachloride fail to induce the usual synthesis of drug-metabolising enzymes. There is a decrease in total microsomal protein, mixed function oxidases and in particular, cytochrome P-450 responsible for the hydroxylation of many drugs. There is also an absolute decrease in the activity of liver microsomal enzymes. The V_{max} per mg of microsomal protein acting on ethylmorphine and aniline was found in one study of protein deficient rats to be only 65% of normal.

Human studies

A number of studies have been undertaken in humans which show that hepatic microsomal enzyme activity is reduced in malnutrition. Many such studies have employed the drug antipyrine, which is well absorbed after oral administration. It is relatively free of toxic effects, so that it can be used in healthy volunteers and its fate in the body can be followed easily since most of the drug is excreted in the urine. In humans, four urinary metabolites have been identified, namely hydroantipyrine, norantipyrine, 3-hydroxymethylantipyrine, and 3-carboxyantipyrine. There is reason to believe that a different enzyme in the MFO complex controls the metabolism of antipyrine to yield each metabolite. Therefore the urinary metabolite profile provides information concerning changes in the activity of the different types of oxidising enzymes in MFO. Another reason why antipyrine is used for these studies is that not more than 10% of the drug is bound to serum protein. Therefore antipyrine kinetics are not seriously affected by serum protein binding.

Krishnaswamy & Naidu (1977, see Krishnaswamy 1983) found that the $t_{1/2}$ of antipyrine was between 13 and 88% longer in adult Indians suffering from nutritional oedema than in normal well fed adults. The authors concluded that the long $t_{1/2}$ of antipyrine was due to reduced MFO activity rather than to hepatic dysfunction or fatty infiltration of the liver. These latter conditions are commonly encountered in children with kwashiorkor, but not in adults suffering from nutritional oedema. Buchanan et al (1980) studied antipyrine pharmacokinetic profiles in five black South African children suffering from severe kwashiorkor before and after nutritional rehabilitation. The authors found that during the acute phase of the disease, the children excreted a large amount of unchanged antipyrine in urine. After nutritional rehabilitation, the amount of unchanged drug diminished. As can be seen from Table 7.4, $t_{1/2}$ is longer on admission than after nutritional rehabilitation. Clearance is also much larger after nutritional rehabilitation. The changes were attributed to reduced activity of MFO in kwashiorkor. Though the concentration of antipyrine metabolites in urine was much lower on admission than after recovery, the metabolite ratios were similar in the two conditions, suggesting that acute kwashiorkor affected the four oxidative enzymes equally. The significance of this finding is that since the phase I metabolism of most drugs and chemicals may involve oxidation, demethylation, hydroxylation, etc. by MFO enzymes, PEM is likely to affect the metabolism of a wide range of drugs adversely.

Table 7.4 *Half life, apparent volume of distribution, and clearance of antipyrine in five children with kwashiorkor*

$t_{1/2}$ (h)		V_d (L kg^{-1})		Clearance (mL min^{-1} kg^{-1})	
A	R	A	R	A	R
9.9	6.8	0.50	0.62	0.62	1.07
NS		NS		P = 0.05	

A = values on admission; R = values after nutritional rehabilitation; NS = not significantly different; P = probability level.

Glucuronidation of antipyrine metabolites (Phase II metabolism) is also depressed in malnourished children. Impaired metabolism of several other drugs such as chloramphenicol, salicylates and acetanilide has been documented in kwashiorkor and maramus children and in adults suffering from severe malnutrition. On the other hand, drug metabolism in moderately malnourished adults is either normal or even increased.

Wharton & McChesney (1970) found that in East African children suffering from kwashiorkor, the proportion of chloroquine excreted unchanged was higher than it was in normal well fed children. Again this was attributed to reduced activity of hepatic microsomal enzymes.

These kinds of results have led some investigators to suggest that drug dosage needs to be adjusted in kwashiorkor. This can only be done with great care. The amount of drug in circulation after a given dose may be less in PEM patients than in normal individuals, but because of hypoalbuminaemia, more of the absorbed drug is in the free form. There is therefore no sound basis for increasing dosage in kwashiorkor simply because absorption might be reduced. On the other hand, although MFO activity is reduced, for plasma-bound drugs the rate of excretion of unmetabolised drug may be greater in kwashiorkor because of reduced binding. Dosage adjustment must therefore be on an individual patient basis after taking the pharmacokinetic parameters of a given drug and the severity and duration of malnutrition into account.

7.4   MISCELLANEOUS DIETARY FACTORS
Micronutrients

Micronutrients such as vitamin A, E, riboflavin, niacin, pyridoxine, selenium and zinc are required for various essential coenzyme functions. Their deficiency can therefore affect drug metabolism. Vitamin A deficiency predisposes rats treated with aflatoxin B_1, a mycotoxin elaborated by the common food contaminant *Aspergillus flavus*, to colonic carcinoma and liver cancer. Vitamin A is required in the normal differentiation of intestinal mucosal and ciliated cells from basal cells. A deficiency in this nutrient and consequent change in the pattern of differentiation might render the cells more sensitive to the mutagenic effect of aflatoxin B_1. Alternatively, the absence of vitamin A in the diet could lead to formation of a harmful metabolite from aflatoxin B_1. Since acute aflatoxin poisoning can reduce serum and hepatic levels of vitamin A, chronic consumption of aflatoxin could set up a vicious cycle. It is known that vitamin A deficiency can depress MFO activity. This can occur in the absence of other signs of vitamin A deficiency such as night blindness. The implications are that those who suffer overtly from vitamin A deficiency (and there are many in parts of the tropics) must have severely depressed MFO activity. Riboflavin is a constituent of flavoprotein reductase, an enzyme in the MFO complex. Nicotinamide is a constituent of two enzyme cofactors, namely nicotinamide adenine dinucleotide (NAD, coenzyme I, DPN), and nicotinamide adenine dinucleotide phosphate (NADP, coenzyme II, TPN). These enzymes are important for hydrogen and electron transfer, aerobic oxidation and drug metabolism.

Food-derived intoxicants: cyanide and ataxic neuropathy

Many of the foods eaten in the tropics – cassava, beans, yams, millet, maize – contain cyanogenetic glycosides e.g. linamarin (Fig. 7.1) which on hydrolysis yield the highly toxic hydrocyanic acid (HCN). The fresh tuber of the bitter variety of cassava (*Manihot esculenta*) contains as much as 38 mg% of cyanogenetic glycoside and hydrocyanic acid. Cassava is the staple carbohydrate of millions of Africans. The preparation of cassava for food involves complex processing during which most of the cyanide is removed. In Nigeria, the popular cassava meal, *gari*, is prepared by grating the peeled cassava tuber on raspers and pressing the pulp to remove as much of the poisonous juice as possible. During the pressing which lasts 2 – 3 days, fermentation induced by *Pseudomonas* or *Corynebacterium manioc* takes place. These organisms break down starch to produce organic acids thereby decreasing the pH. Under these conditions cyanogenetic glycosides hydrolyse, yielding HCN. The pulp is next sieved and then fried in open iron pans, during which process the high temperature drives off fumes of volatile HCN, so that *gari* powder usually contains no more than about 1 mg % cyanide. In some parts of Nigeria, water is added to the grated cassava pulp before pressing in raffia bags and the starch, *usi*, extracted from the pulp. *Usi* is virtually free of cyanide as the latter is present in solution in the supernatant which is thrown away. Other forms of cassava meal are *funfun, akpo,* and *purupuru.* The cyanide content varies according to the mode of preparation. Since HCN is volatile, *gari* and other cassava meal processors are at risk of cyanide intoxication through inhalation.

The neurological disease called ataxic neuropathy (AN) or tropical neuropathy, described by Osuntokun (1968) is attributed to chronic cyanide intoxication. AN comprises bilateral optic atrophy, bilateral nerve deafness, ataxic gait, weakness and thinning of legs below the knees. The predominant pathological lesion is demyelination of the long tract fibres – optic, auditory, and spinal nerves especially of the lower limbs.

Part of the evidence for the theory that AN is caused by chronic cyanide intoxication from cassava is that the endemic focusses of the disease correspond with places where cassava is intensely cultivated and consumed as the major source of carbohydrate. The people of Epe and Ejirin studied by Osuntokun eat *purupuru* as well as *gari. Purupuru* contains as much as 4 – 6 mg % of cyanide. It is estimated that an adult male may consume 750 g of cassava a day, equivalent to a daily cyanide intake of 35 mg or more depending on the cassava meal. These

Fig. 7.1. Structure of linamarin, a cyanogenetic glycoside found in cassava.

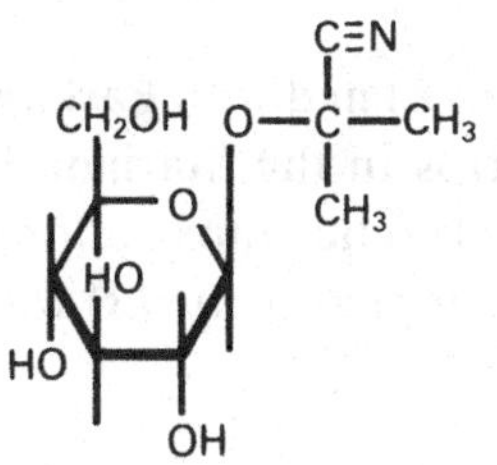

Linamarin

amounts are not lethal outright, but are enough over time to cause chronic intoxication.

Cyanide is detoxified in the body by conversation to (a) thiocyanate, (b) 2-aminothiazoline-4-carboxylic acid, or (c) incorporation into 1-carbon metabolic pool. Thiocyanate formation is the major pathway and plasma thiocyanate levels are valid indices of cyanide exposure. In AN patients, plasma thiocyanate is about 4-fold higher than in controls. High plasma thiocyanate is not due to reduced clearance, direct absorption of thiocyanate from foods containing it, but is a reflection of the cassava-derived cyanide load.

If other tropical foods also contain cynogenetic glycosides, the question is why is cassava blamed for AN in the tropics? It seems that cyanogenetic glycosides differ in the ease with which they can be hydrolysed to release HCN, and different enzymes are responsible for the hydrolysis of different glycosides. The cassava glycoside, linamarin, hydrolyses relatively easily. The enzyme, linase, present in the integument of the cassava catalyses hydrolysis of the glycoside. This enzyme is easily released when the cassava is bruised as in peeling. The other point to note is that not everyone exposed to a high cyanide load suffers overtly from AN. This is partly because nutritional deficiencies in vitamins and high quality proteins exacerbate cyanide toxicity. There may also be other unknown predisposing factors such as a defect in the detoxification of HCN in susceptible cassava consumers.

Other neurological syndromes associated with cyanide intoxication
Lathyrism
This is a pyramidal neurological disorder without optic nerve atrophy or deafness believed to be due to nitrile compounds in lathyrus peas or cyanogenetic glycosides in the seeds of the common vetch (*Vicia sativa*) which usually contaminates the lathyrus peas. The latter are eaten in parts of India where lathyrism is common.

Parkinsonism and dementia
Another neurological syndrome associated with Parkinsonism and dementia occurs among the Chamorros in the Mariana Islands. This illness is thought to be caused by chronic intoxication with a cyanogenetic glycoside from the cycad nut (*Cycas circinalis*) which is a major carbohydrate source for the islanders.

Other diseases engendered by cyanide
Goitre
This is caused by thiocyanate which is the major product of cyanide metabolism. Throughout the tropics and subtropics, among island populations and in parts of Europe, the occurrence of endemic goitre has been found to be closely associated with cyanogenetic glycosides.

Retarded growth and mental development
Exposure of children to a high cyanide load at an early age may affect physical and mental development if this exposure is accompanied by nutritional deficiencies such as lack of high quality protein and micronutrients.

Aflatoxin
Aflatoxins (see Fig. 7.2) are a group of substituted coumarins synthesised by moulds, e.g. *Aspergillus* and *Penicillium* species which commonly contaminate tropical foods especially when these are not properly stored. The characteristic physicochemical feature of these compounds is their intense fluorescence under ultraviolet light. Several aflatoxins and derivatives of parent aflatoxins are known. These mycotoxins were discovered in 1960 in England as a result of large-scale death of farm turkeys fed on contaminated groundnuts from Brazil; the birds died from liver damage. These toxins have since been recognised as constituting a health hazard to man and domestic animals and a threat to the economy of tropical countries who depend on

Fig. 7.2. Structure of aflatoxin B₁ produced by a common tropical food contaminant *Aspergillus flavus*.

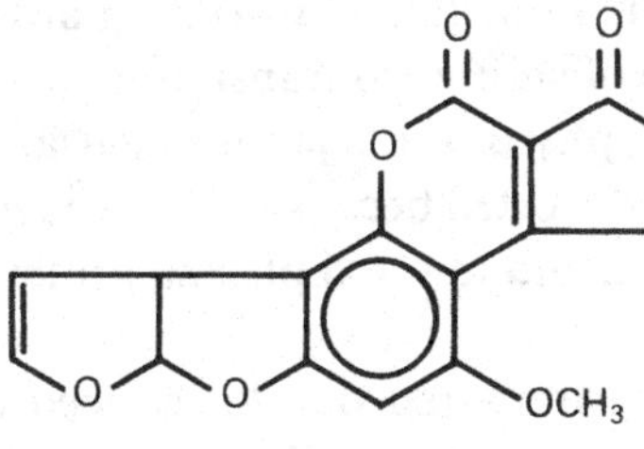

export of agricultural produce such as groundnut and cocoa for foreign-exchange earnings.

Bassir and his colleagues (see Bababunmi 1980) over a period of twenty years studied aflatoxin contamination of Nigerian foods; they found that virtually everything we eat and drink can support the growth of *Aspergillus flavus* and be contaminated by mycotoxins. Examples are dry fish, dry meat, palm-wine, soyabeans, paw-paw, banana, groundnuts, cocoa, red pepper, millet, rice, corn, yams and *gari*. American and European importers of tropical produce consider an aflatoxin content of 0.25 parts per million (ppm) as dangerously unacceptable whereas Bababunmi (1980) stated that the aflatoxin content of Nigeria's principal food crops which are hawked and sold in town markets is not less than 0.5 ppm. Obviously therefore Nigerians, most of whom obtain their foods from open town markets, are exposed to dangerously high levels of aflatoxin as well as being deprived of export earnings from certain crops due to aflatoxin spoilage.

The most vulnerable organ in chronic aflatoxin intoxication is the liver. There is evidence that these toxins or their metabolites can induce cancer in experimental animals. Liver tumours occur in rats fed on mouldy peanut meal and aflatoxins are the carcinogenic agents. Studies in Kenya, Thailand, Mozambique and Swaziland show a highly positive correlation between aflatoxin intake and the incidence of liver cancer in the communities studied, males being more susceptible than females. The incidence of liver cancer in these countries and in Nigeria is among the highest in the world. At the cellular level, aflatoxins are mutagenic, can cause chromosomal aberrations and DNA breakage. As with other neurotoxins of food origin, the toxicity and carcinogenicity of aflatoxins increase with undernourishment.

7.5   SUMMARY

(i) In severe protein energy malnutrition (PEM) drug absorption may be impaired because of shortened transit time in the gastrointestinal tract and atrophy of the jejunal mucosa.

(ii) Drug distribution may be distorted because of expanded extracellular fluid compartment, and lowered plasma protein binding.

(iii) Renal elimination may be impaired due to reduced cardiac output and reduced rate of glomerular filtration.

(iv) Reduced plasma binding, particularly of acid drugs, is

observed. But there is no consistent evidence that the resultant increase in unbound fraction of drugs is sufficient to alter drug action, or to accelerate drug elimination.

(v) Hepatic microsomal enzymes are reduced and the rate of biotransformation of many drugs is depressed.

(vi) The question whether bioavailability of drugs is altered to the extent where adjustment in therapeutic dosage is indicated in PEM cannot be answered with a firm generalisation on the basis of present knowledge.

(vii) In the tropics, where, because of the warm weather and high relative humidity, many foods support the growth of *A. flavus*, aflatoxin intoxication is thought to be associated with a high incidence of liver cancer.

(viii) Many tropical foods such as cassava contain cyanogenetic glycosides. In communities where such foods constitute the major source of carbohydrate, especially in association with protein and vitamin deficiency, chronic cyanide intoxication may occur. The neurological syndrome, ataxic neuropathy is common in such communities and this is attributed to chronic cyanide poisoning. The latter may also be responsible for goitre, and mental retardation in children.

(ix) Chronic intoxication with aflatoxin and cyanide may adversely affect drug response in complex ways.

FURTHER READING

Bababunmi, E.A. (1980). Biochemical research on the aflatoxin molecule. In *Toxicology In The Tropics* ed. R.L. Smith & E.A. Bababunmi, pp. 93–107. Francis & Taylor, London.

Buchanan, W., Davis, M., Danhof, M. & Breimer, D.D. (1980). Antipyrine metabolic formation in children in the acute phase of malnutrition and after recovery. *Br. J. Clin. Pharmac.10*, 363–8.

Campbell, T.C. & Hayes, R.H. (1974). Role of nutrition in the drug-metabolising enzyme system. *Pharm. Rev.* 26. 171–97.

De Leve, L.D. & Piafsky, K.M. (1983). Clinical significance of plasma binding of basic drugs. In *Drug Metabolism and Distribution*, Current reviews in Biomedicine 3, ed. J.W. Lamble, pp. 177–80. Elsevier Biomedical Press, Amsterdam, New York, Oxford.

Edozien, J.C. (1957). The serum proteins of healthy adult Nigerians. *J. Clin. Path.* 10, 276–9.

Edozien, J.C. (1960). The serum proteins in kwashiorkor. *J. Paediatrics.* 57, 594–603.

Krishnaswamy, K. (1983). Drug metabolism and pharmacokinetics in malnutrition. *Trends Pharmacol. Sci.* 4. 295–9.

Osuntokun, B.O. (1968). An ataxic neuropathy in Nigeria. A clinical, biochemical and ectrophysiological study. Brain **91**, 215–48.

Roe, D.A. (1984). Nutrients and drug interactions. *Nutr. Rev.* **42**, 141–54.

Wharton, B.A. & McChesney, E.W. (1970). Chloroquine metabolism in kwashiorkor. *J. Trop. Paediat.* **16**, 130–2.

8

Genetic factors affecting drug action

8.1   INTRODUCTION

Some drugs cause side effects which are not predictable from their known pharmacological properties. Such unusual toxicities called *idiosyncratic reactions* are also usually unrelated to dose. A familiar example is the anti-malarial chloroquine pruritus. In about 1 in 10 Nigerians, this drug, by an unknown mechanism, causes an extremely unpleasant itch, likened to sharp pin pricks occurring unexpectedly in any part of the body at frequent but irregular intervals accompanied by an irresistible urge to scratch the spot. Idiosyncratic drug reactions may be due to the operation of hereditary factors which mediate abnormal metabolism of the drug in the affected individual. Abnormal drug metabolism can also be responsible for wide variabilities in the optimum dosage for the drug involved. It is obvious that if one knew beforehand that an individual had a genetic predisposition to metabolise or respond to a given drug in an unusual way, the prescriber can adjust the dose appropriately to achieve optimum benefit or choose another drug.

The study of the influence of inheritable factors in drug action is now a special branch of pharmacology known as *pharmacogenetics*, defined by Kalow as 'pharmacologic responses and their modification by hereditary influences'. Pharmacogenetics is a wide subject and would include consideration of problems such as inherited characteristics which enable some micro-organisms to metabolise or survive in the presence of otherwise lethal doses of antimicrobial agents (see Chapter 13). In this chapter however, genetic factors which influence the action of selected groups of drugs in man only are considered.

8.2   THE IMPORTANCE OF PHARMACOGENETICS IN THE TROPICS

The frequency of different inheritable characteristics which influence drug action varies between ethnic populations. This is because some of these characteristics are evolutionary adaptations in particular environments. For example, as we shall see later in this chapter, G6PD deficiency appears to be an adaptation for survival in regions where *P. falciparum* was endemic, and is therefore highly prevalent among peoples of African and Mediterranean origin. Unfortunately, however, this deficiency also leads to severe haemolytic anaemias when the affected individuals take certain drugs. It is important that students, physicians, pharmacists and others concerned with drugs in the tropics should be particularly aware of this point. This is because the drugs used in these countries have been developed and tested clinically in populations *genetically different* from the ones where the drugs are used. In tropical countries, not much, if any, post-marketing surveillance is conducted on important drugs. The extent of drug-induced toxicity in the tropics (some of it due to genetic factors) is probably alarming, but we do not know because in the poorly doctored populations of these regions, and in the face of extensive self-medication, detection of toxicity is a serious problem (see also page 14).

8.3   DEFINITION OF TERMS

Simple definitions of some terms used in pharmacogenetics are given below.

Polygenic and monogenic control of drug response

To study the genetic control of a given drug response, e.g. the rate of acetylation of isoniazid, the response is measured in a number of individuals selected at random from the population and a frequency–response curve is plotted. The frequency response curve may show only one peak (Fig. 8.1A), in which case, the response is regulated by a number of genes and is said to be under *polygenic* or *multifactorial* control. The variations among individuals in their response to the drug is said to be *continuous* or *unimodal*. The response rates are normally distributed throughout the population. If the curve is discontinuous (Fig. 8.1B), that is, there are two or more peaks, only one gene regulates the response. Each peak represents a single *phenotype* and the existence of more than one phenotype represents a *polymorphism* in the drug response. The control is said to be *monogenic* and as in Fig. 8.1B above, it is bimodal. If several genes are involved in the regulation of the drug response, some individuals in the population would have more and some less of those genes and the drug response would be normally distributed. In monogenic control, however, where only one gene is involved, some individuals would have the gene and some would not or they may have different variants of the gene.

Homozygotes, heterozygotes

In man there are 22 pairs of non sex-linked chromosomes (also called autosomes) and one pair of sex-linked chromosomes (called X-chromosomes). Chromosomes are made up of genes which are arranged like a chain of beads. In human cells, each inheritable characteristic is controlled by two genes which occur in a fixed position (locus) on the chromosome of each parent. There are thus two genes called alleles or allelic genes involved in the control of each characteristic. The characteristic to which the alleles gives rise is called the *phenotype* whereas the actual nature of the genes is known as the genotype. When the two alleles at a locus are identical, the genotype is *homozygous* whereas when the two alleles are different, the genotype is a *heterozygous*. A trait is *dominant* if it is expressed in a heterozygote; when it is expressed only in the homozygote, it is recessive. For example, the acetylation of isoniazid is controlled by two alleic genes–F' (fast) and S' (slow). In heterozygotes (F'S') acetylation is fast; only the homozygotes (S'S') are slow acetylators. Fast acetylation is thus the dominant trait. Since males have only one X-chromosome, all X-

Fig. 8.1. Polygenic (A) and monogenic (B) control of drug response. For isoniazid, people grouped around the median (a) are fast acetylators; those grouped around the median (b) are slow acetylators.

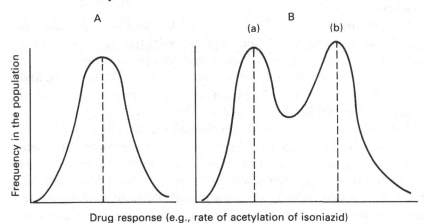

Drug response (e.g., rate of acetylation of isoniazid)

linked traits are expressed in male subjects. G6PD is an example of a sex-linked trait. The defect is fully expressed in male hemizygotes and female homozygotes and only partially expressed in female hetero-zygotes (see later in this chapter).

8.4   EXAMPLES OF DRUGS WHOSE RESPONSE OR METABOLISM IS AFFECTED BY INHERITED FACTORS

Antihypertensive drugs

Clinical observations suggest that there are ethnic variations in the response of hypertensives to diuretics and beta-blockers. Freis and his colleagues at the Veterans Administration Medical Centre in Washington conducted short-and long-term studies in which they compared beta-blockers (propranolol and nadolol) and hydro-chlorothiazide (diuretic) in the treatment of hypertension in black and white patients. The diuretic was consistently more effective than beta-blockers in black hypertensives. Other studies on black Zimbabweans and on a population of Zulus in South Africa also showed the beta-blocker, atenolol, to be relatively ineffective in lowering raised arterial blood pressure and it was suggested that 'beta-blockers should not be used as baseline treatment for hypertension in blacks'. On the other hand, studies in Ibadan (Olatunde, Akinkugbe & Carlisle, 1977; Falase & Salako, 1979) and elsewhere in Nigeria have shown that pro-pranolol, pindolol, timolol, and sotalol are effective antihypertensive agents in Nigerians with mild to moderate hypertension. There is therefore reason to believe that in general, black hypertensives are more likely to respond to diuretics than to beta-blockers and that among blacks there may also be ethnic differences in response to beta-blockers.

The reasons for these differences are not known. One explanation is that the first pass hydroxylation of propranolol (pp. 113, 184) is more extensive in blacks than in whites. A first pass phenomenon may not explain the relative failure of all beta-blockers in blacks as Salako and his colleagues found that the pharmacokinetic profile of pindolol in Nigerians was similar to its profile in other races.

The differences may also be explained on the basis of possible differences in the aetiology of hypertension among white and black populations. Hypertensive blacks tend to have higher plasma volumes (PV) and lower plasma renin activity (PRA) than white hypertensives. It has been proposed that patients with high PV have a *volume-depen-dent* hypertension which will respond to a reduction of extracellular and plasma volume with diuretics while those with high PRA and low PV should respond to beta-blockers. The clinical observations seem to be in agreement with this hypothesis. Also in line with this hypothesis is the finding in the Veteran Administration Medical Centre study that the antihypertensive response to captopril (angiotensin converting enzyme inhibitor) alone was less in black than in white subjects who tend to have high PRA.

Isoniazid acetylation

Many monosubstituted hydrallazines are inactivated by the enzyme N-acetyltransferase. Evans first showed (see Evans, 1977) that the acetylation of isoniazid is bimodally distributed so that subjects can be classified as fast or slow acetylators. The differences between slow and fast acetylators were not due to differences in intestinal absorption, protein binding, renal glomerular filtration or renal reabsorption but to a polymorphism in the activity of the soluble liver enzyme N-acetyltransferase. Slow inactivation is inherited as an autosomal recessive trait. In fast acetylators, the $t_{1/2}$ of isoniazid is about 1 h, whereas in slow acetylators it is more than 2 h. Acetylator phenotypes occur with different frequencies in different ethnic groups of the human race. Table 8.1 shows the frequencies of the gene controlling slow acetylation among different ethnic groups.

Clinical significance of acetylation polymorphism

(i) Isoniazid is used for the treatment of tuberculosis. The drug can cause peripheral neuropathy and hepatotoxicity. Slow acetylators are more likely to suffer toxic peripheral neuropathy than fast acetylators because the parent compound is responsible for this effect. (Fig. 8.2.) It can be prevented by concomitant administration of pyridoxine. On the other hand, fast acetylators are more liable to suffer isoniazid-induced hepatotoxicity because the acetylhydrazine formed from isoniazid is hydroxylated by cytochrome P-450 to a product that is highly toxic to liver cells.

(ii) Isoniazid inhibits the hydroxylation of phenytoin when the two drugs are administered simultaneously. This inhibition is more pronounced and phenytoin toxicity more marked in slow than in fast acetylators.

(iii) There is a higher incidence of antinuclear antibodies and of systemic lupus erythematosus (SLE)-like syndrome in slow than in fast acetylators.

Table 8.1   *Global frequency (q) of allele controlling slow acetylation*

Ethnic group	Location collected	q	(SE)
Japanese	Japan	0.34	0.01
Koreans	Korea	0.33	0.06
Chinese	Singapore	0.46	0.02
Thais	Thailand	0.54	0.04
Philippinos	Cebu	0.82	0.04
Burmese	Rangoon	0.61	0.04
Indians	Madras	0.80	0.04
Libyans	Benghazi	0.81	0.05
Egyptians	Cairo	0.91	0.03
Sudanese (non-Arab)	Khartoum	0.81	0.03
Kenyans)			
Ugandans)			
Tanzanians)	East Africa	0.74†	0.02
Zambians)			
Northern Nigerians	Zaria	0.70	0.03
Southern Nigerians	Nsukka	0.64	0.04
Italians	Rome	0.74	0.03
British whites	Liverpool	0.81	0.03
Swedes	Stockholm	0.82	0.02
Eskimos	Hudson and Jones Bay	0.22	0.03
American Indians	Denver	0.47	0.05
Shuara Indians	Ecuador	0.47	0.05

† Random selection from 953 patients in 35 tuberculosis treatment centres in East Africa.

From Gilles, H.M. (1984). Pharmacogenetic factors in anti-malaria drug testing. In *Handbook of Experimental Pharmacology*, vol. 68, ed. W. Peters & W.H.G. Richards, p. 418. Springer–Verlag, Berlin, Heidelberg.

Fig. 8.2. Acetylation of isoniazid.

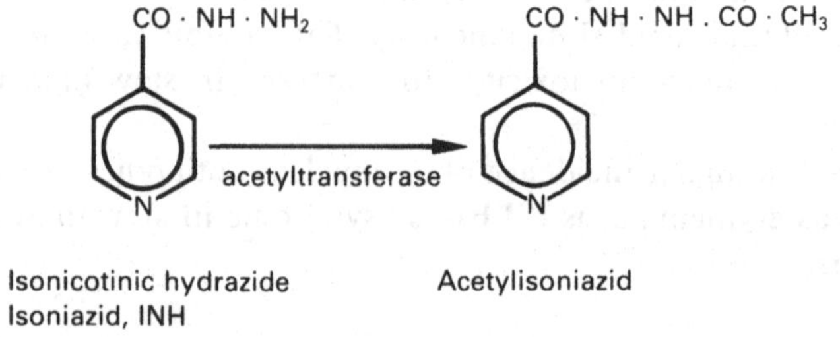

Isonicotinic hydrazide
Isoniazid, INH   Acetylisoniazid

Other drugs metabolised by N-acetylation

Other drugs whose metabolic acetylation shows polymorphism are shown in Fig. 8.3.

Procainamide

Many patients on long-term procainamide therapy develop antinuclear antibodies. This happens more quickly in slow acetylators than in fast acetylators and the SLE-like syndrome is encountered more frequently in slow acetylators.

Hydrallazine

The majority of patients who develop SLE syndrome during hydrallazine treatment are slow acetylators. Fast acetylators require higher doses of hydrallazine to control blood pressure.

Phenelzine

The antidepressant effects and the degree of monoamine oxidase inhibition caused by phenelzine are greater in slow acetylators after a standard dose of the drug.

Fig. 8.3. Examples of common drugs metabolised by acetylation.

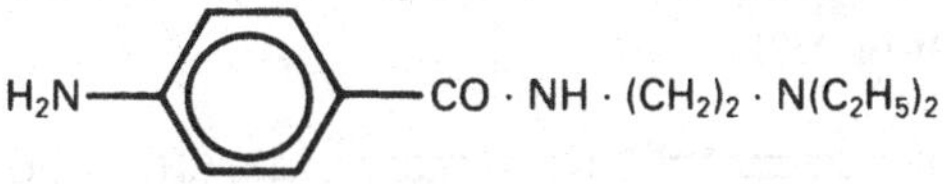

Procainamide

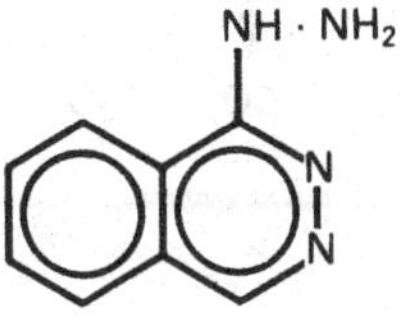

Hydrallazine

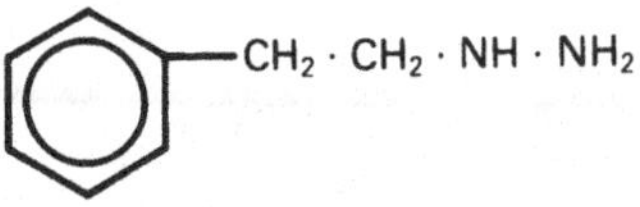

Phenelzine

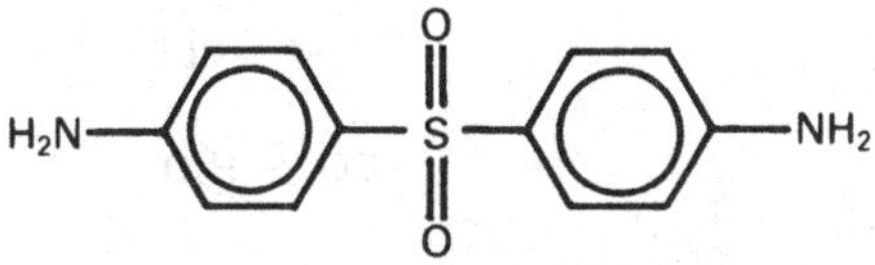

Dapsone

Alcohol dehydrogenase

Primary alcohols are oxidised by the liver microsomal enzyme, alcohol dehydrogenase as in Fig. 8.4. It is worth noting here that in the oxidation of ethanol to acetic acid and then to water and carbon dioxide, the rate-limiting step is the conversion of ethanol to acetaldehyde. Since the rest of the reaction occurs at a faster rate, acetaldehyde and acetic acid do not accumulate in the body. In contrast, the rate-limiting step in the oxidation of methanol is its conversion to formic acid and carbon dioxide. Furthermore, the whole process of methanol breakdown is several times slower than that of ethanol. Thus, the toxic metabolites, formaldehyde and formic acid, accumulate in the body. The retina is particularly vulnerable to them because high amounts of alcohol dehydrogenase are present in this organ for the physiological conversion of vitamin A (retinol, a primary alcohol) to vitamin A aldehyde. This is the explanation for the optic atrophy (blindness) associated with chronic methanol consumption. This point is of particular interest because many locally distilled alcoholic liquors in the tropics e.g. *ogogoro* in Nigeria and *apetesi* in Ghana contain variable amounts of methanol. Chronic consumers of these liquors suffer grades of optic atrophy, but unless they become

Fig. 8.4. Oxidative metabolism of ethanol and methanol. RLS = rate-limiting step.

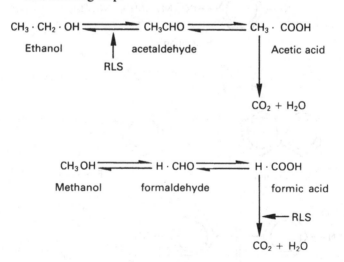

totally blind, one cannot know because many of the people do not read.

Knowledge of alcohol metabolism is applied in the treatment of alcoholism. The drug disulfiram is converted in the liver to diethyldithiocarbamic acid which, by chelating cupric ions, inhibits both aldehyde dehydrogenase and dopamine-β-hydroxylase with resultant accumulation of acetaldehyde and dopamine. This gives rise to mild but unpleasant symptoms of intoxication i.e. vasodilation, skin flushing (a false transmitter action of dopamine), palpitations and headache. This makes it unpleasant for the alcoholic to take even small quantities of ethanol.

Alcohol dehydrogenase shows polymorphism in its activity among different ethnic groups. The rate of alcohol metabolism varies accordingly. Caucasians metabolise ethanol one and half times as fast as Eskimos and Canadian Indians. It is claimed that these differences in the rates of ethanol metabolism correlate with observed differences in susceptibility to the effect of ethanol. The Canadian Indian is about 1.5 times as likely to be inebriated as a Caucasian after a tot of whisky. The variability is due to the existence of different variants of the enzyme having different affinities for the substrate. Certain oriental ethnic groups (Japanese, Taiwanese and Koreans) experience marked facial flushing after ethanol consumption despite normal alcohol dehydrogenase activity. The toxicity is thought to be due to accumulated acetaldehyde whose metabolism is abnormal due to a deficiency of aldehyde dehydrogenase.

Debrisoquine 4-hydroxylation

Debrisoquine is an antihypertensive agent which lowers blood pressure by preventing the release of noradrenaline from adrenergic neurones. The drug is metabolised by hydroxylation at the 4-position and to a lesser extent by aromatic hydroxylation at positions 5, 6, 7 or

Fig. 8.5. 4-Hydroxylation of debrisoquine.

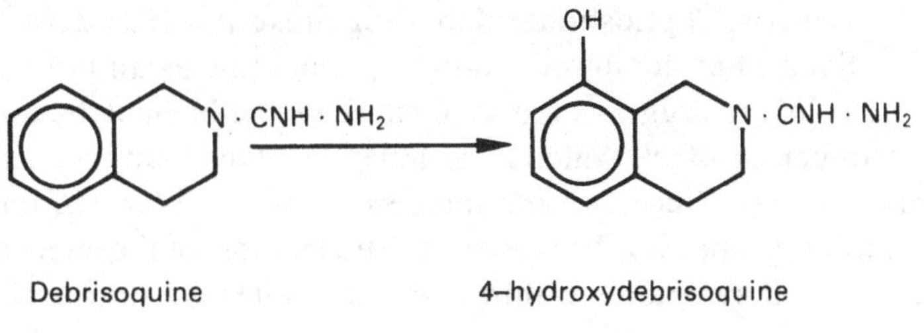

Debrisoquine   4–hydroxydebrisoquine

8. There is a large interpatient variability (up to 40-fold) in the dose required for effective therapy. This variability is due to the existence of a polymorphism in the hydroxylation of debrisoquine to 4-hydroxydebrisoquine. Hydroxylation is controlled by two alleles at a single gene locus. There are thus two distinct phenotypes, namely, poor metabolisers (PM) who excrete the drug unchanged in urine, and extensive metabolisers (EM) who excrete the drug as the hydroxylated metabolite. PM are homozygous for the autosomal recessive gene. Studies among different ethnic groups have demonstrated pronounced inter-ethnic variations in the frequency of PM phenotype: 6–8% of caucasians are PM whereas up to 15% of Nigerians are PM. On the other hand only about 1% of Egyptians are PM. PM are more sensitive to the hypotensive effects of debrisoquine than EM. Other drugs which are hydroxylated and appear to be under genetic control are diphenylhydantoin, phenacetin, nortriptyline, and propranolol. PM of debrisoquine are also PM of these drugs.

Plasma cholinesterase

The neuromuscular blocking drug, succinylcholine is rapidly hydrolysed by plasma cholinesterase (figure 8.6). The usual duration of action of the drug is 2 min. In a small proportion of individuals, an atypical variant of the enzyme is formed with 100 times lower affinity for the drug. In such individuals, the duration of action of the drug can be several hours with consequent prolongation of muscle relaxation and failure in respiration (apnoea). Family studies have shown that individuals with the atypical pseudocholinesterase inherit a rare gene from both parents. The original study carried out in a Canadian population showed that about 4% of the population were heterozygous for the atypical esterase gene and about 1 in 3000 were homozygous.

Another variant of the enzyme has virtually no activity against succinylcholine. The frequency of the gene for atypical esterase varies between ethnic groups, but appears to be absent in Japanese and extremely rare in Africans and peoples of African descent.

Glucose-6-phosphate dehydrogenase (G6PD) deficiency

Soon after the introduction of pamaquine as an antimalarial drug in 1926, the drug was found to cause severe haemolytic anaemia in a number of black Americans. Later, another 8-aminoquinoline, primaquine, introduced during the Second World War was found to have similar properties. The characteristic features of the effect are the appearance of symptoms within a few days after the start of therapy.

The urine turns dark in colour, jaundice develops and the haemoglobin content of the blood drops sharply. In severe cases massive destruction of red blood cells leads to death. It is now known that the susceptibility to this drug-induced haemolytic anaemia is an X-linked hereditary trait – found in Africans and peoples of African and Mediterranean descent and among Jews and Asiatics. The abnormality is associated ith a deficiency of glucose-6-phosphate dehydrogenase (G6PD) enzyme.

The gene responsible for regulation of G6PD production is located on the X-chromosome. Therefore among males there are two distinct phenotypes, those with G6PD deficiency and those with normal erythrocytes. Thus all males having the deficiency are hemizygous. On the other hand, females may be normal homozygous, heterozygous and deficient homozygous. The incidence of dangerous deficiency is higher among males than females.

G6PD genotype

In Nigeria there are three common variants of G6PD: A and B have normal activity and A⁻ is the enzyme associated with deficiency. The corresponding genes are called Gd^A, Gd^B and Gd^{A-}. The Mediterranean variant of the enzyme gives rise to a far more dangerous

Fig. 8.6. Hydrolysis of succinylcholine.

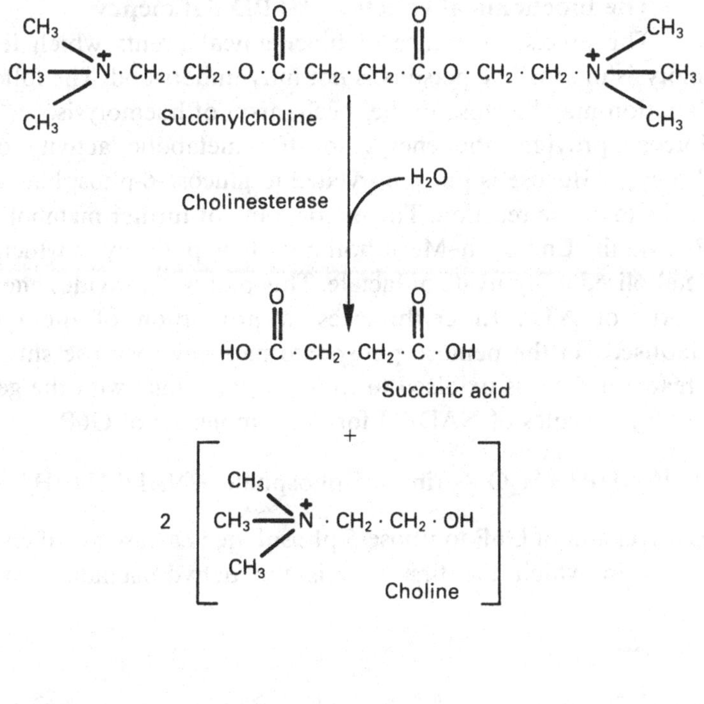

disease. A great many more variants are now known (see Luzzatto, Sodeinde & Martini, 1983).

Evidence that the deficiency resides in the erythrocyte

It was established early that the defect resided in the erythrocyte of susceptible individuals; red cells from primaquine-sensitive individuals were labelled with radioactive chromium (^{51}Cr) (since chromium is exclusively taken up by the red cells, the presence of radioactivity in serum after treatment with primaquine is evidence of haemolysis). The labelled cells were infused into non-sensitive individuals who were then given primaquine. The labelled red cells underwent haemolysis, but not the red cells of the non-sensitive recipient. Next, erythrocytes from a non-sensitive individual were labelled with ^{51}Cr and infused into recipients known to be sensitive to primaquine. When the latter received primaquine, their red cells suffered haemolytic damage, but there was no loss of label from the infused red cells. These observations established firmly that the genetic defect responsible for primaquine idiosyncrasy is intrinsic to the red cells of sensitive individuals. Experiments with the ^{51}Cr-labelling technique have shown that primaquine and other 8-aminoquinolines are only one of several groups of compounds which can haemolyse these 'abnormal' red cells (see Tables 8.2 and 8.3).

The biochemical effects of G6PD deficiency

The precise sequence of biochemical events which lead to haemolysis in sensitive persons is not fully understood. The following explanation may be close to the mechanism of haemolysis.

Glucose provides the energy for the metabolic activity of the erythrocyte. Glucose is phosphorylated to glucose-6-phosphate (G6P) in the hexokinase reaction. The major route of further metabolism of G6P is via the Emboden–Meyerhoff glycolytic pathway in which G6P is metabolised to pyruvate or lactate. This pathway provides energy in the form of ATP. In erythrocytes, a proportion of the G6P is metabolised via the pentose phosphate pathway (pentose shunt). In this reaction, G6P is oxidised to ribose-5-phosphate with the generation of 2 molecules of NADPH for every molecule of G6P:

$$G6P + 2NADP^+ + H_2O — ribose\text{-}5\text{-}phosphate + 2NADPH + 2H^+ + CO_2.$$

The conversion of G6P to ribose-5-phosphate is a cascade of enzymic reactions in which the first step is the dehydrogenation of G6P

Table 8.2   *Drugs to be avoided in G6PD deficiency*

Antimalarials	*Analgesics*
Primaquine	Acetylsalicylic Acid (aspirin) –
Pamaquine	moderate doses can be used
Chloroquine (may be used under	Acetophenetidin (phenacetin)
surveillance when required for	Acetanilide
prophylaxis or treatment of	safe alternative – paracetamol
malaria)	
Sulphonamides and sulphones	*Antihelminthics*
Sulphanilamide	β-naphthol
Sulphapyridine	Stibophan
Sulphadimidine	Niridazole
Sulphafurazone (gantrisin)	
Sulphacetamide (salazopyrin)	
† Dapsone	*Miscellaneous*
Sulphoxone	Vitamin K analogues (1 mg of
Thiazosulphone	menaphthone can be given to
Glucosulphone sodium (promin)	babies)
Septrin	† Naphthalene (moth balls)
	Probenecid
Antibacterial compounds	Dimercaprol (BAL)
Nitrofurans – nitrofurantoin	Methylene blue
– furazolidone	† Arsine
– nitrofurazone	† Phenylhydrazine
Chloramphenicol	† Acetylphenylhydrazine
p-aminosalicylic Acid	Toluidine blue
	Mepacrine

This list is compiled on the basis of data available for patients with the 'MEDITERRANEAN' variant of G6PD. It is probably applicable to most patients from Southern Europe and the Middle East. It would seem cautious to refer to the same also for patients from S.E. Asia and the Far East.

† These drugs may cause haemolysis in normal individuals if given in large doses. Many other drugs may produce haemolysis in particular individuals.

List supplied by Professor Lucio Luzzatto and included here by kind permission.

catalysed by the enzyme *glucose 6-phosphate dehydrogenase* (G6PD). The pentose shunt is the only source of NADPH in erythrocytes. Hence the production of NADPH is diminished in erythrocytes deficient in G6PD.

A shortfall in the amount of NADPH in turn causes a deficiency in the level of another essential cofactor, *glutathione*. Erythrocytes synthesise glutathione which in its reduced form (GSH) has the following critically important functions in red cells:

Table 8.3   *Drugs to be avoided in G6PD deficiency*

Antimalarials
Primaquine (can be give at
  reduced dosage, 15 mg daily
  or 45 mg twice weekly under
  surveillance)
Pamaquine
	Analgesics
	Acetylsalicylic acid (aspirin) –
	  moderate doses can be used.
	Acetophenetidin (phenacetin)
	  Safe alternative – paracetamol

Sulphonamides and Sulphones Sulphanilamide Sulphapyridine Sulphadimidine Sulphacetamide (albucid) Salicylazosulphapyridine (salazopyrin) † Dapsone † Sulphoxone Glucosulphone sodium (promin) Septrin	*Anthelmintics* β-naphthol Stibophan Niridazole

Other antibacterial compounds
Nitrofurans – nitrofurantoin
          – furazolidone
          – nitrofurazone
Nalidixic acid
	Miscellaneous
	Vitamin K analogues (1 mg of
	  menaphthone can be given to
	  babies)
	† Naphthalene (moth balls)
	Probenecid
	Dimercaprol (BAL)
	Methylene blue
	† Arsine
	† Phenylhydrazine
	† Acetylphenylhydrazine
	Toluidine blue

This list is compiled on the basis of data available for patients with the 'A' variant of G6PD deficiency. It can be generally assumed to be applicable to patients from Africa and of African descent.

† These drugs may cause haemolysis in normal individuals if given in large doses. Many other drugs may produce haemolysis in particular individuals.

List supplied by Professor Lucio Luzzatto, and included here by kind permission.

(i) GSH acts as a sulphydryl buffer preventing the oxidation and denaturation of haemoglobin and other erythrocyte proteins.

(ii) It helps to maintain the integrity of erythrocyte membrane; erythrocytes with lowered GSH are more liable to haemolysis than normal cells.

(iii) GSH plays a role in detoxification by reacting with hydrogen peroxide and organic peroxides which are normally toxic to the cell

$$2GSH + R\text{--}OOH \rightarrow GSSG + H_2O + ROH$$

Normally, GSH tends to be oxidised to GSSG. This must be reduced in order to maintain the required level of GSH; the reduction requires glutathione reductase and NADPH. This system generates GSH continuously so that in the normal erythrocyte more than 99% of the total glutathione is in the form of GSH (Figure 8.7).

In G6PD-deficient erythrocytes, NADPH production is diminished and GSH generation from GSSG is impaired. The erythrocyte in this state is susceptible to haemolytic damage.

How drugs damage G6PD-deficient erythrocytes

It is not clear why exposure of G6PD-deficient erythrocytes to certain drugs should cause haemolytic damage in these cells. The mechanism of haemolysis is obscure, but probably involves the following.

(i) The level of GSH, lower than normal in G6PD-deficient erythrocytes, is reduced further by drugs such as primaquine.

(ii) With lowered levels of GSH, the haemolytic drugs may distort the red cell membrane and render the cells liable to removal and destruction by the spleen.

(iii) Haemolytic drugs or their reactive intermediates may interact directly with sulphydryl groups which are no longer protected against oxidative attack because of low levels of GSH.

(iv) As erythrocytes age (life expectancy, 120 days) their content of

Fig. 8.7. Reduction of GSSG to GSH.

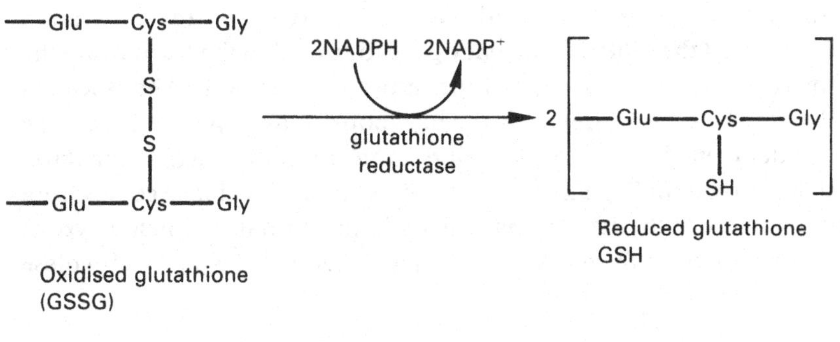

Glu——Cys——Gly
|
S
|
S
|
Glu——Cys——Gly

Oxidised glutathione
(GSSG)

2NADPH   2NADP⁺

glutathione
reductase

2 [Glu——Cys——Gly]
                |
               SH

Reduced glutathione
GSH

G6PD decreases. This decrease is even more marked in cells originally having low G6PD values. Hence in G6PD deficiency, old erythrocytes are more susceptible to damage than young cells. Even in G6PD deficiency, young cells usually have enough enzyme to protect them against haemolytic drugs. That is why the haemolytic anaemia in certain types of deficiency prevalent among peoples of African origin is self-limiting after about one week. The haemoglobin level rises to normal in spite of continuation of therapy with the haemolytic drug. Even so, drug-induced haemolytic anaemia could be a serious problem in an environment where the patient is undernourished and anaemic owing to parasite infestation.

8.5   INTERACTION BETWEEN GENETIC FACTORS

Dapsone and sulphonamides such as sulphamethazine have been known to cause haemolytic damage in some, but not all, G6PD-deficient individuals. It has now been demonstrated that acetylated dapsone is not haemolytic. Thus G6PD-deficient *fast acetylators* are somewhat protected from the haemolytic effect of the drug, whereas G6PD-deficient *slow acetylators* are more vulnerable.

8.6   G6PD DEFICIENCY PROTECTS AGAINST
P. FALCIPARUM MALARIA

It is a widely held view that G6PD deficiency protects the individual from *P. falciparum* malaria though not from other malarias. The hypothesis is controversial but it is supported by three kinds of evidence. Firstly, G6PD deficiency is found among people who live, or whose ancestors lived, in regions of the world where *P. falciparum* malaria is, or has been, endemic. Thus G6PD deficiency is of high frequency in Africa (south of the Sahara), the Middle East (Arabia and Iran), the Mediterranean basin (Turkey, Greece, Italy and Sicily), the Indian subcontinent, and South East Asia. Slave trade and emigration have caused the G6PD-deficiency gene to spread to the Caribbean, the Americas and Northern Europe especially Britain. The socalled 'Geographical coincidence' is the backbone of the hypothesis that the gene deficiency was an evolutionary protective device against malaria (cf. haemoglobin S, page 326). The second line of evidence comes from comparison of the level of parasitaemia in normal and heterozygous females suffering from malaria. A typical study is one on 445 Togolese females where it was found that the level of parasitaemia was significantly lower in heterozygotes that in normal females. Thirdly, at the cellular level, Luzzatto compared the rate of parasitisation of normal and G6PD-deficient erythrocytes within the blood of heterozygous females; it was found that normal erythrocytes uniformly had more parasites than deficient erythrocytes. It seems that the deficiency gene Gd^{A-} protects against *P. falciparum*. On the other hand, however, males who were hemizygous for Gd^{A-} were not protected although those who were hemizygous for Gd^A were. Therefore it would appear that the protection is not a simple function of the amount of enzyme. It has also been shown that the growth of *P. falciparum in vitro*, is significantly inhibited in erythrocytes from female heterozygotes, male hemizygotes and in artificial mixtures of hemizygote and normal red cells showing that protection is directly related to enzyme deficiency.

Mechanism by which G6PD deficiency protects against malaria

It is not known how G6PD deficiency protects the erythrocyte from *P. falciparum* parasitisation. One suggestion is that the parasite lacks its own G6PD and therefore needs the erythrocyte enzyme to complete its pentose phosphate metabolism of glucose. An alternative view is that *P. falciparum* development is abrogated in a G6PD-deficient erythrocyte due to the fact that the latter is unable to withstand the oxidative stress imposed by the presence of the parasite. Neither of these propositions can account for the observation that parasite development can be normal in G6PD-deficient male hemizygotes and why, *in vivo*, resistance to parasitisation occurs more frequently in female heterozygotes. Luzzatto proposed that the protective effect of G6PD deficiency lies in the presence within the heterozygote female of the mosaic of both deficient and normal erythrocytes (see Luzzatto, Sodeinde & Martini, 1983).

Ethnic differences in drug response cannot in all cases be attributed to genetic factors. The decision as to whether a particular difference in drug metabolism between two populations is environmental (e.g. due to diet or other cultural practices) or is genetic in origin is a hard one to make. The examples discussed in this chapter are those for which there is good evidence that the differences between peoples in their response to drugs are due to inheritable characteristics. The drugs discussed are of particular interest in the tropics, but the list is by no means comprehensive. Hopefully, by giving the subject a prominent chapter in this book, students of pharmacology in the tropics will become even more aware of the problem of ethnic variability in drug response and add to this list of drugs as they come across other examples in the course of their reading. Then, it is important for the practitioner always to exercise caution when prescribing or dispensing drugs likely to produce serious toxicities in a high proportion of the population as a result of known or likely genetic characteristics.

FURTHER READING

Bienzle, U., Lucas, A. O., Ayeni, O. & Luzzatto, L. (1972). Glucose-6-phosphate dehydrogenase and malaria. Greater resistance of females heterozygous for enzyme deficiency and of males with non-deficient variant. Lancet 1, 107–10.

Boobis, A. R. (1979). Genetic factors affecting side effects of drugs. In *Drug Toxicity*, ed. J. W. Gorrod, pp. 51–89. Taylor & Francis Ltd., London.

Evans, D.A.P. (1977). In *Drug Metabolism from Microbe to Man*, ed. D. V. Parke & R. L. Smith. Taylor & Francis, London.

Falase, A. O. & Salako, L. A. (1979). Beta-adrenoceptor blockers in the treatment of hypertension. *Afr. J. Med. Sci.* 8, 13–18.

Freis, E. D., Materson, B. J. & Flamenbaum, W. (1983). Comparison of propranolol or hydrochlorothiazide alone for treatment of hypertension. *Am. J. Med.* 74, 1029–41.

Gilles, H. M. (1984). Pharmacogenetic factors in antimalaria testing. In *Handbook of Experimental Pharmacology*, vol. 68, ed. W. Peters & W.H.G. Richards, pp. 411–20. Springer-Verlag, Berlin, Heidelberg.

Lamble, J. W. (1983), ed. *Drug Metabolism and Distribution. Current Reviews in Biomedicine 3*. Elsevier Biomedical Press, Amsterdam.

Luzzatto, L. (1979). Genetics of red cells and susceptibility to malaria. *Blood* 54, 961–76.

Luzzatto, L., Sodeinde, O. & Martini, G. (1983). Genetic variation in the host and adaptive phenomena in *Plasmodium falciparum* infection. In *Malaria and the Red Cell*, pp. 159–73. Pitman, London. (Ciba Foundation Symposium 94).

Olatunde, I. A., Akinkugbe, O. O. & Carlisle, R. (1977). Beta-adrenergic blockers in the treatment of hypertension. Experience with propranolol in Ibadan, Nigeria. *E. Afr. Med. J.* 54, 194.

PART V

Selective Toxicity

9

Antimicrobial drugs

9.1   INTRODUCTION

Progress in the development of drugs used in the treatment of infections caused by micro-organisms has been due to a detailed understanding of the metabolic processes which enable these organisms to multiply in the host. Such biochemical studies reveal particular vulnerable pathways which can be blocked by drugs to kill the organism or inhibit its growth. The aim in this chapter is to present some of the important sites of action of antimicrobial drugs. The two groups of micro-organisms dealt with in this chapter are bacteria and fungi. The emphasis is on sites of action and the mechanisms by which drugs selectively harm these micro-organisms. Accounts of therapeutic usage which the student should encounter in the clinic are discussed only briefly.

We saw in Chapter 4 that drugs produce their beneficial effects by first binding to specific receptors; the usefulness of the drug depends on its specificity. This general principle applies also in the chemotherapy of infectious diseases. Indeed, the idea of receptors was first proposed by Ehrlich and was originally applied in chemotherapy of parasitic diseases. It is useful to state some of Ehrlich's basic ideas here:

  (i) In every microorganism there are discrete and specific sites
       called receptors which bind chemicals. When bound, the
       chemical may be harmful to the cell. In chemotherapy the aim
       is to use chemical substances which bind and kill invading
       organisms, but are harmless to host cells. The chemical thus
       acts like a 'magic bullet' seeking out only the pathogenic
       organisms for destruction.
 (ii) The safety of the chemical (i.e., its therapeutic index) depends

on its relative affinities for binding to invading organisms and host cells.

(iii) Chemicals need not kill the parasite. It is sufficient to prevent multiplication, then normal body defences (the immune system and phagocytosing cells) would cope with non-dividing organisms.

(iv) Microorganisms can become resistant to chemicals. Ehrlich discovered this phenomenon in trypanosomes treated with the dyes, parafuchsin and trypan blue, and he suggested that the receptors in the resistant organisms had diminished affinity for the dye.

As we shall see in the course of this chapter and the rest of this Part, these ideas are as valid today as when they were first formulated.

9.2   EXPLANATION OF BASIC TERMS
Antibiotics
The term *antibiotic* is used to refer to chemical substances such as penicillin which are obtained from cultures of microorganisms and which are toxic to other microorganisms in low concentrations.

Antimicrobial agent
Is used more frequently in this book to refer to antibiotics as well as synthetic agents such as sulphonamides which are used to treat infections caused by a range of microorganisms including bacteria and fungi.

Selective toxicity
Antimicrobial agents interfere with vital pathways in the biochemistry of microorganisms. Since the biochemistry of mammalian cells differs from that of microorganisms in many essential details, it is possible to kill the invading organism or prevent its growth without interfering with the cellular functions of the host. This idea is referred to in the text as selective toxicity.

Selective toxicity is achieved when the process to be inhibited: (a) occurs in the microorganism but not in the cell; (b) occurs in both host cells and microorganisms but the process in the microbe is by far more sensitive to inhibition by the antimicrobial agent than that in the host; (c) occurs in both host and microbe, but the microbe concentrates the drug preferentially; or (d) when the invading organisms, but not the host cells, possess a mechanism which converts a nontoxic compound to a metabolite toxic to the organism.

Examples of the different ways by which selective toxicity is achieved will be met in the course of the following discussion.

Antimicrobial agents which are effective in curing infections either kill the invading bacterium or prevent its growth. In the former case, the action is *bactericidal* and in the latter *bacteriostatic*. In bacteriostasis the number of organisms is not increasing and the body's defences are able to remove the non-growing organisms.

9.3   SITES OF ACTION OF ANTIMICROBIAL DRUGS
Anti-microbial agents can kill microorganisms or inhibit their growth by blocking:

(1) cell wall synthesis
(2) cell membrane function
(3) protein synthesis
(4) nucleic acid synthesis
(5) synthesis of essential metabolites.

Cell wall synthesis
Bacterial cell walls are a target for drug action because these walls encase the cytoplasmic membranes and protect the cells from rupturing under the influence of osmotic pressure, the interior of the cell being hypertonic in relation to its external surroundings. Mammalian cells do not have such special walls. A drug blocking cell wall synthesis is therefore selectively toxic to bacteria.

The nature of bacterial cell walls
The detailed structure of the cell wall differs from one type of bacterium to another. In Gram-positive bacteria, such as *Staphylococcus aureus*, up to 50% of the wall mass consists of a polymer called peptidoglycan. The polymer is made up of units of disaccharides having decapeptide side chains (Fig. 9.1). The amino acids in the side chain are glycine, alanine, glutamic acid and lysine. Several disaccharide decapeptide units are linked through the 4-hydroxyl group of an N-acetylglucosamine residue to form the large linear peptidoglycan polymer. This structure is water soluble and not rigid. Toughness and rigidity are introduced by a process called cross-linking which means that the side chains of adjacent peptidoglycan units become joined. The reaction is known as transpeptidation and is catalysed by an enzyme called peptidoglycan transpeptidase (Fig. 9.2).

Cross-linking of this type is a well known process in the plastics industry where it is used also to increase the strength of the product.

The purpose of cross-linking can be emphasised by saying that the concrete wall in a building would not be a strong protective structure if the individual blocks were not cemented together. Linked to the peptidoglycan are acidic (teichoic or teichuronic acid) polymers. These add strength to the wall and may comprise 40–45% of the wall mass. The rest of the wall (5–10%) consists of proteins.

Gram-negative bacteria such as *Escherichia coli* have an outer membrane consisting of lipopolysacharides, phospholipids, fatty acids and proteins (see Fig. 9.3). This outermost layer provides additional protection by restricting access of potentially harmful substances to the cell membrane. The presence of this outer coat is the reason why some penicillins though active against Gram-positive organisms are inactive against Gram-negative bacteria (see page 205). The walls in mycobacteria (*Mycobacterium tuberculosis* and *M. leprae*) are different again. The cell walls in these organisms contain large amounts of complex lipids, the most important of which is mycolic acid. This acid is unique to this class of organisms and partly explains the resistance of mycobacteria to a large number of antimicrobial agents. The important target for drug action in fungal cells is the membrane. This is discussed on page 206.)

Sites of drug action for inhibition of cell wall synthesis

There are several possible sites at which drugs can act to inhibit cell wall synthesis. Of these, four are of practical importance.

Fig. 9.1. A peptidoglycan unit consisting of a disaccharide linked to a decapeptide.

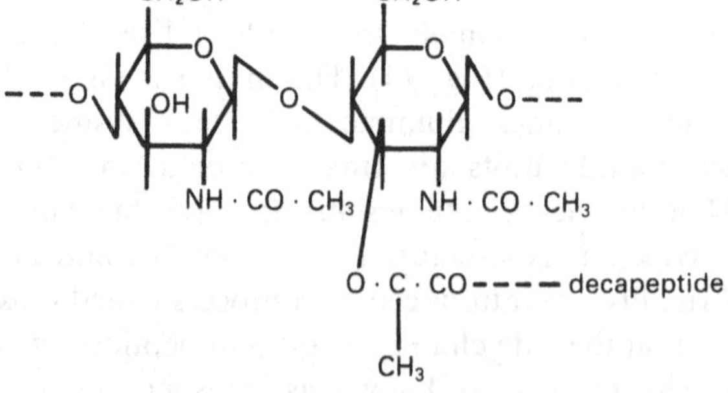

Disaccharide decapeptide

Fig. 9.2. Cross-linking of two linear peptidoglycan units catalysed by peptidoglycan transpeptidase.

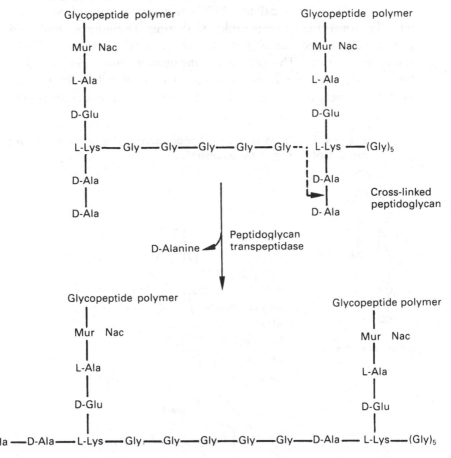

Fig. 9.3. Diagrammatic representation of (A) Gram-positive, e.g. *Staph.aureus* and (B) Gram-negative, e.g. *E.coli*, cells.

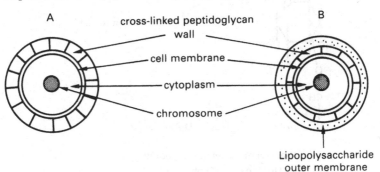

(a) *D-alanyl–D-alanine synthetase*

The peptidoglycan polymer unit (Fig. 9.1) is formed from a smaller building block called UDP-N-acetylmuramic acid pentapeptide. To form the pentapeptide, L-alanine, D-glutamic acid and L-lysine are joined successively to the carboxyl group of UDP-N-acetylmuramic acid. The synthesis of the pentapeptide is completed by the addition, not of an amino acid, but of D-alanyl-D-alanine. To make this dipeptide, the naturally occurring L-alanine is converted to

Fig. 9.4. Synthesis of UDP-N-acetylmuramyl pentapeptide and the site of action of cycloserine*.

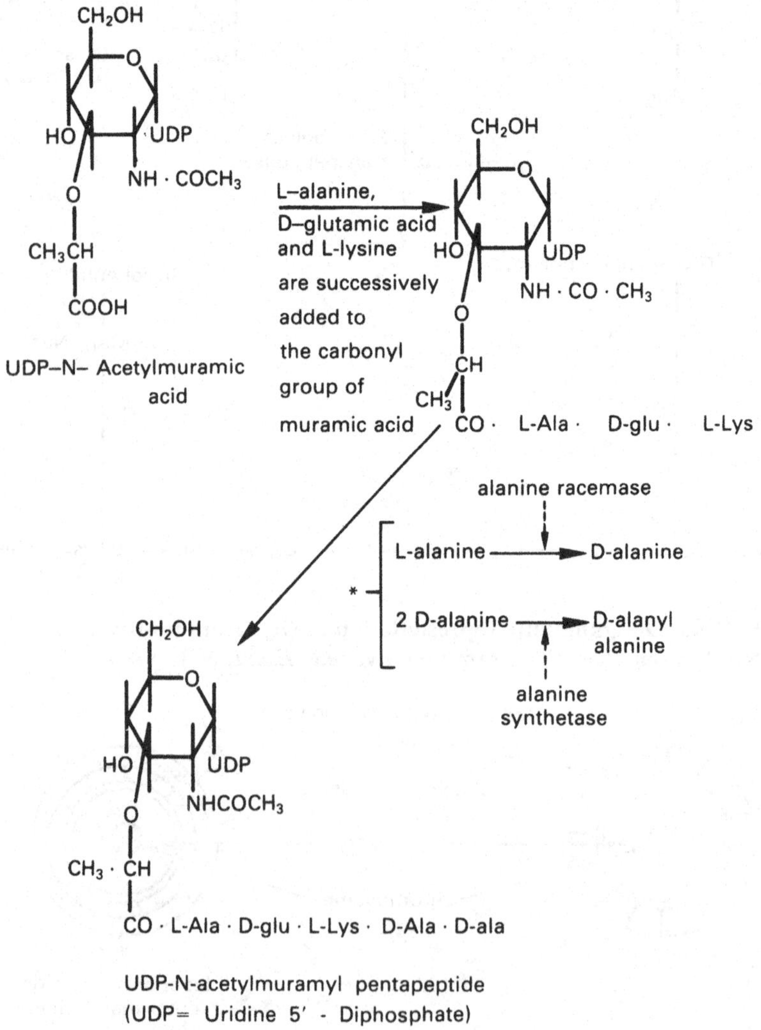

UDP-N-acetylmuramyl pentapeptide
(UDP= Uridine 5' - Diphosphate)

D-alanine by a racemase; another enzyme, D-alanyl–D-alanine synthetase, then joins two D-alanine molecules. The drug *D-cycloserine* is a competitive inhibitor of alanine racemase and D-alanyl–D-alanine synthetase (see Fig. 9.4). It therefore prevents the formation of the pentapeptide. The evidence, listed below, concerning the mode of action of cycloserine suggests that the drug binds to the enzymes in place of the natural substrate, a sort of competitive antagonism.

(i) Structural resemblance between cycloserine and D-alanine (Fig. 9.5) can be demonstrated by molecular modelling. The inhibition can thus be attributed to displacement of D-alanine from binding sites on the enzyme.

(ii) D-cycloserine binds more strongly to the synthetase than the natural substrate D-alanine, the ratio of K_m (for D-alanine) to K_i (for D-cycloserine) being about 100.

(iii) The action of cycloserine is specifically antagonised by addition of D-alanine to the growth medium.

As well as competing with alanine for binding sites on the enzymes, cycloserine also enters the bacterial cell interior by a transport mechanism which uses the same carrier protein as alanine. Therefore, while the selective toxicity of the drug is due to inhibition of cell wall synthesis, its known high toxicity to humans may be due to inhibition of alanine transport and thus a deficiency of this amino acid in host cells.

Cycloserine is employed in the treatment of tuberculosis where resistance to other drugs makes its use imperative.

(b) *Inhibition of peptidoglycan formation*

We have seen that the peptidoglycan polymer consists of disaccharide decapeptide units. Each is made by adding a hexosamine unit to the UDP-N-acetylmuramic acid pentapeptide (Fig. 9.4) to form a disaccharide pentapeptide. Next, five glycine units are added successively to the lysine of the pentapeptide to complete the disaccharide decapeptide. This stage in the synthesis is inhibited by the antibiotic

Fig. 9.5. Structures of cycloserine and alanine.

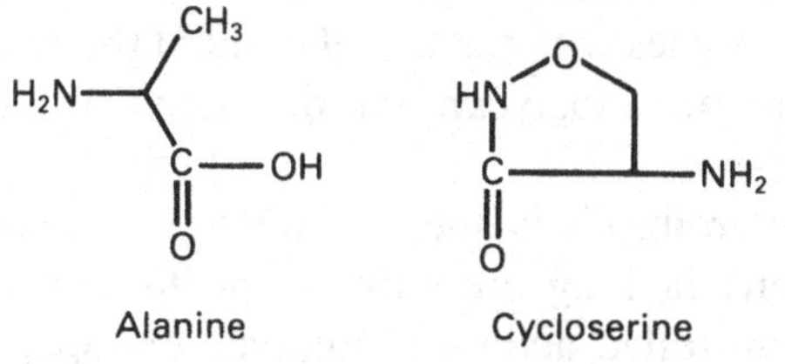

Alanine   Cycloserine

vancomycin which specifically binds to the D-alanyl-D-alanine residue thereby preventing formation of a complete peptidoglycan unit.

Vancomycin is a large molecular weight bactericidal antibiotic, useful in the treatment of severe *Streptococcus epidermidis*, *Staphylococcus aureus* and *Clostridium difficile* infections. The latter organism causes severe super infections when broad-spectrum antibiotics kill off most other organisms in the gut.

(c) *Inhibition of peptidoglycan transpeptidase*

The cross-linking of side chains catalysed by peptidoglycan transpeptidase (Fig. 9.2) is strongly inhibited by penicillins and cephalosporins. These drugs, also known as beta-lactam antibiotics, inhibit transpeptidation by binding covalently to the enzyme. This reaction between drug (I) and enzyme (E) may be written as

$$E+I \; \underset{k_2}{\overset{k_1}{\rightleftharpoons}} \; EI \; \overset{k_3}{\longrightarrow} \; EI* \; \overset{k_4}{\longrightarrow} \; E + \text{degraded inhibitor.}$$

The first reaction is a reversible binding to the enzyme. The second stage involves chemical modification of the enzyme with covalent binding to the inhibitor, and is irreversible. The final stage releases the enzyme after degradation of the inhibitor. The characteristic feature of the beta-lactam antibiotics is that k_3 is high thereby ensuring that the inhibitor is not released and the natural substrate is occluded. k_4 is low thereby ensuring that the period during which the enzyme is in the inactive form is long. This explains the outstanding effectiveness of the beta-lactam antibiotics.

Several lines of evidence support this mode of action for these drugs. The most direct is that particulate enzyme preparations from *E. coli* can, in the presence of the nucleotide pentapeptide and alanine, carry out the whole peptidoglycan synthesis *in vitro*, including the final cross-linking. In the presence of a beta-lactam, the synthesis is not completed but stops with the formation of what are called Park nucleotides such as disaccharide decapeptides. It seems that normally the section of the peptidoglycan that binds to the enzyme is the D-alanyl-D-alanine residue of the side chain. The CO-N bond of the beta-lactam ring apparently competes with the CO-N bond of the D-alanyl-D-alanine residue of the peptidoglycan for the active site of the transpeptidase enzyme.

The killing effect of the antibiotic is due not only to simple osmotic damage sustained by cells lacking cross-linked peptidoglycans; in addition there is an uncontrolled action of autolytic endopeptidases which normally work in harmony with the synthetic enzymes to allow insertion of portions of newly made peptidoglycan into the wall. A deficiency of autolysins has been used to explain cases of tolerance to beta-lactam antibiotics.

(d) Inhibition of mycolic acid synthesis

Cell walls of mycobacteria contain mycolic acids which are unique to this class of organism. This partly explains why many antibiotics which are effective against most other organisms are useless against mycobacteria. Mycolic acid is made up of long-chain hydroxy-fatty acids. Cell walls deficient in this material are structurally weak and can rupture under osmotic pressure. These acids are not constituents of mammalian cells, so a drug which prevents their synthesis is selectively toxic to pathogens.

Isoniazid is an example of such a drug. It is used in the treatment of diseases caused by *M. tuberculosis*. A summary of drugs inhibiting cell-wall biosynthesis is given in Table 9.1.

9.4   THE PENICILLINS AND CEPHALOSPORINS (FIG. 9.6)

Penicillin was discovered by Fleming in 1928 when he accidentally found that the mould *Penicillium notatum* which had contaminated agar plates seeded with *S. aureus* had produced a substance which inhibited growth of the bacteria. The substance was eventually identified as penicillin. Benzylpenicillin (penicillin G) was obtained

Fig. 9.6. Structural formulae of penicillins.

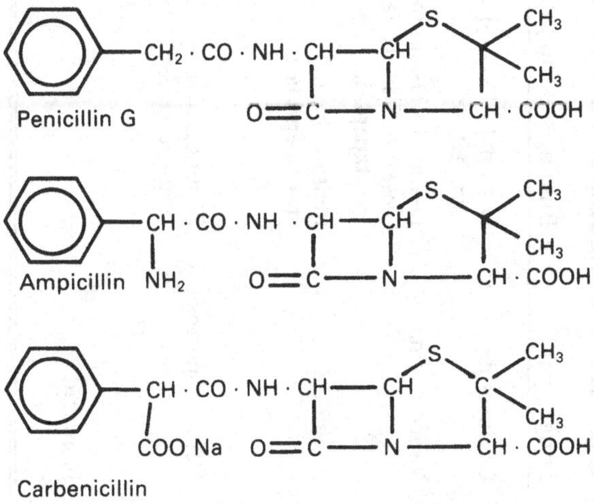

Table 9.1 *Inhibition of cell-wall biosynthesis*

Drug (type)	Binding site/Enzyme	Mechanism of action	Effect on bacteria	Organism treated
Cycloserine	D-alanyl – D-alanine synthetase	Blocks formation of D-alanyl – D-alanine	Bactericidal	*M. tuberculosis*
Vancomycin	D-alanyl – D-alanine residue of disaccharide pentapeptide	Blocks biosynthesis of peptidoglycan units	Bactericidal	*S. aureus, C. difficile*
Penicillin	Peptidoglycan transpeptidase	Inhibition of transpeptidation (cross-linking of peptidoglycan polymers	Bactericidal	Most Gram-positive and Gram-negative organisms
Cephalosporins	Peptidoglycan transpeptidase	Inhibition of transpeptidation (cross-linking) of peptidoglycan polymers	Bactericidal	Most Gram-positive and some Gram-negative organisms
Isoniazid	–	Inhibition of mycolic acid synthesis	Bactericidal	*M. tuberculosis*

by adding phenylacetic acid to the fermentation medium during penicillin production. Penicillin G was the first penicillin preparation to be used on a large scale but its clinical usefulness is limited; it is unstable in acid and destroyed in the stomach. It cannot be taken by mouth. When phenoxyacetic acid is used in fermentation instead of phenylacetic acid, phenoxymethylpenicillin (penicillin V) is formed. Penicillin V is acid-stable and active orally. These penicillins are active against Gram-positive organisms and are used in the treatment of pneumonia and streptococcal and staphylococcal infections. They are also active against gonococcal and meningococcal infections. They are largely inactive against the majority of Gram-negative bacilli. When workers in Beecham discovered that the benzyl side chain can be removed from penicillin to yield 6-aminopenicillamic acid, the way was open for three major types of improvement. Semi-synthetic compounds were produced which were:

(i) acid resistant
(ii) penicillinase resistant
(iii) active against both Gram-positive and Gram-negative organisms.

Cephalosporin C is obtained from a different source but is similar in structure to penicillin in having a β-lactam ring. Cephalosporin C can be modified. The side chain is removed to give 7-aminocephalosporanic acid which can be used to produce semisynthetic derivatives. Cephalothin is a clinically useful derivative although not active orally. Cephalexin is active orally. Cephalosporins are active against Gram-positive and Gram-negative organisms (Fig. 9.7).

Broad-spectrum penicillins

Penicillin G and many other penicillins are not effective against infections caused by most Gram-negative organisms. Those penicillins which are effective against Gram-positive *and* Gram-negative organisms such as ampicillin and carbenicillin are called broad-spectrum penicillins. In this sense 'broad spectrum' does not have the same meaning as it has when applied to the truly broad-spectrum antibiotics such as the tetracyclines which act against a wide variety of organisms. The reason narrow-spectrum penicillins do not kill Gram-negative organisms is that the drugs are unable to penetrate the restrictive lipopolysaccharide-containing outer membrane of these organisms. Ampicillin and carbenicillin have slightly modified structures which enable them to penetrate the outer coat to reach the transpeptidase enzyme in the cell.

Cell membrane

Apart from the cell wall, the cytoplasmic membrane also contributes to bacterial cell integrity by acting as a sieve to prevent unwanted molecules from diffusing passively into the cell. Chemical substances which alter this function of the cell membrane can be toxic to the cell. Such drugs have very limited systemic use clinically because they are toxic to both mammalian and bacterial cells. We can hazard four ways in which drugs can act to alter membrane function.

(a) Interaction with membrane components to alter membrane permeability

Many antiseptics (e.g. phenol and phenol derivatives) and cationic detergents (e.g. chlorhexidine) used externally as disinfectants interact chemically with membrane components to change membrane permeability. They cause leakage of cytoplasmic components such as nucleotides, amino acids and phosphates and eventually kill the organism.

An example of an antibiotic used systemically that causes disorganisation of bacterial cell membrane is *polymixin B*. This is a cyclic polypeptide antibiotic active chiefly against Gram-negative

Fig. 9.7. Structural formulae of cephalosporins.

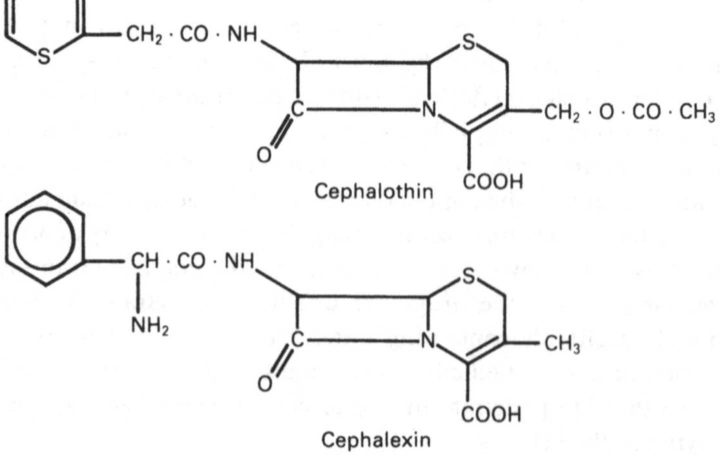

7-aminocephalosporanic acid

Cephalothin

Cephalexin

bacteria, e.g. *Pseudomonas aeroginosa*. The clinical use of this drug is limited because of its toxicity to man.

(b) Ionophores

These are large molecular weight linear or cyclic polypeptide antibiotics which facilitate the passage of inorganic ions across the cell membrane by forming lipid-soluble complexes with metal ions. These are then carried from regions of high to regions of low ion concentration. An example is *cyclosporin*. Ionophoric antibiotics can be highly specific for Na^+, K^+ or Ca^{2+} ions. These types of compound are widely used experimentally to define the role of ions in cell function, but they are not used clinically because their action is not specific for bacterial cells.

(c) Initiation of pore-formation

Some antibiotics create channels (pores) in the cytoplasmic membranes of pathogens thereby allowing free passage of ions. An example of a pore-forming antibiotic is *gramicidin A* (others are gramicidins B and C).

(d) Interaction with sterols in fungal cell membranes

The cell membranes of fungal cells differ from those of bacterial cells in including large amounts of sterols. This accounts for the resistance of fungal infections to most bacterial antibiotics. Chemicals which interact with sterols are selectively toxic to fungal cells. The most important group of drugs with high affinity for sterols in fungal cell membranes are the polyene antibiotics. Examples are *amphotericin B* and *Nystatin*. They are called 'polyene' because these large molecules contain several conjugated double bonds. The drugs are used in the treatment of fungal infections particularly those caused by *Candida albicans*. Superinfection with *Candida* organisms occurs when antibacterial therapy unbalances the microbial flora in the gut, resulting in fungal overgrowth (opportunistic fungal infection). Some fungal organisms are pathogenic.

Polyene antibotics are produced by actinomycetes. The drugs bind to the ergosterol of fungal membranes and thus alter membrane permeability. The affinity of the drugs for the fungal sterol is much greater than their affinity for the cholesterol of mammalian membranes. This allows sufficient selective toxicity for, e.g. amphotericin B, to be administered intravenously in the treatment of systemic mycoses such as *albicans* and *Histoplasma capsulatum*. Nystatin is less selective and is used for topical treatment of cutaneous mycoses. It can also be used orally since the drug is not absorbed from the gut.

Inhibition of protein synthesis

A detailed treatment of the complex process of protein synthesis is beyond the scope of this book. The interested reader who is not already familiar with the subject should consult standard texts in biochemistry. Here only certain critical terms relevant to the sites of drug action will be defined.

Protein synthesis takes place on ribosomes which are the machines in which aminoacids are linked together to form polypeptides.

Ribosomes are spherical particles with molecular weights of more than a million. They sediment in the Svedberg centrifuge at a rate expressed as, e.g. 70S (Svedberg units). Three main classes of ribosomes are common in mammalian and bacterial cells:

(a) 80S, confined to mammalian cells
(b) 70S, found in bacterial cells, and
(c) 55S, found only in mammalian mitochondria. 55S ribosomes resemble bacterial 70S ribosomes in functional organisation and antibiotic sensitivity.

These large peptides dissociate into smaller subunits and recombine under appropriate conditions:

$$80S \rightarrow 60S + 40S$$
$$\text{and } 70S \rightarrow 50S + 30S$$

80S and 70S ribosomes consist of proteins and ribonucleic acids (RNA) in approximately equal proportions.

Important features in protein synthesis

The code for protein synthesis contained in deoxyribonucleic acid (DNA) is transmitted by a special ribonucleic acid, called messenger RNA (mRNA). The transmission of genetic information from nuclear DNA to mRNA is known as *transcription*. The interpretation of the transmitted code into the required aminoacid sequence for the protein to be synthesised (*translation*) is undertaken by another RNA known as transfer RNA (tRNA). There is at least one type of tRNA for each of the 20 basic aminoacids. The function of tRNA is to ensure that the aminoacid specified by the code is incorporated in its correct place in the aminoacid sequence. The aminoacid to be incorporated is activated by a specific enzyme known as *aminoacyl-tRNA synthetase*.

At the start of protein synthesis in bacterial cells, 70S ribosome dissociates into two subunits, 30S and 50S. Protein synthesis is initiated when mRNA attaches to the 30S subunit. Then, tRNA, complexed to the initiation aminoacid (*formylmethionine*), making N-formyl-methonine-tRNA complex, becomes bound to 30S.

The initiation complex is recombined with 50S to reconstitute the functioning 70S ribosome where other aminoacids are linked together to form the growing polypeptide. Under the influence of mRNA and the specific tRNAs *enlongation* of the polypeptide proceeds until a *termination* signal from mRNA announces that the protein chain is complete. The completed protein is released from the ribosome which then dissociates into 50S and 30S subunits ready for use in the next cycle. See Fig. 9.8 for a schematic representation of these events.

Antibiotics with receptor sites on 30S ribosome
(a) Aminoglycosides (Fig. 9.9)
Aminoglycoside antibiotics are obtained from different species of *Streptomyces*. Examples are streptomycin, gentamicin, neomycin and kanamycin. They are polycationic compounds consisting of aminosugars linked together by glycosidic bonds. They are major drugs in the treatment of tuberculosis.

Site of action Aminoglycoside antibiotics bind to the P10 protein (called P10 as reference to its migration on gel electrophoresis) of 30S ribosomal subunits. The drugs do not bind to mammalian 80S ribosomes. They are therefore selectively toxic to sensitive bacteria. Toxicity of aminoglycosides in humans is not due to inhibition of protein synthesis but to the ability of the drugs to chelate divalent cations such as calcium. Binding to 30S has two major consequences. First, although the initiation complex is formed, successive addition of amino acids to the complex (elongation) is prevented. Thus protein synthesis is blocked at the stage of initiation complex formation. The bactericidal action of these antibiotics is due to their high affinity for the P10 protein; in certain types of resistance to streptomycin, the affinity of the drug for P10 is greatly reduced. Secondly, the aminoglycoside bound to 30S, causes mRNA to misread the code for amino acid sequence, so that tRNA transfers the wrong amino acids. Therefore, if protein synthesis takes place at all, the wrong sort of protein is made. Aminoglycosides are bactericidal. Other antibiotics such as chloramphenicol and the tetracyclines which also inhibit protein synthesis are however, bacteriostatic. The difference is probably the

Fig. 9.8. Protein synthesis (redrawn from Pratt, 1977).

(A) The initiation complex consisting of 70S ribosome, formyl-methionine-tRNA and two ribosomal acceptor sites, A and P.

(B) A second tRNA carrying another aminoacid (AA') becomes bound to the A site. The two aminoacids are juxtaposed in the 50S.

(C) Under the influence of peptidyl transferase the two aminoacids are linked by a peptide bond. Peptidyl transferase is one of the proteins of the 50S subunit. The dipeptide becomes attached to the site A.

(D) Translocation. tRNA for formylmethionine is released from site P. The tRNA with the dipeptide moves from A to P. A site is now free ready to receive the next aminoacyl tRNA. The process of enlongation continues with the sequential addition of single aminoacid units until synthesis is terminated by mRNA.

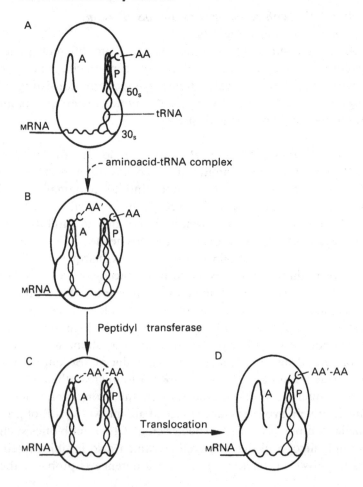

fact that aminoglycosides bind firmly to the receptor site, (dissociation constant 94 nM) whereas other protein synthesis inhibitors dissociate easily.

Pharmacological properties of aminoglycosides unrelated to antibacterial action Aminoglycosides cause a non-depolarising type of neuromuscular block. They may therefore cause skeletal muscle paralysis in patients under ether anaesthesia or those being treated with muscle relaxants. Patients suffering from myasthenia gravis are at risk. The effect is presynaptic on acetylcholine release and involves calcium since it can be reversed by administration of calcium gluconate or an anticholinesterase drug such as neostigmine. Aminoglycosides also cause ototoxicity affecting both hearing and balance. The effect is exerted directly on the peripheral sensory nerve to the inner ear. The action also seems to involve calcium chelation in the nerve by these polycationic antibiotics.

Fig. 9.9 Streptomycin.

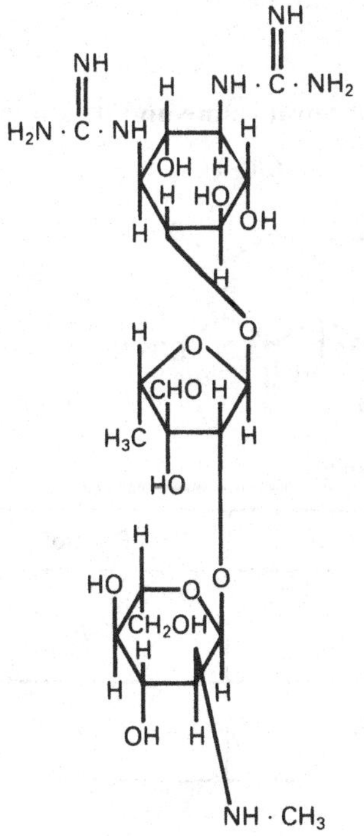

(b) *Tetracyclines*

The tetracyclines (Fig. 9.10) are obtained from various species of *Streptomyces*. These antibiotics are active against a wide range of bacteria and are therefore referred to as broad-spectrum. The antimicrobial action of the drugs is due to their ability to inhibit protein synthesis. Unlike the aminoglycosides, the tetracyclines bind to both bacterial 70S and mammalian 80S ribosomes but protein synthesis on 70S is more sensitive to block by tetracyclines. This difference, and the fact that the drugs are selectively concentrated in sensitive bacteria by a facilitated transport mechanism, constitute the basic for selective toxicity.

The drugs bind to the 30S subunit of the 70S ribosome and prevent binding of aminoacyl-tRNA to the A site on the ribosome. The transfer of individual aminoacids to the growing polypeptide is blocked. The drugs may also inhibit peptide-chain termination. The ability of the drugs to chelate divalent cations may be important here since Mg^{2+} plays a role in the dissociation of ribosomes. Their action is bacteriostatic. The structural requirements for optimum activity are complex as they relate not only to direct inhibition of protein synthesis but also to transportation into the bacterial cell.

Fig. 9.10. Structural formulae of tetracycline and its analogues.

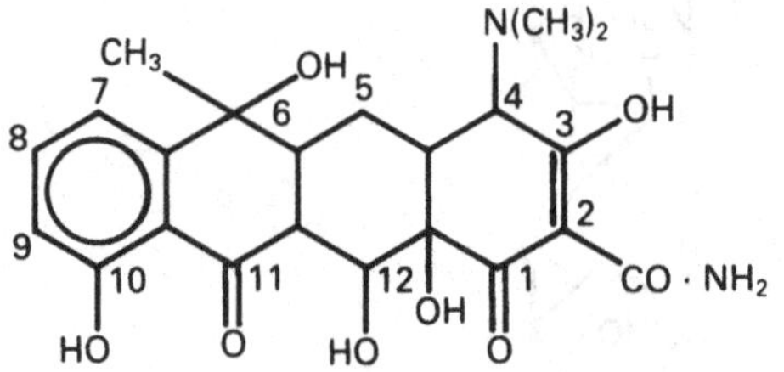

Tetracycline

Analogue	Substitution	Position
Chlortetracycline	- Cl	7
Oxytetracycline	- OH	5
Doxycycline	-OH,-CH₃	5,7

Antibiotics with receptor sites on 50S
(a) Chloramphenicol (Fig. 9.11)

Chloramphenicol is a broad spectrum antibiotic like the tetracyclines. Among its important clinical uses is the treatment of typhoid fever. Although originally obtained from a species of *Streptomyces*, it is now produced by synthesis.

Site of action Chloramphenicol binds exclusively to 50S subunits of 70S ribosomes and blocks peptidyl transferase. Peptide-bond formation and enlongation are prevented and protein synthesis blocked.

The binding to 50S is reversible. Therefore bacterial cells inhibited by chloramphenicol can resume protein synthesis and growth when the concentration of the drug falls below effective level. The drug is thus bacteriostatic.

Chloramphenicol has no effect on protein synthesis taking place on 80S ribosomes. Since mammalian protein synthesis takes place on 80S ribosomes, chloramphenicol is selectively toxic to bacteria. However, some protein synthesis takes place on 55S ribosome in mammalian mitochondria. This ribosome has functional similarity to bacterial 70S and is inhibited by chloramphenicol. The major toxic effect of chloramphenicol, namely bone-marrow depression, presenting as thrombocytopoenia is attributed to inhibition of mitochondrial protein synthesis.

(b) The macrolide antibiotics

The macrolides are a group of large molecular weight antibiotics with complex structures containing lactone rings linked to aminosugars through glycosidic bonds. Erythromycin is the only useful member of the macrolide group of antibiotics. It is particularly effective against Gram-positive organisms and used where an alternative to penicillin is indicated. Erythromycin inhibits protein synthesis on 70S but not on 80S ribosomes. It binds exclusively to prevent peptidyl-tRNA from gaining access to the donor site (site P) during translocation, thereby interfering with chain elongation. 50S ribosome subunits from *E. coli*

Fig. 9.11. Chloramphenicol.

O_2N—⬡—$CH \cdot CH \cdot NH \cdot CO \cdot CHCl_2$

with CH_2OH above the first CH and OH below it.

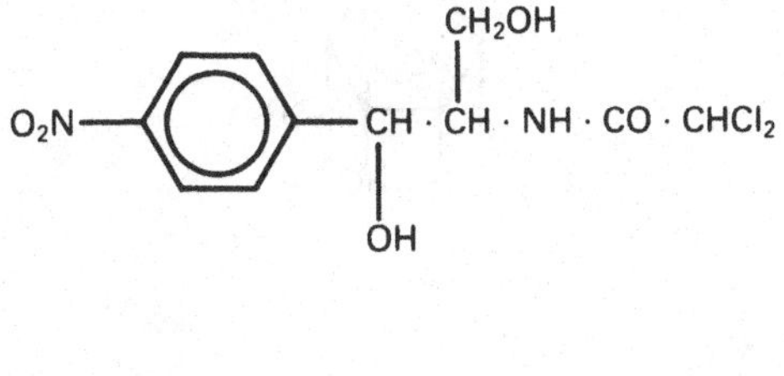

strains resistant to erythromycin do not bind the drug. This is due to an alteration, in the resistant mutants, of the receptor protein in 50S which binds the drug. Chloramphenicol also binds to the resistant mutants with decreased affinity, suggesting that both chloramphenicol and erythromycin bind to similar receptor sites on 50S subunits. The binding of erythromycin to 50S is reversible. The action is therefore bacteriostatic. Other macrolide antibiotics having a similar mode of action though not used clinically are carbomycin, oleandomycin and spiramycin.

(c) Lincosamide antibiotics

Two clinically useful lincosamide antibiotics are lincomycin and clindamycin (see Fig. 9.12). Lincomycin is obtained from *Streptomyces lincolnesis*. Clindamycin is a synthetic derivative of lincomycin. The lincosamides are active against Gram-positive but not Gram-negative organisms. The antibiotics inhibit protein synthesis in Gram-positive bacteria by binding to 50S subunits of 70S ribosomes.

Protein synthesis on 80S ribosomes is insensitive to the inhibitory action of the lincosamides. 50S from Gram-negative organisms are also resistant to lincosamides. The drugs appear to inhibit protein synthesis at the stage of peptide-chain synthesis directed by peptidyl transferase. They probably inhibit peptide bond formation by interfering with the correct positioning of aminoacyl-tRNA and peptidyl-tRNA at the A and P sites (see Fig. 9.8). The receptor proteins on 50S which bind the lincosamides are similar to those which bind chloramphenicol and erythromycin. Cross-resistance between the three classes of antibiotics may thus occur. A summary of antibiotics which inhibit protein synthesis is shown in Table 9.2.

Fig. 9.12. Lincosamide antibiotic: clindamycin.

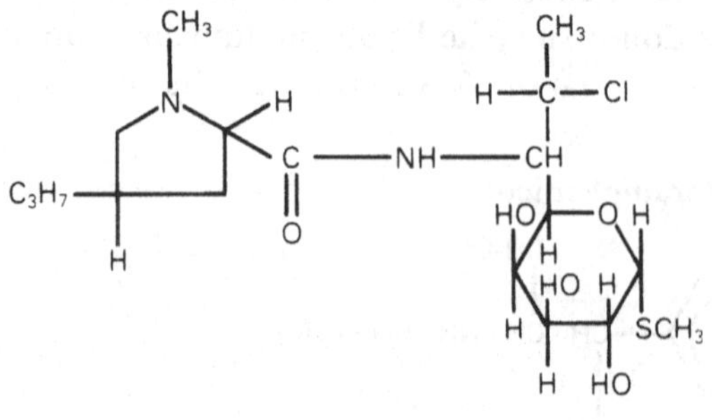

Table 9.2 *Anti-microbial agents inhibiting protein synthesis*

Drug	Binding site	Mechanism of action	Effect on bacteria	Organism treated
Aminoglycoside (streptomycin)	P10 of 30S subunit	Inhibition of elongation process and misreading of aminoacid sequence code by mRNA	Bactericidal	*M. tuberculosis*, broad spectrum
Tetracyclines	30S subunit and selectively concentrated in bacteria	Prevention of aminoacyl-tRNA access to the A site and block of elongation	Bacteriostatic	Broad spectrum
Chloramphenicol	50S subunit	Blocks peptidyl transferase. Peptide bond formation and elongation inhibited	Bacteriostatic	Broad spectrum, but especailly typhoid fever
Macrolides (erythromycin)	50S subunit	Occludes peptidyl-tRNA from site P, blocks translocation and peptide chain elongation	Bacteriostatic	Gram-positive organisms
Lincosamides (clindamycin)	50S	Peptide chain elongation blocked by interference with the correct positioning of aminoacyl- or peptidyl-tRNA at A and P sites	Bacteriostatic	Gram-positive organisms

Inhibition of nucleic acid synthesis

The code for the sequence of aminoacid incorporation in any given protein is contained in the nuclear DNA. The code is *transcribed* by mRNA and *translated* by tRNA during protein synthesis. We have seen that a large number of antibiotics bind to ribosomal subunits and interfere with translation. Other drugs interfere with transcription and thereby ultimately prevent protein synthesis.

DNA consists of two nucleotide chains joined together by bases. The two chains of the DNA are twisted about each other in the form of a double helix. During transcription, the two strands of the double helix separate; one strand serves as a template upon which a complementary RNA is synthesised under the influence of the enzyme *RNA polymerase*. A drug can interfere with the transcription process by (a) preventing DNA separation, (b) introducing an incorrect component into the replicating RNA, or (c) by blocking RNA polymerase. Of the large number of chemical agents which are known to have these sorts of actions, only a few are of clinical use.

Rifampicin

Rifampicin is a semisynthetic member of the rifamycin group of antibiotics produced by *Streptomyces mediterranei*. The drug is active against most Gram-positive bacteria and mycobacteria, but not against Gram-negative bacteria due to the presence of a permeability barrier in the latter. Its efficacy in the treatment of tuberculosis is well established, usually in combination with isoniazid or ethambutol. The drug inhibits RNA synthesis by binding very strongly to DNA-dependent RNA polymerase (dissociation rate constant, 3 nM). The drug has extremely weak binding affinity for mammalian polymerases which are up to 2000 times less sensitive to the drug than bacterial enzymes. This is the basis of the selective toxicity of rifampicin: because of the strong binding of the drug to bacterial RNA polymerases, the action is bactericidal.

Inhibition of synthesis of essential metabolites

Folic acid is required for the growth of bacteria and of mammalian cells. Mammalian cells take up folic acid from dietary sources by a special active energy-dependent transport mechanism. This transport process does not occur in bacterial cells, which must therefore synthesise folic acid *de novo*, intracellularly. This difference is the basis of the selective toxicity of antimicrobial agents which inhibit folic acid biosynthesis. Folic acid is reduced to tetrahydrofolic acid which functions as a coenzyme in reactions in which one-carbon units are transported from one molecule to another. Tetrahydrofolic acid is required for the biosynthesis of thymidine, purines and aminoacids. Thymidine and the purines are required for nucleic acid (DNA and RNA) synthesis and aminoacids are necessary for the biosynthesis of proteins. Hence, inhibition of folic acid synthesis leads to inhibition of cell growth.

Biosynthesis of folic acid

The biosynthesis of folic acid is illustrated in Fig. 9.13. p-Aminobenzoic acid is a natural intermediate in bacteria folic acid biosynthesis. It does not occur in mammalian cells. The reduction of dihydrofolic acid to tetrahydrofolic acid is directed by the enzyme dihydrofolate reductase (DHFR).

Inhibitors of dihydropteroate synthetase
(a) The sulphonamides

The therapeutic value of the sulphonamides was recognised in 1935 when Domagk demonstrated that the dye, prontosil, was effective in treating mice infected with streptococci. Prontosil was later shown to be metabolised in the body to p-aminobenzene sulphonamide which is the active part of the molecule. The sulphonamides are structurally analogous to p-aminobenzoic acid (PABA). The compounds differ from one another according to the substitutions on the sulphonamide group (see Fig. 9.14).

The therapeutic efficacy of the different sulphonamides depends mainly on the pKa of the —SO₂NH— group of the molecule. The concentration of sulphonamides required to produce 50% inhibition of dihydropteroate synthetase is directly proportional to the pKa over the range 5.8 to 9.3. A similar relationship exists between pKa and antibacterial activity. The most active compounds are those with pKa of about 6.5. Those with lower pKa are highly ionised at body pH and inactive, since only the unionised form readily penetrates the bacterial cell membrane.

The sulphonamides compete with PABA for binding to dihydropteroate synthetase. The sulphonamides become alternative substrates giving rise to 'dihydropteroate-like' products in which PABA is replaced by sulphonamide. The product cannot be used for folic acid synthesis. The binding affinity of the sulphonamides for dihydropteroate synthetase is greater than is the affinity of the PABA which is displaced. PABA does competitively antagonise sulphonamide action. The inhibition of bacterial growth by sulphonamides can also be pre-

Fig. 9.13. Biosynthesis of folic acid in microorganisms.
Stage (I): *para*-aminobenzoic acid (PABA) is linked to pteridine to form dihydropteroic acid. This stage is catalysed by dihydropteroic acid synthetase. Sulphonamides and sulphones inhibit this enzyme or act as 'false substrates'. Stage II: glutamic acid is linked to dihydropteroic acid to form dihydrofolic acid. Stage III: Dihydrofolic acid is reduced to tetrahydrofolic acid (tetrahydrofolate). This stage is catalysed by dihydrofolate reductase (DHFR). Trimethoprim, pyrimethamine, proguanil and dapsone inhibit this enzyme. (Folinic acid is formyltetrahydrofolate.)

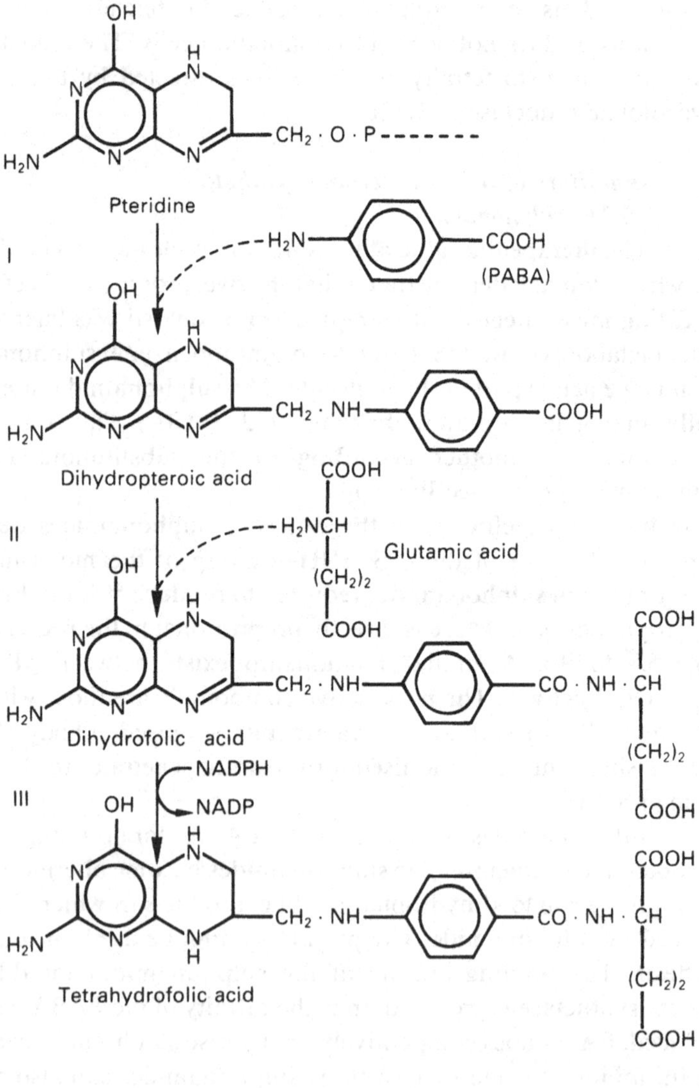

vented by products of one-carbon transfer mechanisms such as thymidine, purines and aminoacids. One important clinical significance of this is that in purulent infections, the pus may contain large amounts of these substances as a result of cell breakdown. These can reduce the efficacy of the sulphonamides in these circumstances, in which case the causative organisms may then be mistaken for resistant mutants.

(b) The sulphones (Fig. 9.15)

Sulphones are the drugs of choice in the treatment of leprosy. Examples are (diaminophenylsulphone) dapsone, sulphoxone, glucosulphone, and acetosulphone. Dapsone is also used in combination with other drugs in the treatment of malaria.

The sulphones are structural analogues of PABA and they bind to

Fig. 9.14. Molecular structures of sulphanilamide and its analogues.

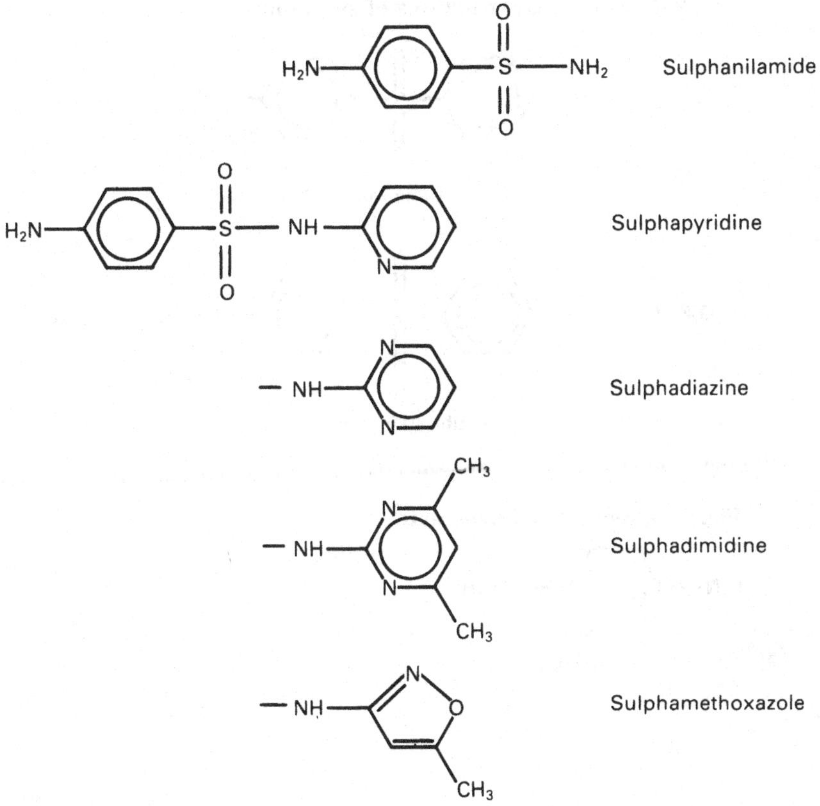

the active site of dihydropteroate synthetase. Like the sulphonamides, the sulphones are utilised in the production of sulphone-containing folate analogues which cannot lead to the biosynthesis of folic acid.

(c) p-Aminosalicylic acid (PAS) (Fig. 9.16)

PAS is a toxic substance sometimes used in the treatment of tuberculosis. The newer drugs such as rifampicin and ethambutol are now more frequently used alone or in combination with isoniazid. The drug inhibits the growth of *M. tuberculosis* by binding to dihydropteroate synthetase, thereby preventing the biosynthesis of folic acid. Its bacteriostatic action is blocked by PABA.

The susceptibility of dihydropteroate synthetases from different bacteria to inhibition by antimicrobial agents

We have seen that the three groups of drugs just described inhibit folic acid synthesis by displacing PABA from binding sites on

Fig. 9.15. Molecular structures of sulphones.

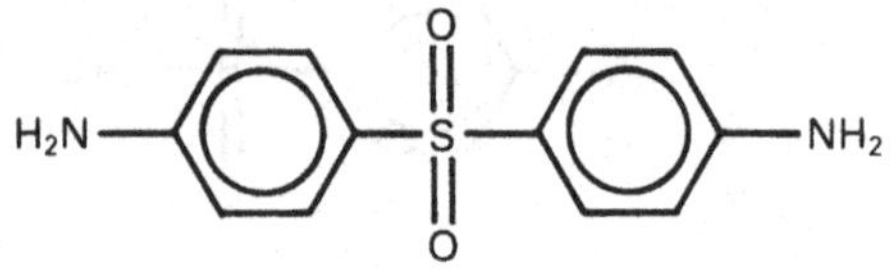

Dapsone

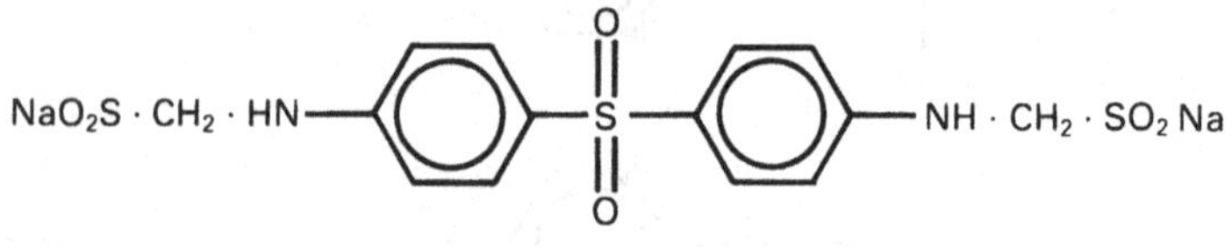

Sulphoxone sodium

Fig. 9.16. p-aminosalicylic acid.

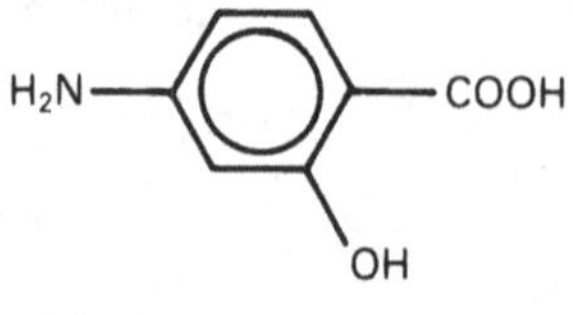

dihydropteroate synthetase. Why then are bacteria not equally susceptible to inhibition by the three classes of antimicrobial agents? The
reason for this is that the binding site on the enzyme varies from one
bacterium to another. The receptor configuration in the enzyme from
M. tuberculosis is suitable for binding PABA and PAS but not for binding sulphonamides. On the other hand, dapsone binds dihydropteroate synthetase from *M. leprae* and *Plasmodium facciparum*, but not the
enzyme from other bacteria. The sulphonamides can displace PABA
from enzymes in many bacteria but not those in *M. tuberculosis* and *M.
leprae*. These structural differences in the enzymes could have arisen as
a result of selection pressure exerted by toxic substances normally
present in the environment of different bacteria.

Inhibitors of dihydrofolate reductase

Folic acid cannot be used by the bacterial cell until it has been
reduced to tetrahydrofolic acid (folinic acid) by dihydrofolate
reductase (DHFR). This enzyme is blocked by diaminopyrimidines.
These compounds are structural analogues of the aminohydroxy-
pyrimidine moiety of the folic acid molecule (see Fig. 9.17).

(a) Pyrimethamine

Pyrimethamine is a diaminopyrimidine used extensively in
the treatment of malaria. The drug inhibits DHFR enzyme of malaria
parasites. Plasmodia synthesise dihydrofolic acid *de novo* as do bacteria.
Pyrimethamine inhibits DHFR isolated from *Plasmodium burghei* 3600
times more effectively than it does the enzyme from humans. The drug
thus acts quite selectively on plasmodial dihydrofolate reductase.
Pyrimethamine is bound to body tissues and has a t½ of about 4 days
after a single oral dose. For prophylaxis the drug is given once weekly.
Pyrimethamine is sometimes used in combination with dapsone or
sulphadoxine. Even though dapsone and the sulphonamides are not
effective antimalarial drugs on their own, they can potentiate the
action of pyrimethamine as the drugs attack two separate steps in the
biosynthesis of tetrahydrofolic acid.

(b) Proguanil

Proguanil is an antimalarial drug active against the asexual
erythrocytic forms of *Plasmodium falciparum*. Proguanil itself is inactive,
but becomes active after metabolic conversion in the liver to a
dihydrotriazine.

The metabolite inhibits the conversion of dihydrofolic acid to tetrahydrofolic acid by binding to the dihydrofolate reductase of plasmodia. Mammalian reductase is not affected, which accounts for its selective toxicity. The $t_{1/2}$ is shorter than that of pyrimethamine; for prophylaxis the drug has to be taken daily, and can also be used in combination with dapsone.

(c) Trimethoprim

Trimethoprim is also structurally analogous to the amino-hydroxypyrimidine moiety of the folic acid molecule, and it inhibits dihydrofolate reductase of bacteria.

Fig. 9.17. Inhibitors of dihydrofolate reductase.

Trimethoprim

Pyrimethamine

Cycloguanil

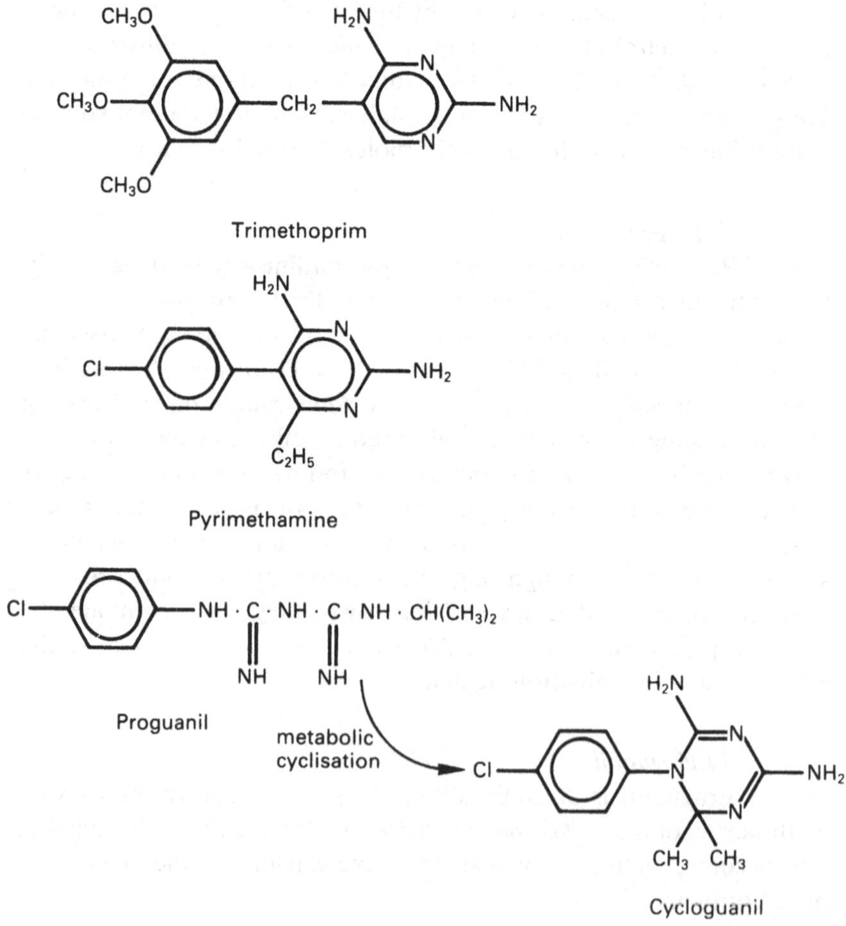

The action is bacteriostatic. The basis of selective toxicity is that animal reductase is far less sensitive to trimethoprim than the bacterial enzyme. Hitchings showed that 60000 times more trimethoprim is required to inhibit the human enzyme than to inhibit the enzyme from *E. coli*. Folic acid deficiency in patients given trimethoprim is thus not a serious problem.

Onset of action Although sulphonamides rapidly block folic acid synthesis, bacteria can continue to grow for several generations by using the existing pool of folic acid since dihydrofolate reductase is not affected. There is therefore a lag in the onset of antibacterial action with the sulphonamides. With trimethoprim, tetrahydrofolate is rapidly depleted and dihydrofolic acid is trapped in its unusable form. There is thus no time lag in the onset of inhibition of cell growth.

(d) Methotrexate

Several folic acid analogues have been tested for anti-bacterial activity. Most of these compounds were found to be toxic to mammalian cells. This is because folic acid, in contrast to PABA, is important for mammalian cell function. Folic acid analogues interfere with folic utilisation. The cytotoxic action of some folic acid analogues in man has been exploited in the treatment of some cancers such as leukaemia. For example, see methotrexate (Chapter 12).

9.4 COMBINATION THERAPIES

In the drug treatment of malaria the dihydrofolate reductase inhibitors, pyrimethamine and proguanil can each be combined with dihydropteroate synthetase inhibitors such as dapsone or a sulphonamide. Such combinations are *synergistic, that is, the effect of the two drugs used together is greater than the sum of the effects of the individual components*.

The combination of trimethoprim and a sulphonamide has provided the most dramatic example of synergism in combination. The combined formulation frequently used is trimethoprim and sulphamethoxazole (TMP–SMZ).

The synergism is due to the fact that the drugs inhibit two different enzymes – dihydropteroate synthetase and dihydrofolate reductase in the same biosynthetic pathway. This is an example of sequential blockade.

Apart from synergism, combination therapy confers other clinical advantages, listed below.

(i) In the case of TMP–SMZ the combination has a broader spectrum of antimicrobial action than trimethoprim or sulphamethoxazole alone.

(ii) The combination reduces the rate of emergence of resistant organisms. *Plasmodium falciparum* parasites resistant to pyrimethamine alone can be killed by pyrimethamine combined with dapsone or a sulphadoxine.

(iii) The combination is more consistently bactericidal whereas the drugs used alone are bacteriostatic.

(iv) Lower doses of each drug are used, thereby minimising toxic effects of the individual drugs.

FURTHER READING

Franklin, T. J. & Snow, G. A. (1981). *Biochemistry of Antimicrobial Action*, 3rd edn. Chapman & Hall, London, New York.

Hitchings, G. H. (1973). Mechanism of action of trimethoprim – Sulphamethoxazole I. *J. Infect. Dis.* **128**, suppl. S433.

Izaki, K., Matsuhashi, M. & Strominger, J. L. (1968). Biosynthesis of the peptidoglycans of bacterial cell walls: peptidoglycan transpeptidase and D-alanine carboxypeptidase: penicillin sensitive enzymatic reaction in strains of *E. coli. J. Biol. Chem.* **243**, 3180.

Pratt, W. B. & Fekety, R. (1986). *The Antimicrobial Drugs*. Oxford University Press, New York.

Pratt, W.B. (1977). Chemotherapy of Infection. Oxford University Press, New York, Oxford.

Strominger, J. L., Blumberg, P. M., Suginaka, H., Lmereit, J. & Wickins, G. G. (1971). How penicillin kills bacteria. Progress and problems. *Proc. Roy. Soc. Lond.* **179**, 369.

Woods, D. D. (1962). The biochemical mode of action of the sulphonamides. *J. Gen. Microbiol.* **29**, 2905.

10

Anti-protozoal drugs

10.1   INTRODUCTION

Protozoa are unicellular organisms in which the single cell performs all the functions necessary for its existence. The protozoa are eukaryotes, that is, the DNA is located in well defined chromosomes contained within a nucleus separated from the rest of the cytoplasm by a nuclear membrane as distinct from prokaryotes e.g. bacteria, which have their DNA in chromosomes lying free in the cytoplasm. In the tropics, protozoa are responsible for a large number of diseases in man and animals. Some major pathogenic protozoa are listed in Table 10.1.

In this chapter, some important drugs used in the treatment of protozoal parasitic diseases are discussed. As in previous chapters, the emphasis is on the sites of action of the drugs. Detailed life cycles are not dealt with. These can be found in standard texts on parasitology some of which are listed at the end of this chapter. The life cycle of the malaria parasite is described since knowledge of this is critically important for understanding malaria chemotherapy.

In the last few years, researches in molecular biology and biochemistry of protozoal parasites have revealed peculiar pathways and enzymes which can be exploited in the development of selectively toxic antiprotozoal agents. Some of these new possibilities are described to emphasise the new approach in the search for useful drugs.

10.2   RESEARCH AND DEVELOPMENT PROBLEMS
(a) Costs

Until recently, not much was known of the metabolism of protozoal parasites. Consequently, the biochemical basis for the selective action of even very effective antiprotozoal drugs is poorly understood;

Table 10.1   *Major pathogenic protozoa*

Disease	Pathogenic protozoa
Amoebic dysentery	*Entamoeba histolytica*
Leishmaniasis	*Leishmania donovani*
	Leishmania tropica
	Leishmania braziliensis
African trypanosomiasis	*Trypanosoma gambiense*
	T. brucei, T. vivax
	T. rhodesiensis
South American trypanosomiasis	*T. cruzi*
Malaria	*Plasmodium vivax*
	P. falciparum
	P. ovale
	P. malariae
Toxoplasmosis	*Toxoplasma gondii*
Trichomoniasis	*Trichomonas vaginalis*

and the development of new drugs has been slow. In the past, the search for new drugs consisted of screening large numbers of possible agents for antiprotozoal activity. When a compound with reasonable activity was found (the lead compound), as many structural analogues of it as possible were made and studied in detail. This approach yielded drugs whose mechanism of action sometimes remained unknown even after several years of clinical usage. The method was also tedious and slow. It is said, for example, that mefloquin (page 239) is the only successful compound out of 300000 screened for antimalarial activity by American Scientists during the Vietnam War. The drug is still not available for general use and its mechanism of action remains obscure.

The new method of search is to identify an enzyme or metabolic pathway which is peculiar to the parasite and then to produce compounds which can interfere with the enzyme or pathway. This approach is now possible because of recent and continuing advances in the understanding of the biochemistry of protozoal parasites. In theory such a rational approach should yield useful drugs more rapidly than the empirical approach. Whether it will be so in practice remains to be seen.

There are two main reasons why developments in the chemotherapy of protozoal diseases have been slow. Firstly, *in vitro* cultures are critically important for the detailed investigation of parasite biochemistry under conditions in which host factors do not interfere. Unfortunately, the technology for establishing and maintaining *in vitro* cultures of protozoal parasites is much more complex than that applicable in bacteriology. It is only recently, for example (see Trager & Jensen 1976), that it has been possible to culture *Plasmodium falciparum in vitro*. Now, scientists are able to undertake some important biochemical and pharmacodynamic studies of this clinically important parasite.

Secondly, the basic technology and manpower needed to mount the necessary research effort into protozoal parasites are not available in those countries where the need for such research is greatest; and because of high cost, research and development of drugs, for application, in tropical diseases is not a priority for most European and American multinational drug companies. Newton (1983) has stated the position as follows:

> Research and development costs continually rise (in 1979 $US 6–8 million was thought to be a realistic estimate for putting a new drug on the market; development costs for the latest antimalarial, mefloquin have recently been put at $US 15 million) and the poverty of the less developed countries makes them an unattractive market. The result is that only a small and diminishing number of pharmaceutical companies are now actively searching for new drugs to treat these diseases; the number of drug companies with an antimalarial programme is reported to have fallen from 15 to 5 in recent years.

Ten years on, development costs are much higher and third world countries much poorer. In contrast, drug companies in industrialised nations devote large proportions of their research and development budgets to drugs used in the treatment of diseases such as rheumatism, gout, travel sickness and anxiety! It is a remarkable fact that all the principal developments in antimalarial drugs took place during major wars (first and second World Wars and Vietnam war) when European and American forces *had* to be deployed in malaria zones. Consequently, most of the drugs presently available for the treatment of major protozoal infections have been in use for 20 years or longer. Many of them are dangerously toxic and are used only because safer alternatives are not available.

In recognition of the dilemma in which third world countries found themselves the World Health Organisation set up a Special Programme for Research and Training in Tropical Diseases (TDR) to focus research effort on important diseases peculiar to the tropics. However, it is clear that the solution to some of the socalled tropical diseases problems lies as much in medical as in political (or military) action in providing improved standards of life.

Adaptability of protozoal parasites

For various reasons one would expect the drug therapy of protozoal diseases to be relatively easy to achieve. For one thing the primary cause of the disease can be exactly known, and the metabolic deficiencies which underline the parasitic nature of the causative organisms should render a specific disease particularly amenable to drug treatment. Furthermore, the organisms should be prone to attack by the host's immunological and phagocytic defence mechanisms.

The truth, however, is that protozoal parasitic diseases have proved extremely elusive to pharmacological and immunological manipulations. Some of the remarkable adaptations which enable these organisms to survive in the presence of otherwise lethal concentrations of antimicrobial agents are discussed in chapter 13. Moreover, protozoal parasites overcome host defence mechanisms by exceedingly high rates of growth and complex life cycles. For instance, the organisms may exist in different morphological and biochemical forms (e.g. erythrocytic and exo-erythrocytic forms of plasmodia, and extracellular and intracellular forms of *Trypanosoma cruzi*) thereby confusing the host defence mechanisms. Drugs may be effective against one form but not against others. In the case of the African trypanosoma (page 246) which is entirely extracellular, the organism can change its antigenic identity in response to the host's immunological challenge.

In this chapter the emphasis of the discussion is on the mechanism of action of the drugs used in the treatment of protozoal parasitic diseases. The reader will notice that the drugs are grouped under diseases rather than mechanisms as is the case with the other chapters in this section. This is because in the chemotherapy of protozoal parasitic diseases, there is much less overlap in drugs and their mechanisms of action than is the case with bacterial, helminth and cancer chemotherapy.

10.3   MALARIA

Malaria, the dreaded fever which earned West Africa, the frightening epithet of *the White man's grave*, also had the distinction of having prevented adventurous Europeans of the 19th century from settling on a permanent basis in West Africa with consequent dissimilarities in the sociopolitical development of West, East and Southern Africa. Until the late 19th century, malaria was thought to be due to 'the emanation of foul air from decomposing vegetation'. In 1880, Alphonse Laveran of Algeria showed that the malaria parasite in the red blood cell of humans was the cause of malaria fever, and in 1898, Ronald Ross, an Englishman, proved that malaria parasites were transmitted by anopheline mosquitoes.

The term malaria applies to all infections caused by parasites belonging to the genus *Plasmodium*. More than 40 species are known which can infect man, primates, rodents and birds. Of these, only 4 species, *P. vivax, P. falciparum, P. ovale* and *P. malariae* can cause infection in man. The characteristic clinical symptom of malaria infection is fever, the time interval between febrile episodes being typical of the species of parasite. *P. falciparum* infection is the most severe and can be fatal. It is therefore described as malignant tertian malaria. The disease in Africa and South East Asia is caused most frequently by *P. falciparum* and is responsible for large-scale morbidity and mortality in those regions. *P. ovale* infections occur in Africa but very rarely.

Life cycle of the malaria parasite

Knowledge of the life cycle of the malaria parasite is important for understanding malaria chemotherapy because different stages in the cycle are affected by different drugs.

The malaria parasite has life cycles in two hosts, namely the vertebrate, e.g. man, and the invertebrate, the anopheline mosquito (*Anopheline arabiensis*).

Life cycle in man

When a female anopheline mosquito infected with malaria parasites bites, sporozoites in its saliva are injected into the bloodstream. Within a few minutes, the sporozoites disappear from the circulation and about 48 h later malaria parasites are found in the liver cells. During the next three days these sporozoites undergo nuclear division to form *exoerythrocytic schizonts*. The schizont consists of several daughter parasites called merozoites. The number of merozoites produced by *one* mature schizont is estimated to be more than 30000 in *P. falciparum*. The infected hepatocyte eventually bursts, releasing the merozoites into the bloodstream. This liver stage is called the pre- or exo-erythrocytic stage and takes 5½ days in *P. falciparum* (Fig. 10.1).

The erythrocytic cycle begins when the merozoites enter red blood cells a few minutes after their release from hepatocytes. It is now thought that merozoites invade erythrocytes after recognising and attaching to a specific receptor on the erythrocyte membrane. This receptor is thought to be a membrane protein called glycophorin. Or, according to Okoye & Bennett (1985), it is a band 3 (on gell electrophoresis) membrane protein. Inside the erythrocyte, the merozoite undergoes complex morphological changes, developing into a ring form (the parasite becomes shaped like a ring) called a *trophozoite*. The nucleus of the trophozoite divides to produce up to 32 daughter nuclei each of which eventually becomes surrounded by cytoplasm to form a

Fig. 10.1. Life cycle of a primate malaria parasite (from Bray & Garnham, 1982, with permission: *Br. Med. Bull.* (1982), 38, 117.

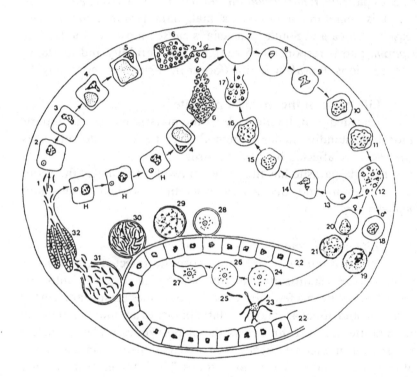

1: sporozoites injected into skin by the mosquito; 2: 2-day-old exoerythrocytic form in a hepatocyte; 3, 4, 5: growing exoerythrocytic schizonts; H: hypnozoites in hepatocytes; 6: mature exoerythrocytic schizonts bursting, releasing merozoites into the blood; 7: erythrocyte; 8, 9: growing trophozoites; 10, 11: growing schizonts; 12: mature schizont releasing merozoites; 13, 14, 15, 16, 17: erythrocytic cycle repeated; 18, 19: growth of the microgametocyte; 20, 21: growth of the macrogametocyte; 22: mosquito has taken gametocytes up into its midgut; 23: exflagellation of the microgametocyte; 24: macrogametocyte escapes from erythrocyte to become a macrogamete; 25: microgamete; 26: macrogamete about to be fertilized; 27: zygote or oökinete; 28, 29, 30: oöcyst growth on the mid-gut surface; 31: oöcyst bursting, releasing sporozoites; 32: sporozoites in the mosquito salivary glands.

merozoite. The parasite at this stage is known as the *erythrocytic schizont*. The schizont in the red blood cell is pigmented and can be seen and identified in a thin smear of infected blood. The mature schizont occupies all or most of the infected red cell which eventually bursts, releasing merozoites into the bloodstream. This is the stage when clinical signs of malaria appear. The large number of red blood cells destroyed by malaria parasites accounts for the anaemia which is characteristic of the disease. The maturation of the erythrocytic schizont and the release of merozoites occupy an interval of time characteristic of different species of malaria. In *P. falciparum* infection, the cycle occupies 48 h and the disease is called malignant tertian malaria.

The merozoites invade fresh red blood cells and either undergo another erythrocytic schizogony (develop into a schizont) or develop into male (microgametocyte) or female (macrogametocyte) forms. It is not known what causes the merozoites to develop into sexual forms.

Life cycle in the mosquito

The sexual cycle is completed in the mosquito when the latter bites an individual in whose blood mature gametocytes are circulating. In the mosquito, the female macrogametocytes escape from the red blood cell as free macrogametes. The male microgametocyte undergoes nuclear division to form eight microgametocytes which also leave the erythrocyte as free microgametes. All this takes place in the stomach wall of the mosquito. Male and female gametes then fuse to form a *zygote* which eventually comes to rest as an *ookinete* in the epithelial cell layer of the gut. Here the ookinete undergoes meiotic division giving rise to 10000 daughter cells called *sporozoites*. When the ookinete disintegrates, the sporozoites are released into the haemocoelomic fluid of the mosquito and eventually find their way into the salivary gland where they mature into infective sporozoites.

Relapse and recrudescence

It is common experience that a clinical attack of malaria may occur several months after an infection has been successfully treated and without further exposure to the parasite. This is called a relapse. Garnham has defined *true relapse* as renewed parasitaemia following a period in which the blood contained no parasites and no reinfection had occurred. Relapse should be differentiated from *recrudescence* which is renewed infection after treatment with a drug like chloroquine. After the cessation of treatment, surviving erythrocytic forms of the parasite undergo erythrocytic schizogony until the disease

is reestablished. Malaria parasites that cause relapses are *P. ovale* and
P. vivax. In these species some of the sporozoites injected by the
mosquito differentiate into *hypnozoites* ('sleeping' sporozoites) which
remain dormant for long periods (8–10 months for *P. vivax*) in the liver.
At a predetermined time for relapse, the hypnozoites undergo
exo-erythrocytic schizogony, forming merozoites which, on release,
invade red blood cells. *P. falciparum*, the parasite of African and South
East Asian malaria, does not form hypnozoites and does not cause
relapses. Renewed *P. falciparum* infection results from recrudescence.

Immunity to malaria

Many inhabitants of regions where malaria is endemic are
partially immune. In such people a malaria attack, if it does take place,
is mild. The state of partial immunity is sustained by repeated exposure to the parasite. After prolonged absence from a malaria zone, the
level of immunity is reduced. Should partially immune individuals resident in malaria regions take prophylactic treatment? Some malari-
ologists recommend that such individuals need only take prompt treatment for acute attack, but individuals must consider their personal
experience and consult their physician.

Up to six months after birth, children born to immune mothers and
who are fed on breast milk are resistant to malaria. This is due partly
to immunity conferred by the mother and partly (it is claimed) because
breast milk, the main diet of the infant, contains no p-aminobenzoic
acid which the parasite needs for FH$_4$ synthesis. Older children and
pregnant women or malnourished people are particularly vulnerable.
For this group, prophylactic treatment is imperative.

Inherited factors which protect against P. falciparum malaria
(a) Sickle cell haemoglobin

It has been postulated that the possession of the sickle-cell
haemoglobin (Hbs) affords protection against falciparum malaria.
Parasitisation of an Hbs erythrocyte by *P. falciparum*, increases the
tendency of the erythrocyte to sickle possibly due to loss of potassium
ions from the cell. Parasitised sickled cells are removed from the circulation more effectively than normal parasitised cells. The Hbs-contain-
ing red blood cell is thus not a suitable environment for the parasite to
develop; heterozygotes have a selective advantage against falciparum
malaria (see page 326).

(b) Glucose-6-phosphate dehydrogenase deficiency

There is also evidence that glucose-6-phosphate dehydrogenase (G6PD) deficiency affords protection against falciparum malaria. The mechanism of this protective effect is less clear. Luzzatto has shown that in the same G6PD-deficient individuals, parasites occur more frequently in non-deficient than in enzyme-deficient cells indicating that G6PD-deficient red blood cells are invaded less than are normal ones. It has also been suggested that since enzyme-deficient cells are sensitive to oxidant stress, then parasitisation of these cells could lead to their premature lysis, and they would thus be unable to support parasite growth (see page 191).

(c) Other red cell factors

Other red cell 'disorders' thought to protect individuals against *P. falciparum* malaria are:

(i) haemoglobin C (frequency of up to 28% in Northern Ghana);
(ii) haemoglobin F (foetal haemoglobin) may partly explain the resistance to malaria in the first six months of life;
(iii) thalassaemia; and
(iv) haemoglobin E.

(d) Hypergammaglobulinaemia

Edozien has suggested that the ability, in blacks, to synthesise and maintain high concentrations of gammaglobulins is inherited and has probably been selected for the protection it offers against malaria and other parasitic infections (see also page 158).

Development of a vaccine against malaria

Many laboratories are engaged in research towards the development of a suitable vaccine against *P. falciparum* malaria. Antigenic material is being prepared from the different forms of the parasite (gametocytes, sporozoites, merozoites) for active immunisation or for the production of specific antibodies for passive immunisation. The possibilities afforded by genetic engineering are being explored.

Drug treatment for malaria
Traditional remedies

Raised body temperature is a universally recognised symptom that something is functionally wrong in the body. In traditional societies, fever is clearly easily diagnosed. The mother can usually tell when the temperature of the child on her back is raised even only slightly above normal. There are therefore numerous folk remedies for the treatment of fevers. Some of these, e.g. *dongo yaro* or mango bark, are used extensively in rural and urban Nigeria for the treatment of malaria. Since these remedies appear to be clinically effective, there is much research effort to establish their antimalarial activities. Aqueous extracts of *dongo yaro* (*Azadirachta indica*) have been shown to possess anti-inflammatory activity. It is possible that part of the clinical benefit from some of the remedies is due to their content of anti-inflammatory phenolic acids, which by lowering a raised body temperature, allow the immune system (especially in the partially immune) to deal with the parasite. It is also possible that the plants indeed contain antimalarial activities which have not been detected.

Modern remedies
There are three objectives in modern malaria chemotherapy:

- (a) Suppressive (prophylactic) treatment to prevent infection from taking hold;
- (b) Treatment of acute attack to eliminate an infection which has already taken hold; and
- (c) Radical cure to eliminate all forms of the parasite.

Suppressive (prophylactic) treatment
In true prophylaxis, the aim would be to kill the sporozoites injected by the mosquito so that no infection can occur. Unfortunately no drugs are known which affect this stage of the parasite. The socalled prophylactics prevent the development of erythrocytic schizonts and so suppress clinical attack. The drugs most frequently used in prophylactic therapy are the dihydrofolate reductase inhibitors, alone or in combination with sulphones or sulphonamides. The most frequently used DHFR inhibitors are pyrimethamine and proguanil. Examples of combined formulations are: maloprim = pyrimethamine + dapsone; and fansidar = pyrimethamine + sulphadoxine.

The use of these drugs in malaria is based on the same principles as already described for bacteria. Like bacteria, malaria parasites must synthesise folic acid *de novo* using *p*-aminobenzoic acid as essential metabolite. Folic acid is reduced to tetrahydrofolic acid (FH$_4$) under the influence of the enzyme dihydrofolate reductase (DHFR). Thus sulphonamides (inhibitors of dihydropteroate synthetase) and the DHFR inhibitors cause a sequential block of FH$_4$ synthesis and hence inhibit growth of parasite (see also page 217). The combined formulation is synergistic and effective in treating plasmodia that have become resistant to DHFR inhibitors alone or chloroquine.

Chloroquine is effective as a suppressive prophylactic drug. However, since chloroquine is the most effective erythrocytic schizonticide for *P. falciparum*, the drug is best reserved for the treatment of an acute attack of malaria and should not be used in prophylactic treatment. The emergence of chloroquine-resistant falciparum malaria and its spread in Brazil and South East Asia can be attributed to the large-scale use of chloroquine in prophylactic treatment in which the drug was included in table salt.

Prophylactic treatment of P. vivax or P. malariae

In regions where malaria is caused by vivax or malariae parasites, prophylactic treatment with schizonticides is not sufficient. The liver forms of the parasite (schizonts and hypnozoites) are not affected and can give rise to a relapse after the end of prophylactic treatment with the above drugs. To prevent this, primaquine can be used in addition. It should be noted that primaquine can cause severe haemolytic anaemia in persons deficient in G6PD (see page 185).

Treatment of acute attack

Clinical attack of malaria is treated with drugs effective against erythrocytic schizonts and merozoites. The following groups of drugs are effective: I against erythrocytic schizonts:

(i) quinine
(ii) 4-aminoquinolines, e.g. chloroquine, amodiaquine,
(iii) DHFR inhibitors and sulphonamides, e.g. pyrimethamine, proguanil, dapsone, sulphadoxine,
(iv) antibiotics, e.g. tetracycline;

and II against tissue schizonts and hypnozoites: 8-aminoquinoline, e.g. primaquine, pamaquine and pentaquine.

Quinine

Quinine and its dextrorotatory isomer, quinidine (Fig. 10.2), are alkaloids of the bark of the cinchona tree indigenous to South America. Other alkaloids are the isomers cinchonidine and cinchonine. The inhabitants of Peru originally used the bark as a traditional fever remedy. Historical records contain different versions of how the medicinal value of cinchona was discovered by Europeans. One account is that the plant became known as a fever remedy when it was used to treat the wife of the Spanish Viceroy in Peru, Countess

Chinchon, in 1638. Moved by the effectiveness of the treatment, the Viceroy brought the bark to Spain and it was from then on used widely in Europe for the treatment of fevers. In 1677 it was included in the London Pharmacopoeia. The crude drug was used for nearly 200 years before its alkaloids were isolated in 1820. Although quinine can be synthesised, the process is too laborious and expensive to be practical. Quinine is still obtained from its natural source.

Quinine causes a wide variety of unwanted and toxic effects including blurred vision, ringing in the ears, intravascular haemolysis (blackwater fever), and muscle weakness. This cluster of side-effects is called *cinchonism*. The use of quinine as an antimalarial is therefore restricted to emergency treatment of acute severe malaria with or without cerebral involvement. It is given by slow intravenous infusion in these circumstances. Quinine has recently gained prominence because it is effective in the treatment of most chloroquine-resistant falciparum malariae when used alone or in combination with tetracycline.

Primaquine

Primaquine (Fig. 10.3) is the only 8-aminoquinoline antimalarial that is now widely used in areas where *P. vivax* is endemic. The others, pamaquine and pentaquine are obsolete due to unacceptable toxicities. The critical importance of primaquine is that it is the most effective drug available for the *radical cure* of vivax and other relapsing malarias. It is thus very important that the drug is used properly so that resistant strains of vivax parasites do not emerge. So far, resistance to primaquine is not a serious problem. For radical cure it may be combined with chloroquine or other erythrocytic schizonticides.

Primaquine is liable to cause severe haemolytic anaemias in patients whose red blood cells are deficient in the enzyme G6PD. For this reason, and because most of the disease in West Africa is

Fig. 10.2. Molecular structure of quinine.

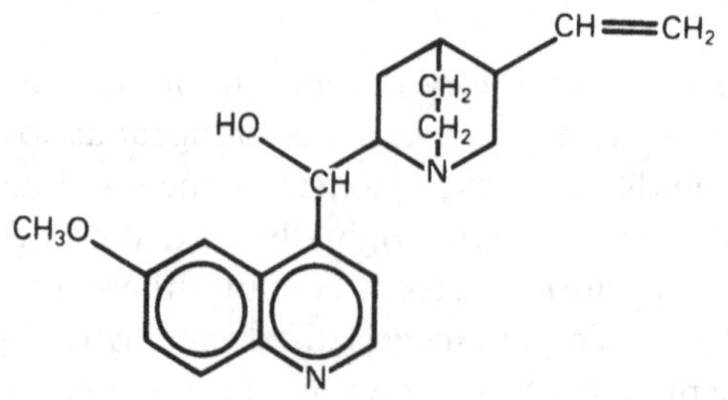

falciparum malaria, the drug is not used in this region. Falciparum malaria does not have latent liver stages requiring the type of action possessed by the 8-aminoquinolines. The severity of primaquine-induced haemolysis is dose-dependent. With low doses the effect is self-limiting because young red blood cells are resistant to drug-induced haemolysis (see also page 187). In areas where G6PD deficiency is endemic, it is advisable to monitor the haemoglobin concentration of patients treated with potentially haemolytic drugs. Their administration should be discontinued if there is a sudden drop in haemoglobin concentration or a marked darkening of the urine.

Fig. 10.3. Molecular of structures of (a) 4-aminoquinolines, and (b) an 8-aminoquinoline.

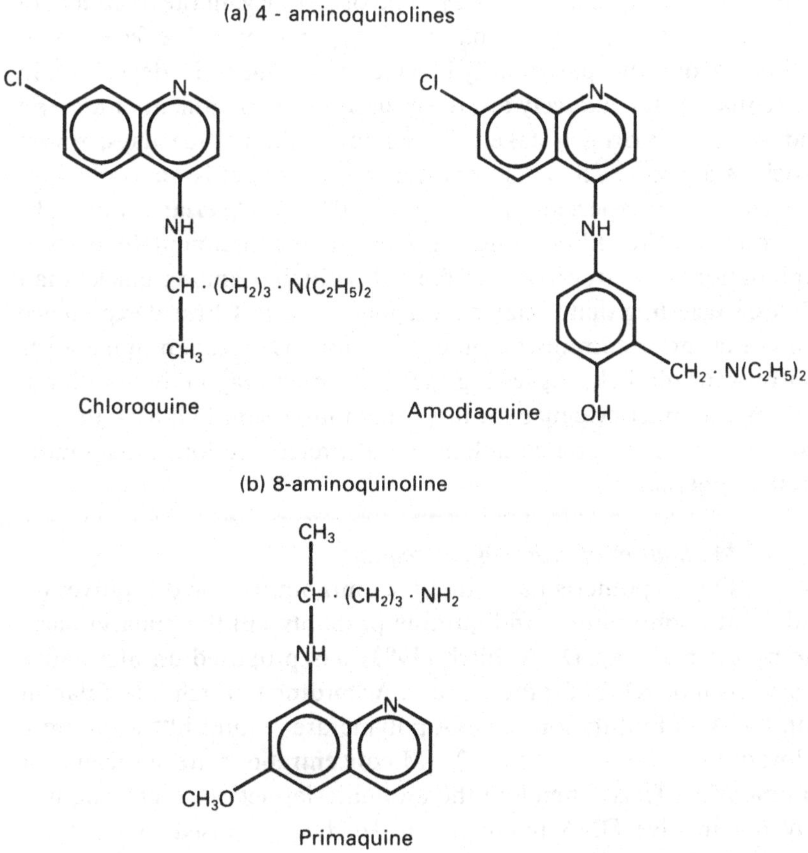

(a) 4 - aminoquinolines

Chloroquine

Amodiaquine

(b) 8-aminoquinoline

Primaquine

Chloroquine

Chloroquine, the most active antimalarial among the 4-aminoquinolines (Figure 10.3) was first investigated in 1934 by the Germans. During the second World War, the necessity to deploy American and European allied troops in malarious zones compelled the Americans in 1943 to synthesise and test thousands of 4-aminoquinolines; in the process, chloroquine was rediscovered. The impetus for the search for synthetic antimalarials was partly the wide range of toxic effects caused by quinine and partly the fact that the major source of quinine, namely, the cinchona plantations of Indonesia, fell under enemy control.

Note the presence of quinoline nucleus in quinine and in the synthetic antimalarials. The 4- and 8-aminoquinolines differ in the position of the side chain. Amodiaquine and chloroquine have chlorine instead of a methoxy nuclear substituent as in primaquine and quinine. Mefloquine (Fig. 10.4) also has a quinoline nucleus.

In large doses and used over a period of time, e.g. in the treatment of rheumatoid arthritis and amoebiasis chloroquine has toxic effects similar to those of quinine, particularly blurred vision due to its deposition in the retina. In the relatively low doses used in the treatment of malaria and where the drug is taken for no more than three days, severe toxicities are rare. The commonest unwanted effect is an unpleasant itch (pruritus) experienced by up to 10% of Nigerians who take chloroquine. The chloroquine itch has defied experimentally derived explanation. The prevalence of the itch is higher among blacks than whites, suggesting that it may have a genetic basis. Clinical experience shows that prior administration of histamine H_1-receptor antagonists can prevent the itch, suggesting that histamine may be involved, but there is no direct evidence for this. This unpleasant itch accounts for much chloroquine non-compliance and preference for amodiaquine among Nigerians.

Mechanism of action of chloroquine

One hypothesis has it that the aminoquinoline derivatives (4- and 8-aminoquinolines) and quinine probably kill the malaria parasite by intercalating DNA. Fitch (1983) has proposed an alternative mechanism of action for these drugs. According to Fitch intercalation with DNA and inhibition of DNA polymerase require 10^{-5}M or more chloroquine, whereas 10^{-9} to 10^{-8}M concentrations are sufficient for antimalaria effects. Therefore the antimalarial action of chloroquine may not involve DNA intercalation. He has proposed that chloroquine becomes toxic to the parasite by binding to ferriprotoporphyrin (FP) which is a component of a pigment produced when the parasite degrades haemoglobin. FP itself is toxic to the cell, but normally, soluble haem produced by the parasite, forms nontoxic complexes with FP. Chloroquine has a higher affinity for FP than the haem binders, thereby preventing the detoxification of FP. The chloroquine-FP is thought to damage parasite cell membrane by interfering with ion conductance. The evidence for this mechanism of action has been discussed by Fitch (1983). Some of the salient points are as follows. (i) Malaria parasites degrade haemoglobin. (ii) It seems that the generation of haemoglobin degradation products is necessary for the sensitivity of the parasite to chloroquine. Parasites that fail to produce pigment are usually resistant to chloroquine; when chloroquine-resistant non-pigmented parasites revert to pigment production, they regain sensitivity to chloroquine. These points support the proposed mechanism of action, but there are examples of non-pigmented parasites which show sensitivity to chloroquine. (iii) FP is toxic to cell membranes and chloroquine-FP complexes are even more toxic.

This approach has some exciting possibilities. It has been known for long that the parasitised erythrocyte concentrates chloroquine 100 times more than normal erythrocytes. A high-affinity binding substance like FP would explain that observation. It is also known that chloroquine-resistant *P. falciparum* takes up much less chloroquine than sensitive parasites. A reduced concentration of FP in such cells would thus explain chloroquine resistance. Furthermore, identification of a chloroquine receptor should enhance predictability in the design of new antimalarial compounds.

Mefloquine

The most promising compound to emerge from the US Army programme on antimalarial drugs initiated during the Vietnam war is mefloquine. The compound which is structurally related to quinine (Fig. 10.4) was one of some 300000 compounds tested in the programme. Mefloquine is a 4-quinoline methanol. It acts on erythocytic schizonts, but not on gametocytes or tissue parasites. The drug was developed as an agent for the treatment of multi-drug resistant falciparum malaria. A single dose of 1500 mg is effective against most malarias including drug-resistant falciparum malaria. Unfortunately, mefloquine-resistant falciparum malaria has been observed. To avoid the spread of resistance to one of the few drugs which can be used to treat chloroquine-resistant malaria, formulations in which mefloquine is combined with pyrimethamine or sulphadoxine are being tested.

The mechanism of action of mefloquine is not known. Unlike quinine and the aminoquinolines, mefloquine does not intercalate with DNA. It seems to share the same mechanism of accumulation in parasitised erythrocytes with chloroquine since the drug interferes with chloroquine-induced clumping of pigment in the parasite and competes with chloroquine for uptake by infected erythrocytes. It is not known why it is that in chloroquine-resistant parasites, there is a change in chloroquine but not in mefloquine uptake and accumulation by parasitised erythrocytes. Mefloquine is undergoing clinical trials.

Quinghaosu (artemisinin)

Quinghaosu (GHS) is an endoperoxide of a sesquiterpine lactone (Fig. 10.5) isolated from the plant *quin hao (Artemisia annua* L.). Quinhaosu roughly means 'active principle of quin hao'. The plant is

Fig. 10.4. Molecular structure of mefloquine.

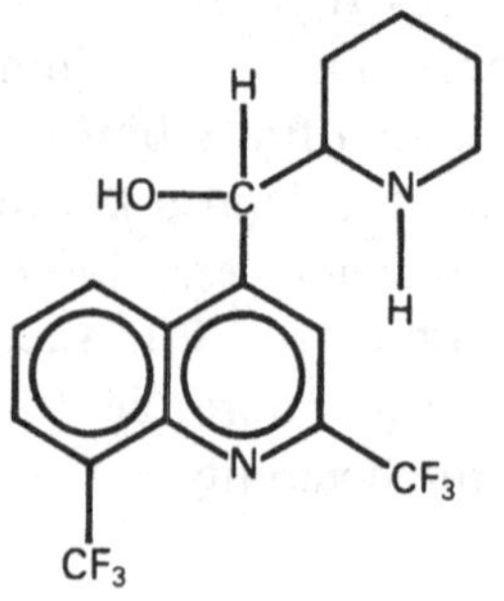

Mefloquine

Fig. 10.5. Molecular structure of quinhaosu (artemisinin).

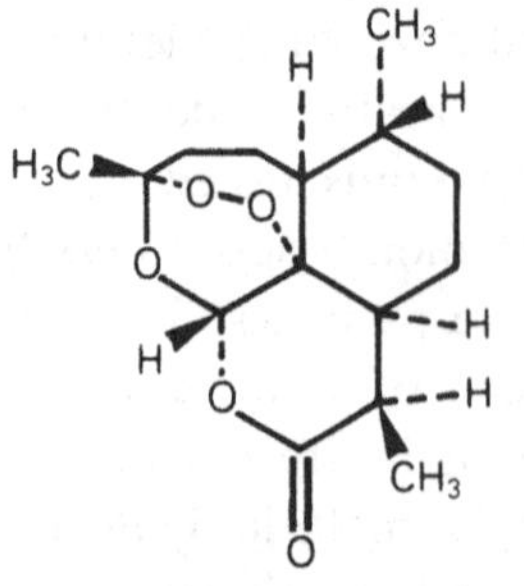

Quinhaosu

mentioned in ancient Chinese manuscripts dating back to 168 BC where 'the bark is recommended for use in haemorrhoids'. In prescriptions written by Ge Hong in 340 AD it is advised that 'to reduce fever one should soak one handful of quinhao in 1 sheng (litre) of water, strain the liquor and drink it all'. Since then it has been known among Chinese traditional practitioners that 'Chills and fever of malaria can be combated by quin hao preparations'. After decades of attempts to confirm the antipyretic and antimalarial activity of water extracts of quin hao, Chinese scientists isolated the crystalline compound QHS from diethyl ether extracts in 1972.

The antimalarial activity of QHS is at least equal to those of chloroquine and mefloquine and QHS is active against the asexual blood forms of *P. vivax* and *P. falciparum* as well as chloroquine-resistant falciparum malaria. QHS is more rapidly acting than chloroquine. It is particularly useful in cerebral malaria – a potentially fatal advanced form of falciparum malaria where more than 5% of the red cells are infected. Clinical trials have shown that the time for recovery from cerebral malaria-induced coma is shorter after QHS than after cloroquine or quinine treatment.

The mechanism of action of QHS is not known. In *in vitro* tests using *P. falciparum* isolates, the combination of QHS and chloroquine is antagonistic. The drug affects polyamine, but not folic acid metabolism.

Several derivatives of QHS, e.g. dihydroquinghaosu (DHQHS) and artemether have been synthesised and are more potent than QHS.

Radical cure

In *P. malariae* and *P. vivax*, some of the merozoites released from disintegrating erythrocytes reinfect liver cells and so begin a second exo-erythrocytic cycle. Also, some of the parasites may develop into hypnozoites and lie dormant in the liver. These liver forms are not affected by the blood schizonticides used in the treatment of acute attack. The objective in radical cure is to kill both blood and tissue forms of the parasite. With *P. falciparum*, there is no reinfection of liver cells by merozoites and there are no hypnozoites. In this case successful treatment of the acute attack with, e.g. chloroquine is equivalent to radical cure. To achieve radical cure in *P. vivax* and *P. malariae* infections, primaquine or other 8-aminoquinolines effective against tissue parasites must be used.

10.4   AMOEBIASIS
Introduction
Amoebiasis (amoebic dysentery) is caused by *Entamoeba histolytica*. The cysts of the protozoa are passed in the faeces of the infected person. When ingested in contaminated food or water, the cysts enter the large intestine where they disintegrate, releasing amoebae or tropozoites. The trophozoites invade the epithelium of the large intestine causing ulcers and developing into cysts which are again passed in the stools. Some trophozoites penetrate the intestinal wall and are carried in the portal circulation to the liver where they cause liver abscesses. Diarrhoea is the usual clinical symptoms of infection but some carriers show no symptoms. There are several species of amoebae living in the human gut lining, most are harmless. Even the species *E. histolytica* is not always pathogenic; there are several races of *E. histolytica* only one of which is pathogenic. It is said that only under certain circumstances does the organism become pathogenic. What triggers this change is not known.

Drugs used in the treatment of amoebiasis
The mechanism of action of most of the drugs used in the treatment of amoebiasis remains uncertain even though some of the drugs are very effective.

Metronidazoles (flagyl)
Metronidazole (Fig. 10.6) is a nitro-imidazole derivative. Other compounds closely related are tinidazole, ornidazole and nimorazole. They act against trophozoites in the intestinal wall and other body tissues but not against cysts in the lumen. Therefore for best results metronidazole should be combined with a luminal amoebicide such as diloxanide.

Fig. 10.6. Nitroimidazole amoebicides.

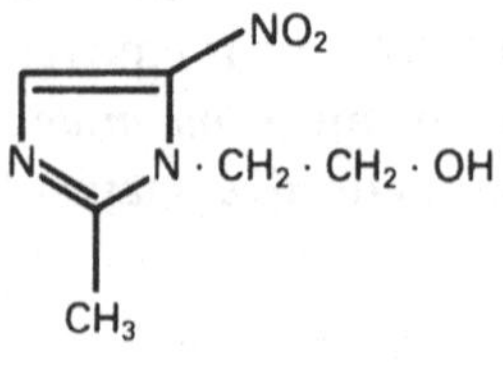

Metronidazole

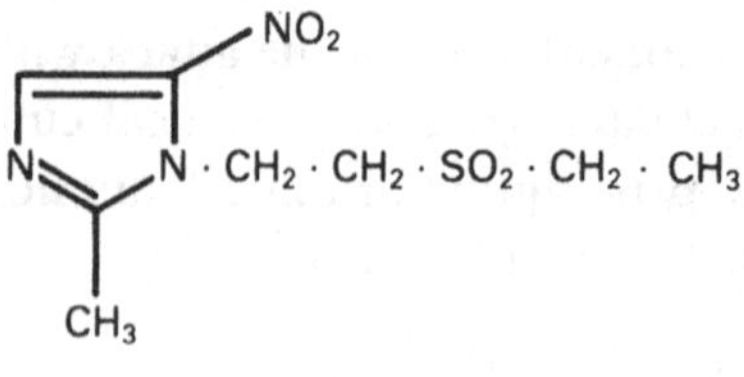

Tinidazole

Mechanism of action

The drug is thought to act as an electron sink by accepting electrons from ferredoxin (the parasite's electron transport protein) and depriving the cell of essential reducing equivalents. Essential coenzymes such as NADH and NADPH are not formed, leading to the death of the parasite. Mammalian cells do not rely on ferredoxin for the production of reducing equivalents. Metronidazole is therefore selectively toxic to *E. histolytica.*

Furthermore the nitro group of metronidazole becomes reduced in accepting electrons from ferrodoxin. The reduced metabolite is said to be toxic to the parasite. It binds to DNA and by distorting its helical structure, prevents DNA from functioning as a template. The parasite thus 'commits suicide' by converting the drug to a metabolite toxic to it. This property is common to nitroaromatics.

Emetine

Emetine (Fig. 10.7) is the methyl ester of cephalin isolated from the plant ipecacuanha. One explanation of the way the drug works is that the drug prevents protein synthesis by inhibiting the translocation of peptidyl-tRNA from the acceptor site to the donor site on 70S ribosomes (see page 210). DNA and RNA synthesis are also inhibited but inhibition of protein synthesis is the primary effect. The basis of its selective toxicity is that emetine has no effect on protein synthesis directed by 80S ribosomes in mammalian cells. Dihydro-emetine has similar effects but is supposed to be less toxic. Emetine is sometimes used in combination with tetracycline. The antibiotic has no amoebicidal action on its own; the beneficial effect arises from a

Fig. 10.7. Emetine.

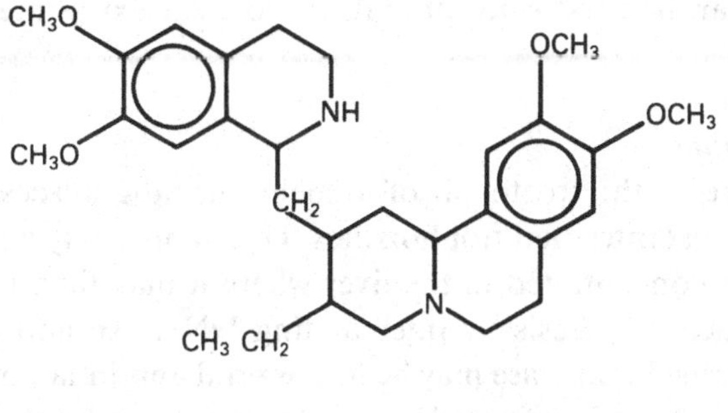

reduction in the population of intestinal bacteria which the parasite needs for survival. An aminoglycoside antibiotic *paromomycin* is directly amoebicidal and can be used on its own for the treatment of intestinal amoebiasis.

Emetine is inactive against hepatic abscesses. To clear the hepatic disease, emetine or dihydroemetine may be combined with chloroquine.

Emetine is cardiotoxic and can cause muscle weakness either by blocking neuromuscular transmission or by directly damaging skeletal muscle cells. Toxicity limits the clinical use of emetine and dihydroemetine.

Diiodohydroxyquin (Iodoquinol)

is an iodinated 8-hydroxyquinoline derivative which can clear the intestine of trophozoites but not tissue of trophozoites or hepatic amoeba. This is probably because the drug is poorly absorbed. The mechanism of action is unknown. Like many other 8-hydroxyquinolines the drug can cause subacute myelo-optic neuropathy (SMON). The Japanese appear to be particularly susceptible to this toxicity. The prevalence of SMON was high in Japan up to 1970. When the trivial use of 8-hydroxyquinoline derivatives, especially iodochlorohydroxyquin (vioform) in the treatment of 'travellers' diarrhoea' was banned in that year, there was a dramatic drop in the incidence of SMON in that country. The use of these drugs is highly restricted in many countries.

Diloxanide

is a derivative of dichloroacetamide. The drug is directly amoebicidal. The mechanism of action is unknown, but it is useful in treating asymptomatic cyst passers, and in clearing intestinal trophozoites. It can be used with other drugs to clear extra-intestinal parasites.

Chloroquine

is effective in the treatment of amoebic hepatic abscess, but has no action against intestinal trophozoites. This is probably because the drug is highly concentrated in the liver where it may then inhibit parasite nucleic acid synthesis by intercalating DNA. An additional benefit of chloroquine in this case may be its powerful anti-inflammatory action. This has been attributed to chloroquine inhibition of prostaglandin production at the level of phospholipase A_2 blockade.

10.5 LEISHMANIASIS
Introduction
There are three types of disease caused by the protozoan parasites called Leishmania in man:

(a) Visceral leishmaniasis (Kala-azar)
is caused by *L. donovani*, a parasite widely distributed in tropical Africa, Asia, the Mediterranean and South America. *L. donovani* is harboured by small mammals and transmitted to man by the bite of sandflies of the genus *Phlebotomus*. The incubation period can be up to six months. The disease is characterised by malaise, headache, fever, enlargement of spleen and liver, abnormality of white blood cells and haemorrhage, and is fatal in a high proportion of cases.

(b) Cutaneous leishmaniasis (oriental sore)
is caused by *L. tropica* and is common in North Africa, Asia and the Mediterranean. The disease is characterised by superficial ulceration of the skin at the site of the bite, often the face. Cutaneous leishmaniasis may not be lethal, but a disfiguring scar is left after spontaneous healing of the ulcer.

(c) Mucocutaneous leishmaniasis
is caused by *L. braziliensis*, found in Africa and Central and South America. The parasites enter the bloodstream and invade mucous membranes of the nose, larynx and face causing ulceration and gross disfigurement.

Drugs used in the treatment of leishmaniasis
The conventional drugs used in the treatment of leishmaniasis are sodium stibogluconate, pentamidine, amphotericin B and cyclouanil. Very little is known of the mechanism of action of these drugs. Sodium stibogluconate (SSb) (Fig. 10.8) is the most important drug; it is a pentavalent antimonial. The drug is active against visceral and cutaneous leishmaniasis and less active against the mucocutaneous form. Like all other pentavalent antimonials, SSb is inactive against schistosomiasis. It could be that SSb is not absorbed by the schistosome or the mechanism for reducing the penta- to a trivalent antimonial is more efficient in leishmania than in schistosoma. Pentamidine is used in the treatment of cutaneous or visceral leishmaniasis. It is particularly useful in places where response to antimonials is poor (e.g. in the Sudan) or where toxicity of the antimonials is unusually high (e.g. in China).

Table 10.2   *Drugs used in the treatment of leishmaniasis*

Drug	Disease
Sodium stibogluconate	Visceral, cutaneous, mucocutaneous
Pentamidine	Cutaneous, visceral
Cycloguanil	Cutaneous, mucocutaneous
Amphotericin B	Mucocutaneous

SSb inhibits the enzyme phosphofructokinase, an essential enzyme in glycolysis. The mammalian enzyme is 100 times less sensitive to inhibition by SSb than the protozoan enzyme. This is the basis of its selective toxicity. Cycloguanil is used in the treatment of cutaneous leishmaniasis and amphotericin B in the treatment of the mucocutaneous form of the disease (see Table 10.2).

10.6   TRYPANOSOMIASIS
Introduction
There are three main types of diseases caused by different species of trypanosoma, discussed below.

Chaga's disease
is caused by *T. cruzi* and occurs in Central America, Mexico and many countries of South America. It is transmitted to man in the faeces of blood-sucking bugs which scratch the parasite into the skin,

Fig. 10.8. Sodium stibogluconate.

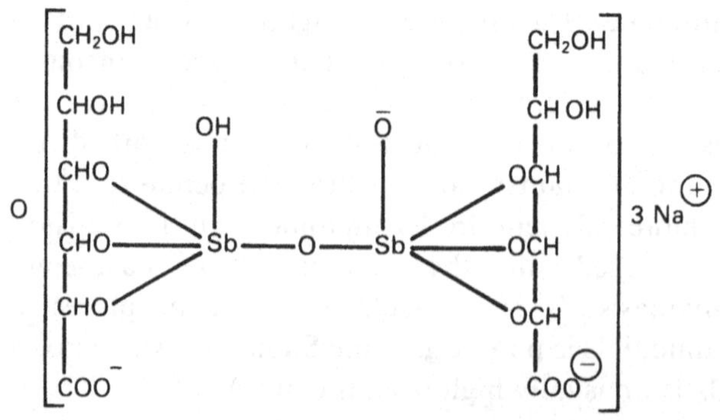

or through transfusion of infected blood. After an incubation period of 7–14 days, an erythematous swelling occurs at the site of the infection. At the same time there is generalised acute illness including headache, fever and myocarditis, oedema, hepatosplenomegaly. The disease can be fatal especially in infants.

African trypanosomiasis (sleeping sickness)

This disease is transmitted by various tse-tse flies (*Glossina*) which are found in the savanna of West, Central and East Africa. The first stage of the illness (haemolymphatic stage) is peripheral and includes parasite invasion of the lymphatic system; fever, dyspnoea, tachycardia, enlargement of the spleen and liver may occur. The second stage is the chronic sleeping sickness stage in which the parasite invades the central nervous system (CNS). There is headache, mental dullness, apathy, and loss of weight. The patient sleeps continually, and coma and death may result. Sleeping sickness is caused by two different types of trypanosoma.

(1) *T. brucei gambiense* is common in West Africa and produces, after an incubation period which can be as long as several years, a slowly-developing disease.

(2) *T. brucei rhodesiense* produces a more abrupt onset and rapidly progressive type of illness after an incubation period of about 3 weeks. This form of the disease is more common in East and Central Africa. Trypanosomiasis is a major disease of cattle and is responsible for the fact that large areas of the African savanna cannot be used for cattle breeding.

Drugs used in the treatment of trypanosomiasis

The drugs used in the treatment of trypanosomiasis are: suramin, melarsoprol, pentamidine, and benznidazole.

Pentamidine

Pentamidine (Fig. 10.9) is a diamidine derivative. Other related drugs with trypanocidal activity are propamidine, stilbamidine and hydroxystilbamidine. Pentamidine is used for the treatment of the haemolymphatic stage of African trypanosomiasis before the parasites have invaded the central nervous system. The drug is also used in pro-phylactic treatment. The mechanism of action of pentamidine is obscure. The trypanocidal action of the drug is probably due to bind-ing of the drug to the DNA of trypanosoma kinetoplast. In trypanosoma, the kinetoplast is a specialised structure that contains its own DNA and is part of the mitochondrial system. The diamidines bind to kinetoplast DNA and appear to interfere with DNA replication.

Suramin

Suramin is a trypanocidal drug with a complex structure. It is used to treat the early stages of sleeping sickness. The mechanism of action is not known. The compound is known to bind to and inhibit a wide variety of enzymes. The basis of its selective toxicity to trypanosoma is that mammalian cells are relatively impermeable to suramin. Even so, suramin when used clinically, causes serious toxic effects including central nervous system effects, peripheral neuropathy, and nephrotoxicity.

Melarsoprol

Melarsoprol (Fig. 10.10) is an organic *trivalent* arsenical whose use is limited to the treatment of the CNS stages of sleeping sickness only, because of severe toxicity. Trypansamide, another arsenical even more toxic than melarsoprol, is a pentavalent arsenical which is converted to the trivalent form *in vivo*. The organic arsenicals probably interact non-specifically with sulphydryl (-SH) groups in proteins thereby inhibiting a wide range of enzymes.

Differences in the permeability of mammalian and trypanosomal cells to the drug is the basis of selective toxicity to trypanosoma. Even so, melarsoprol produces many side effects including hypertension, albuminuria, peripheral neuropathy, muscle pain and oedema.

The critical use of melarsoprol is in the treatment of African trypanosomiasis involving the CNS. The drug can penetrate the blood–brain barrier.

Fig. 10.9. Pentamidine.

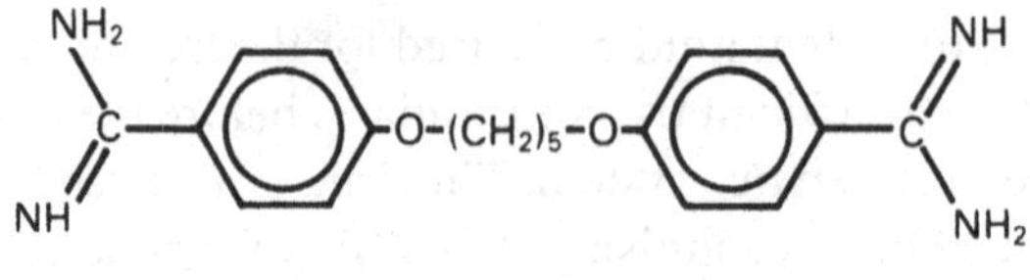

Pentamidine

Nifurtimox

In contrast to the trypanosomes which cause the African sleeping sickness which are extracellular, *T. cruzi*, the organism of Chaga's disease, is both intracellular (amastigote) and extracellular (mastigote).

Nifurtimox, a nitrofuran derivative (Fig. 10.11), is active against both forms of the parasite of Chaga's disease. The mechanism of action is unknown. The drugs active against African trypanosomiasis do not affect the amastigote form of *T. cruzi* and are therefore useless in the treatment of Chaga's disease. Nifurtimox, like most drugs used in the treatment of trypanosomiasis, is toxic and would not be in use if better drugs were available. More than 10% of adults receiving the drug are said to suffer anorexia, nausea, vomiting, stomach pain, nervous excitation, vertigo, headache, myalgia, insomnia, and skin rashes!!

Fig. 10.10. Melarsoprol.

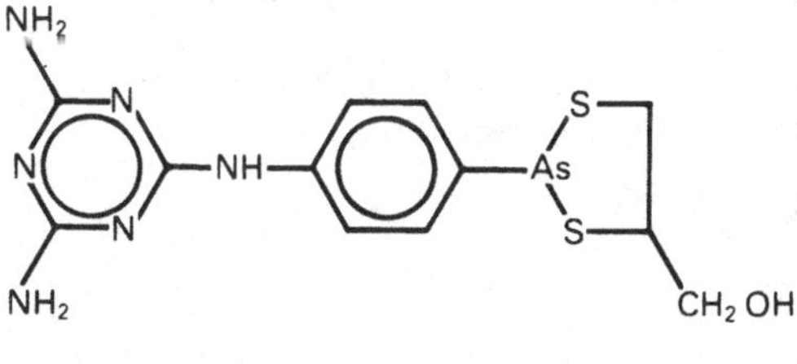

Melarsoprol

Fig. 10.11. Nifurtimox.

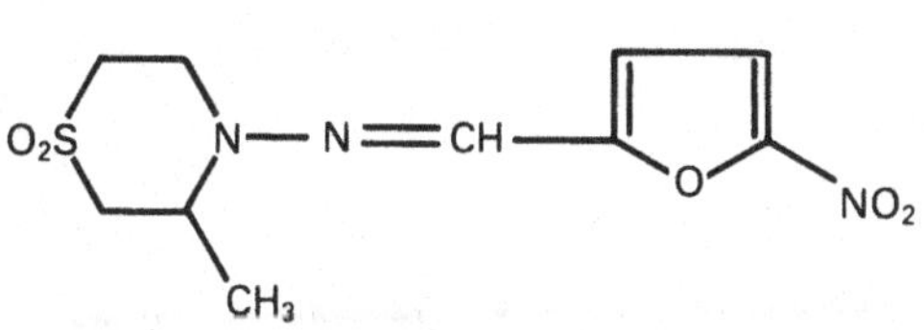

Nifurtimox

FURTHER READING

Alving, C.R., Schneider, I., Swartz, G. M. & Steck, E. A. (1979). Sporozoite-induced malaria: Therapeutic effects of glycolipids in liposomes. *Science* **205**, 1142–4.

Bray, R. S. & Garnham, P.C.C. (1982): The life cycle of primate malaria parasites. *Br. Med. Bull.* **38**, 117–22.

Bruce-Chwatt (1981), L. J., ed. *Chemotherapy of Malaria*, 2nd edn. WHO, Geneva 1981.

Fitch (1983). Mode of action of antimalaria drugs. In *Malaria and the Red Cell*, Ciba Foundation Symposium, pp. 222–32. 94, Pitman, London.

Howells, R. E. (1982). Advances in chemotherapy. *Br. Med. Bull.* 38, 193–9.

James, D. M. & Gilles, H. M. (1985). *Human Antiparasitic Drugs*. John Wiley & Sons, New York.

Luzzatto, L. (1979). Genetics of red cells and susceptibility to malaria. *Blood* 54, 961–79.

Newton, B. A. (1983). New strategies in the search for antiprotozoal drugs. In *Chemotherapeutic Strategies*, ed. D. I. Edwards & H. R. Hiscock, p. 87. Macmillan Press, London and Basingstoke.

Okoye, V.C.N. & Bennett, V. (1985). *P. falciparum* malaria: band 3 as a possible receptor during invasion of human erythrocytes. *Science* 227, 169–71.

Pasvol, G. & Jungrey, M. (1983). Glycophorins and red cell invasion by *Plasmodium falciparum*, in *Malaria and the Red Cell*, Ciba Foundation Symposium 94, p. 174. Pitman, London.

Peters, W. (1980). Chemotherapy of malaria. In *Malaria, Vol. I. Epidemiology, Chemotherapy, Morphology and Metabolism*, ed. J. P. Kresier, pp. 145–283. Academic Press, New York.

Trager, W. & Jensen, J. B. (1976). Human malaria parasites in continuous culture. *Science* 193, 673–5.

Ukoli, F.M.A. (1982). *Introduction to Parasitology in Tropical Africa*. John Wiley and Sons Limited, Cluchester, New York.

11

Anthelmintics

11.1 INTRODUCTION

Serious worm infections are common in Africa, the Middle and Far East, Central and South America and other tropical regions of the world, but less common in the industrialised countries of the West. The diseases caused by helminth infections are often called tropical diseases. They are in fact diseases of underdevelopment since the common feature of the societies in which helminth infections are highly prevalent is low socioeconomic status.

Pathogenic helminths belong to three major classes, namely, Cestodes, Nematodes and Trematodes (Table 11.1). Helminth infections constitute a hazard to human health and a great economic cost in terms of human morbidity and loss of domestic animals. Here are some examples of the effects of helminth infections in man:

(a) *Mechanical obstruction* Large ascaris burden can cause mechanical or spastic obstruction of the intestine and produce serious or fatal illness. A single worm migrating into the pancreatic or biliary ducts, or the appendix, can be responsible for acute obstructive pancreatitis, liver abscess or appendicitis.

(b) *Hypersensitivity* The antigens shed by ascaris larvae as they migrate through the lungs can induce antibody formation and cause severe immediate hypersensitivity or asthma.

(c) *Anaemias* Hookworm infection leads to morbidity by blood loss, iron deficiency anaemia and hypoproteinaemia which can be serious in individuals already malnourished.

(d) *Malnutrition* Helminth infection can have adverse effects on the nutritional status especially of individuals who are already suffering from starvation. The mechanisms by which helminth infection can adversely affect nutritional status are complex

Table 11.1   *Some major pathogenic helminths*

Class	Species	Common name
NEMATODES (roundworms)	*Wuchereria bancrofti* (lymphoreticular)	
	Loa loa	microfilaria
	Onchocerca vulvulus (river blindness)	
	Dracunculus medinensis	guineaworm
	Ancylostoma duodenale	hookworm
	Necator americanus	
	Trichinella spiralis	muscleworm
	Ascaris lumbricoides	roundworm
	Enterobius vermicularis	threadworm
	Stronglyloides stercolaris	
	Trichuris trichiura	whipworm
TREMATODES (flukes)	*Schistosoma haematobium*	
	S. mansoni	bilharzia
	S. japonicum	
	S. intercalatum	
CESTODES (tapeworms)	*Taenia saginata*	beef tapeworm
	Taenia solium	pig tapeworm
	Hymenolepis nana	

but may include: loss of appetite; decreased absorption of essential nutrients such as iron and vitamins; host–parasite competition for food materials; and diarrhoea.

(e) *Upper gastrointestinal haemorrhage* due to portal hypertension caused by *S. mansoni* is a major cause of mortality among adult males in Egypt.

(f) *Carcinoma of the bladder* associated with chronic *Schistosoma haematobium* infection is a common malignancy in Egyptian men.

11.2   LIFE CYCLE OF HELMINTH PARASITES

Helminths have complicated life cycles in which man is either primary or secondary host. The primary (or definitive) host harbours the adult sexually mature worms. The intermediate host harbours other stages in the life cycle. In many cases, man becomes infected by ingesting the parasite in the form of cysterci (encysted larvae) in inadequately cooked flesh (beef, pork or fish) or by ingesting ova deposited by the primary host. For example, in bilharzia, the schistosome embryo develops in a water snail (gastropod) vector. Man is infected by the free-living larvae after penetrating the skin. The microfilariae worms are transmitted by biting flies, etc. For more detailed information on the biology of pathogenic parasites, the reader should consult recent books on the subject. In the rest of this chapter, the two processes most amenable to attack by anthelmintic drugs, namely muscle function and energy production, are described briefly. Then follows a description of the mechanism of action of the important anthelmintic drugs.

The aim in anthelmintic chemotherapy, as in bacterial and protozoal chemotherapy, is to introduce into the infected person or domestic animal drugs which are toxic to the helminth parasite but not to the host. The drugs should selectively interfere with physiological or biochemical processes essential for the functional integrity of the worm. Selective toxicity can also be achieved in the case of helminths residing in the lumen, by using orally active, non-absorbable drugs which affect parasite function by direct contact in the gut.

One difference between helminth and other microbial infections having a bearing on chemotherapy is that most helminth parasites do not multiply in the host as do protozoa or bacteria. Consequently, the severity of helminth infection depends on the number of eggs or larvae entering the host. Therefore, inhibition of *growth*, a good strategy in the chemotherapy of bacterial infections, is not a useful approach in helminth chemotherapy. Rather, the aim here is to weaken the worm and expel it or to kill it.

11.3 PHYSIOLOGICAL BASIS OF ANTHELMINTIC DRUG ACTION

Two processes in helminths most amenable to chemotherapeutic attack are neuromuscular transmission and the reactions that generate metabolic energy (glycolysis).

Innervation and muscle function in helminths

Muscle function in the worm can be a critical target for chemotherapeutic action. If the worm muscle is paralysed, it is unable to maintain its position in the gut against the direction of normal propulsive movement. It is then expelled along with other gut contents by peristalsis. Piperazine acts in this way by causing flaccid paralysis of ascaris muscle. Detailed studies of the mechanism of action of piperazine have shown that the neurophysiology of ascaris muscle is essentially different from that of mammalian muscle; this is discussed below.

Acetylcholine receptors

Acetylcholine contracts ascaris muscle. This effect is competitively antagonised by piperazine. d-Turbocurarine is a weak antagonist of acetylcholine in ascaris muscle, while piperazine has relatively weak neuromuscular blocking action in mammalian skeletal muscle. This accounts for the selective toxicity of piperazine. These facts show that the acetylcholine receptors in ascaris muscle have different pharmacological properties from the receptors in mammalian skeletal muscle. Ascaris muscle cholinergic receptors are thus neither classical nicotenic nor muscarinic.

Muscle innervation

Much of the work on nerve muscle transmission in nematodes has been done on *A. lumbricoides*. The muscles in the body wall are innervated by four sets of nerves running longitudinally in the hypodermis: the dorsal and ventral and two lateral nerves. These nerves originate from the circumpharyngeal commissure (nerve ring) which encircles the pharynx anteriorly, and runs to join a cluster of ganglia near the tail (anal ganglia) (Fig. 11.1). This system of nerves constitutes the *somatic nervous system*, and is responsible for the co-ordination of motor activity in nematodes.

The nerve-muscle junction in ascaris is also different from that in mammalian muscle. It appears that not all ascaris muscle cells are innervated. Rather, the nerve cord is associated with a 'syncytium' in which the individual cells are linked in such a way that impulses generated in one cell can be conducted to adjacent cells. Intracellular recordings show that spontaneous spike potentials occur in the region of the syncytium. Acetylcholine (ACH) released from the nerve cord or applied exogenously depolarises the membrane in the region of the syncytium and increases the rate of firing of spikes. Depolarisation then spreads to other cells which respond by contracting. ACH is not a neurotransmitter in the classical sense, but a modulatory neuro-hormone whose function is to increase the rate of 'impulse' formation in the region of the syncytium and so facilitate muscle contraction. The drug piperazine causes hyperpolarisation and cessation of spike activity in syncytial cells, probably by blocking ACH receptors.

Neurotransmitters

The nerve cord of ascaris contains inhibitory fibres where γ-aminobutyric acid (GABA) is the putative inhibitory neurotransmitter. Part of the evidence for this is that GABA is extremely potent in causing hyperpolarisation and cessation of spike activity in ascaris muscle. In this respect, it is 100 times more potent than piperazine. It is suggested that ascaris muscle has dual innervation, namely excitatory cholinergic and inhibitory (GABAergic) nerves. Not much is known of the innervation and neurotransmitters in other worms. There is evidence that 5-hydroxytryptamine (5-HT) is an excitatory neurotransmitter in Schistosomes. Some anthelmintics, e.g. hycanthone, are thought to act by interfering with the function of 5-HT in Schistosomes. Cholinesterase

Fig. 11.1. The generalised nematode nervous system: (a) whole individual; (b) section through intestinal area. phar, pharynx; cpc, circumpharhyngeal commissure; sm, somatic muscle; int, intestine; vn, ventral nerve; dn, dorsal nerve; ln, lateral nerve; rect, rectum; lg, lumbar ganglion. (Redrawn from Croll & Matthews (1977), p. 39.)

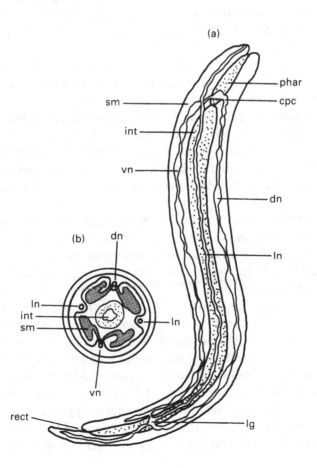

activity seems crucial to the survival of certain worms. Consequently, inhibition of this enzyme is a drug target in the treatment of some helminth infections. For example, the drug metrifonate owes its usefulness in the treatment of *S. haematobium* infections to inhibition of cholinesterase. The severe limitation to its use is that the drug does not differentiate sufficiently between human and helminth cholinesterases.

11.4   METABOLIC ENERGY PRODUCTION IN HELMINTH PARASITES

A sensitive target for anthelmintic chemotherapy is interference with metabolic energy production. In living cells, metabolic energy is derived from the breakdown (catabolism) of macromolecules. In vertebrates, the process takes place in a number of stages. Macromolecules are broken down by digestive enzymes to give monomers, e.g. proteins are broken down to amino acids, carbohydrates to monosaccharides and lipids to fatty acids. The monomers are then broken down further to yield energy as ATP or are used in other essential functions.

Catabolism in parasitic helminths differs from that in mammals in three ways. Firstly, the range of substrates that helminths can use is limited; in most worms, glycogen is the only energy source. Secondly, in helminth parasites, acetyl-CoA is not as important a metabolite as it is in mammals; rather, phosphoenolpyruvate is the key metabolite. Thirdly, instead of degrading metabolites to carbon dioxide and water, many helminths form volatile organic acids such as propionic acid, methylvaleric acid, methylbutyric acid, succinic acid, etc., as end products of metabolism.

Carbohydrate catabolism in helminths has been studied extensively, especially in *Ascaris lumbricoides*. The following features of the process relevant to the mechanism of action of some drugs currently in use are briefly described. A detailed biochemistry of parasitic helminths can be found in Barrett (1981).

The catabolism of carbohydrate in helminths is predominantly anaerobic. Many worms will take up oxygen, but they can survive and produce viable eggs in the absence of oxygen. Carbohydrate is broken down in the helminth cell cytoplasm via the Embden–Meyerhof pathway. The process is similar to that in vertebrates up to the step where phosphoenolpyruvate is formed (Fig. 11.2). In *Ascaris lumbricoides* and in some other intestinal helminths, the enzyme pyruvate kinase is absent or present only in low concentrations. Therefore phosphoenolpyruvate is not converted to pyruvic acid as in vertebrates.

Instead, phosphoenolpyruvate fixes carbon dioxide under the influence of the enzyme phosphoenolpyruvate carboxykinase. The metabolic energy produced by carbohydrate catabolism is stored as ATP. The scheme described in Fig. 11.2 yields 4 moles of nucleoside triphosphate for every hexose unit catabolised. Some of the high-energy triphosphate is initially in the form of inosine triphosphate

Fig. 11.2. Carbohydrate catabolism in *Ascaris* muscle. The numbers symbolise enzymes as follows: (1), phosphoenolpyruvate carboxykinase; (2), malate dehydrogenase; (3), malic enzyme; (4), fumarase; (5), fumarate reductase (succinate dehydrogenase). (Redrawn from Barrett (1981), p. 76.)

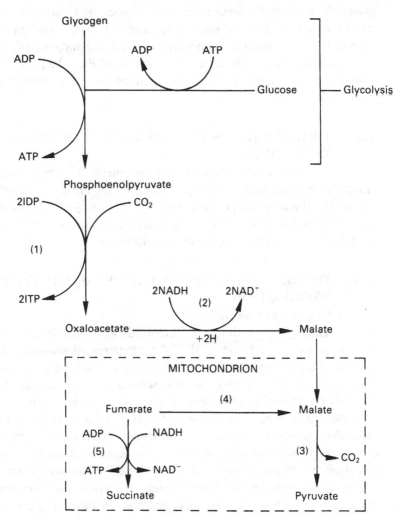

(ITP). However, there is rapid transformation of ITP to ATP by the enzyme nucleoside diphosphate kinase.

$$ITP + ADP \rightarrow IDP + ATP$$

In some helminth parasites where the concentration of pyruvate kinase is high, phosphoenolpyruvate is metabolised in the Embden–Meyerhof pathway via lactic acid to acetyl-CoA, carbon dioxide and water. Such helminths are known as homolactic fermenters, meaning that the final end product of carbohydrate metabolism is lectic acid as is the case in vertebrates. A well known parasite example is the schistosome. Helminth parasites are thus roughly of two types: carbon dioxide fixers such as ascaris which produce volatile acids and the glycolytic homolactic fermenters, e.g. schistosomes. Most intestinal helminths are carbon dioxide fixers, whereas most blood or tissue helminths are homolactic fermenters. In the fermentation pathway of glucose degradation, only about 10% as much ATP can be generated in comparison to a human cell which operates the more efficient citric acid (Krebs) cycle.

11.5   DRUGS USED IN THE TREATMENT OF HELMINTH INFECTIONS

The major drugs used in the treatment of worm infections either cause physiological damage to the parasite muscle or inactivate worms by blocking metabolic energy production. Some drugs affect both systems. Many are effective against a large variety of worms and are referred to as broad-spectrum anthelmintics.

11.6   DRUGS INTERFERING WITH METABOLIC ENERGY PRODUCTION

Organic antimonials

The trivalent antimonial compounds such as antimony potassium tartrate (Fig. 11.3) are used in the treatment of schistosomiasis, whereas the pentavalent antimonials (see page 246) are used against leishmaniasis. The survival of the schistosome in venous blood depends on anaerobic utilisation of glucose; the rate of glycolysis is extremely high. It has been estimated that an adult *S. mansoni* worm catabolises in one hour an amount of glucose equivalent to 20% of its dry weight. As schistosomes are homolactic fermenters, the high rate of glycolysis would compensate for this relatively inefficient pathway of energy generation. Trivalent antimonials in therapeutic doses reduce the rate of glycolysis in intact schistosomes by inhibiting phosphofructokinase (PFK). PFK is a critically important glycolytic enzyme being responsible for the conversion of fructose-6-phosphate to fructose-1,6-diphosphate. Since the schistosomes are critically dependent on glycolysis, the worms are quickly affected and are swept into the liver. It has been shown *in vitro* that the substrate of PFK, fructose-6-phosphate, accumulates under the influence of antimony while the product of PFK activity, fructose-1,6-diphosphate decreases to such low levels that the activity of the subsequent enzyme of glycolysis (aldolase) is shut down as a result of substrate starvation.

It would seem that the inhibition of PFK is caused by a chelation of sulphydryl (-SH) groups at the enzyme site by the heavy metal. However, the binding of antimony to PFK appears to be spontaneously reversible. Worms given sublethal doses of antimony shift to the liver. Shortly after, these lightly 'antimonised' worms return to the original mesenteric site as PFK activity is restored. Some observations suggest that antimony may act by other unknown mechanisms in addition to PFK inhibition. For example it has been found that the drop in schistosome ATP after exposure of the worms to a high dose of antimony was only about 30%; and the PFK of young worms which are generally resistant to antimony shows a greater sensitivity than adult worms to PFK.

Mammalian PFK is only about 100 times less sensitive to organic antimonials than schistosome PFK. This ratio is far from optimal and indicates that a percentage of patients might be expected to react unfavourably to antimony. Clinically, numerous episodes of nausea, vomiting, cardiac irritability or even sudden heart failure following antimony therapy have been reported. Antimony is also unpleasant to administer. Unless it is administered by the i.v. route, it causes local

Fig. 11.3. Antimony potassium tartrate (Tartar emetic).

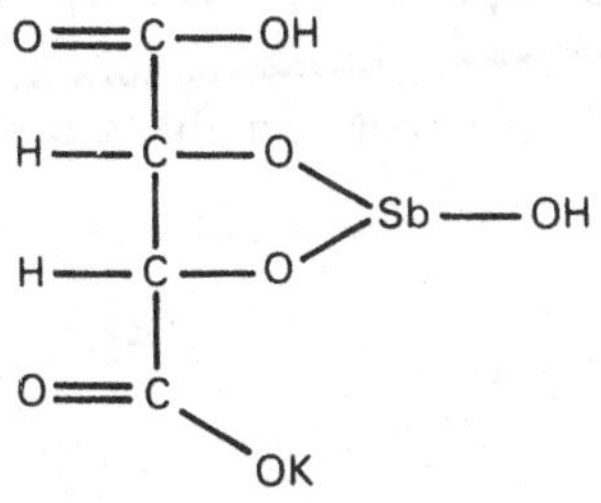

irritant effects. It can be used to treat all forms of schistosomiasis but its application is now limited to S. japonicum.

Niridazole

Niridazole (Fig. 11.4) is effective against diseases caused by S. mansoni and S. haematobium.

The drug does not affect glycolysis directly but increases the rate of breakdown of glycogen. In S. mansoni and S. haematobium glycogen phosphorylase exists in two forms, active and inactive. There is evidence for the interconversion of these two forms. Niridazole inhibits the enzyme glycogen phosphorylase phosphatase which normally converts active to inactive glycogen phosphorylase. In niridazole-treated worms, the glycogen phosphorylase remains permanently active so that the schistosome exhausts its glycogen reserves. Mammalian phosphatase is much less sensitive. Therefore the drug is selectively toxic. It is not clear why schistosomes need to store glycogen, since they live in an intravascular environment (mesenteric vasculature) of virtually constant glucose concentration (about 100 mg%), but they have glycogen stores. Bueding has estimated that the glycogen content of these worms to be 14–29% of dry weight. The store is probably required because of the relatively inefficient glycolytic pathway used by the worm.

Niridazole is taken up as the unmetabolised compound and concentrated about 60-fold in the schistosome. It has been suggested that within the worm, niridazole may be metabolised, although the metabolites have not been identified. It is suggested that the nitro group in the niridazole molecule is reduced in the worm and that this metabolic conversion may overload the nitroreductase system within the worm. In effect, the reduced metabolite may be the toxic agent or niridazole may deprive the worm of the ability to detoxify its own metabolic products. Other studies suggest that niridazole may decrease glucose uptake, possibly by interfering with G6P production as a result of the inhibition of hexokinase.

Thus the mechanism of action of niridazole on the schistosome

Fig. 11.4. Niridazole.

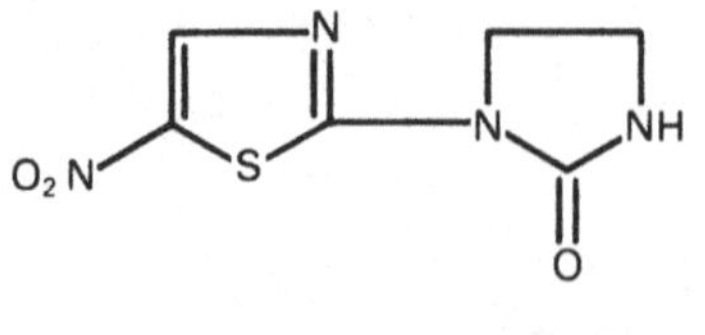

glucose metabolism is not fully understood. It may be inhibition of glucose uptake, glycogen storage and possibly oxidative phosphorylation, but the mechanism is far from being settled. Fundamental research in isolated enzyme systems of the worm might yield many dividends.

The drug also affects the reproductive organs of male and female schistosomes. It appears to cause morphological changes in the sex organs of the worm, e.g. there is a significant shortening of the female worm after niridazole treatment, the ovary and the vitellogenic glands in the female shrink, and in the male, spermatogenesis ceases.

Niridazole has a number of undesirable side effects, the most important of which is the tendency of the drug to induce central nervous system disturbances.

Niclosamide

Niclosamide is a halogenated salicylanilide (Fig. 11.5). The phenolic, amidic and nitro groups are critically important for the anticestode activity of this compound.

Niclosamide is particularly effective in the treatment of tapeworm infections in humans. The drug inhibits anaerobic production of ATP by uncoupling oxidative phosphorylation (preventing the anaerobic incorporation of inorganic phosphate into ADP). The drug also inhibits glucose uptake (see also mebendazole and praziquantel). Tapeworms rely on anaerobic catabolism of carbohydrate for metabolic energy. Niclosamide is not absorbed from the gut; the drug is therefore selectively toxic to the intestinal worms by direct luminal contact. Muscle paralysis by niclosamide has been demonstrated not only in cestodes but also in nematode and trematode worms. It is not known whether this action is linked to the drug's inhibition of phosphorylation nor is the mechanism of paralysis understood.

Fig. 11.5. Niclosamide.

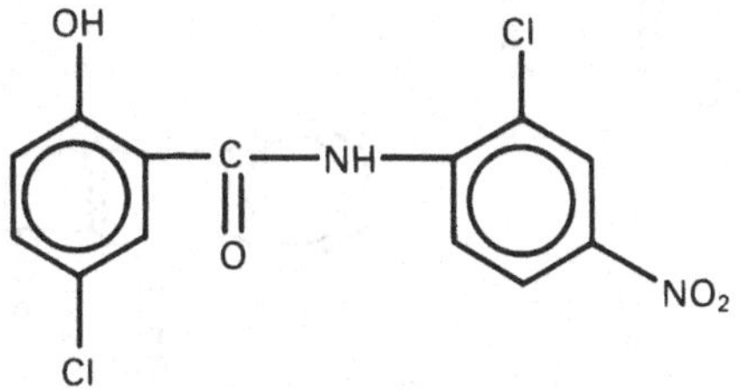

Levamisole

Levamisole (see Fig. 11.6) is the S(−)isomer of tetramisole. The R(+)isomer is inactive. The drug inhibits fumarate reductase of nematode (ascaris) but not of cestode worms. The drug also causes rapid sustained contraction of nematode muscle resulting in spastic paralysis. The effect is apparently due to ganglionic stimulation since it is blocked by conventional ganglion-blocking drugs, e.g. pempidine.

Benzimidazoles

Several benzimidazole derivatives (see Fig. 11.7) are used to treat a number of worm infections. Important drugs in the group are mebendazole, thiabendazole, cambendazole, and flubendazole. The different drugs in the group seem to affect different worms in different ways probably as a result of different pharmacokinetic characteristics. They are effective against *Trichuris trichiura, A. lumbricoides* and *Ancyclostoma duodenale* and are thus described as broad-spectrum.

Mebendazole inhibits glucose uptake in some nematodes, cestodes and trematodes; 80 nM mebendazole inhibits glucose uptake in ascaris by 40%. This is followed by depletion of glycogen stores and eventually by decreased ability of the worms to generate ATP.

Fig. 11.6. Levamisole.

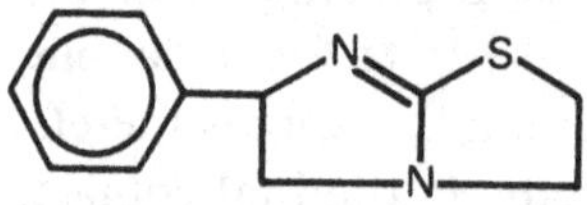

Fig. 11.7. Benzimidazole anthelmintics.

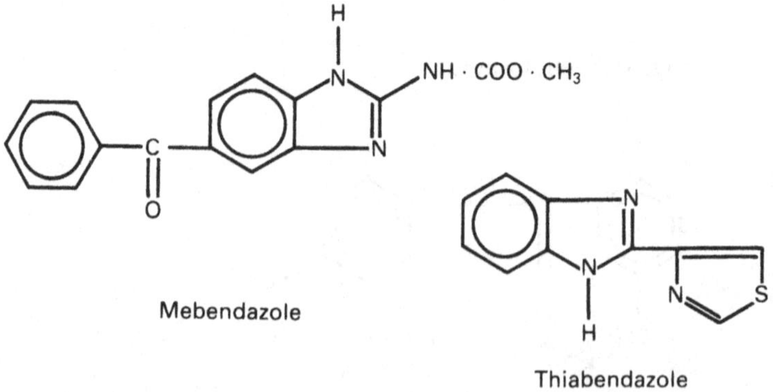

Mebendazole

Thiabendazole

Mebendazole is not absorbed from the gut. The drug is therefore toxic to luminal parasites and almost entirely free of toxicity to humans and domestic animals.

Thiabendazole inhibits fumarate reductase of nematodes. The drug is particularly effective against the nematodes *Strongyloides stercolaris* and guineaworm, *D. medinensis*. Fumarate reductase catalyses the reduction of fumarate to succinate during which ATP and NAD are produced. Fumarate is then a terminal electron acceptor. This critically important reaction is an essential component of the mechanism of energy production in worms but not in the host. Therefore drugs which inhibit it are selectively toxic. Its inhibition by thiabendazole accounts for its broad spectrum of anthelmintic activity. Thiabendazole is relatively toxic to humans. It is widely used in veterinary practice to treat dogs, pigs, horses, cats, and birds. Cambendazole also inhibits the fumarate reductase reaction. Benzimidazoles may also reduce ATP content of worms by uncoupling oxidative phosphorylation and by preventing microtubule formation (see page 287).

11.6.6. Pyrvinium
Pyrvinium (Fig. 11.8) is a cyanine dye. These dyes are potent inhibitors of oxygen consumption. In addition, cyanine dyes block transport of glucose into nematode worms. Since pyrvinium is effective against intestinal nematodes, especially thread worms whose metabolism is anaerobic, the relevant mechanism is possibly inhibition of glucose uptake. Pyrvinium has low solubility and is poorly absorbed from the gut.

11.7 DRUGS INTERFERING WITH MUSCLE FUNCTION
Piperazine
The anthelmintic action of piperazine (Fig. 11.9) has been well studied in *Ascaris* muscle. The mechanism by which piperazine para-

Fig. 11.8. Pyrvinium.

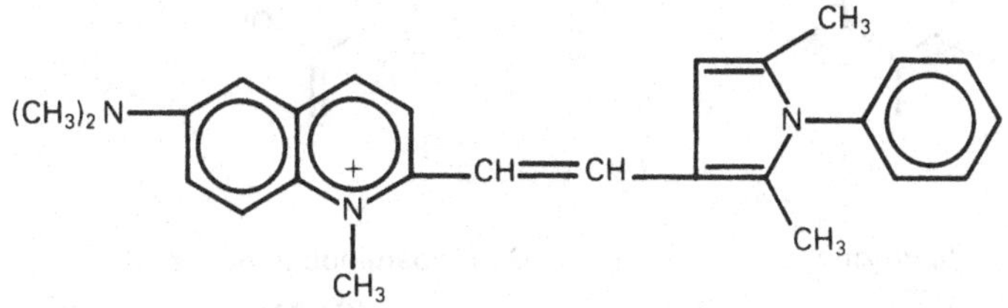

lyses worm muscle is probably complex. It is known that piperazine blocks ACH competitively in ascaris muscle. It is also possible that piperazine mimics the inhibitory neurotransmitter of nematodes which is suspected to be GABA by binding to GABAergic receptors in the region of the synctium (page 254). A GABAergic mechanism would explain why piperazine is relatively weak at paralysing mammalian muscle. Piperazine, by paralysing the worm which is thus unable to maintain its position in the gut, causes the worm to be expelled passively by the normal peristaltic action of the gut.

The perienteric fluid of *A. lumbricoides* contains several volatile acids such as acetic acid, propionic acid, methylbutyric and succinic acid, etc. These are the end products of carbohydrate catabolism involving carbon dioxide fixation. Piperazine drastically reduces the amount of volatile acid excreted by ascaris muscle; this effect can be attributed to inhibition of anaerobic glycolysis. However, it is possible that the reduction in volatile acid formation is not the cause, but the effect of muscle paralysis.

Pyrantel

Pyrantel and the related drug morantel (Fig. 11.10) cause depolarisation and contracture of worm muscle. The drug causes spastic paralysis. The action of pyrantel on nematode muscle (probably acting on the syncytium) is similar to the action of suxamethonium on mammalian skeletal muscle motor end plate. Experimentally, pyrantel behaves like suxamethonium in mammalian skeletal muscle systems. Fortunately, pyrantel pamoate is sparingly soluble and poorly absorbed from the gut. Another reason why the drug paralyses intestinal worms but not mammalian muscle is that worm muscle is about

Fig. 11.9. Piperazine (left) and GABA (right).

Piperazine

Gammaaminobutyric acid
(GABA)

100 times more sensitive to pyrantel than is mammalian muscle. Pyrantel and morantel are effective in ascariasis and other nematode infections (see Table 11.2).

Bephenium

Bephenium is active against *N. americanus, A. duodenale* and *A. lumbricoides* and a number of nematodes infecting livestock. Bephenium has a chemical structure somewhat similar to that of acetylcholine (see Fig. 11.11). The drug is 5 times more potent than acetylcholine in contracting ascaris muscle. The mechanism of worm-muscle paralysis appears to be different from that induced by pyrantel which causes spastic paralysis. Bephenium-induced contraction of worm muscle is followed by relaxation and the worm is paralysed in a flaccid state. The drug is not absorbed from the gastrointestinal tract, which accounts for its relative lack of systemic toxicity. Hookworms, for which infection the drug is now more frequently used in humans, lose their attachment in the gut and are expelled.

Fig. 11.10. Pyrantel (left) and morantel (right).

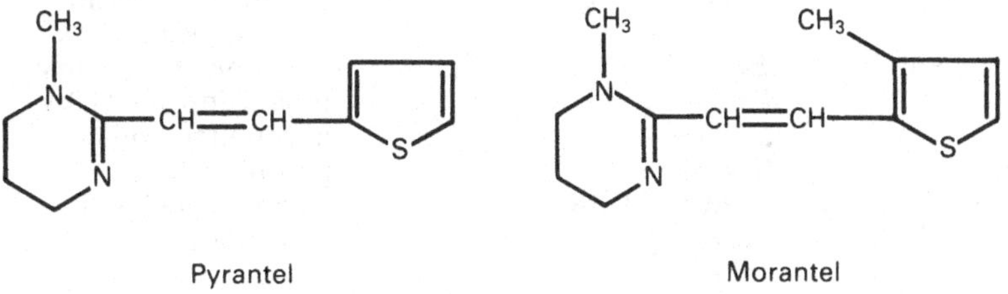

Pyrantel   Morantel

Fig. 11.11. Bephenium hydroxynaphthoate.

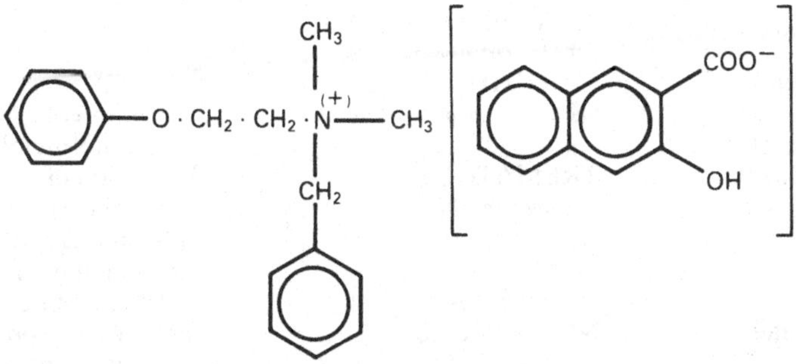

Table 11.2   *Anthelmintic drugs and the worm infections which they are used to treat*

Anthelmintic	Infecting organism	Site of action
Mebendazole	NEMATODES *A. lumbricoides* (Ascariasis) *E. vermicularis* (threadworm) *T. trichiura* (whipworm) *N. americanus* *A. duodenale* (hookworm) CESTODES *Taenia saginata* *T. solium* }tapeworm *H. nana*	Irreversible inhibition of glucose uptake
Thiabendazole	NEMATODES *A. lumbricoides* *T. trichuria* *S. stercoralis* *D. medinensis*	Inhibition of fumarate reductase
Levamisole	NEMATODES *A. lumbricoides* *N. americanus* *A. duodenale*	(a) Inhibition of fumarate reductase (b) Stimulation of ganglia to produce spastic muscle paralysis
Niclosamide	CESTODES *T. saginata* *T. solium* *H. nana*	Inhibition of anaerobic production of ATP by uncoupling oxidative phosphorylation
Diethylcarbamazine	NEMATODES *W. bancrofti* *Loa loa* *O. vulvulus*	Inhibition of filarial cholinesterase
Oxaminiquine	TREMATODE *S. mansoni* *S. haematobium* (in combination with metrifonate)	Unknown
Antimony, potassium tartarate	TREMATODE *S. japonicum*	Inhibition of phosphofructokinase
Niridazole	TREMATODES *S. heamatobium* *S. mansoni* NEMATODE *D. medinensis*	Inhibition of phosphorylase phosphatase leading to depletion of glycogen stores
Pyrantel	NEMATODES *A. lumbricoides* *S. stercoralis* *N. americanus* *A. duodenale*	(a) Muscle depolarisation and spastic paralysis (b) Inhibition of cholinesterase

Anthelmintic	Infecting organism	Site of action
Piperazine	NEMATODES *A. lumbricoides* *E. vermicularis*	Flaccid paralysis of worm muscle. Cholinergic blockade or GABAergic system activation
Bephenium	NEMATODES *N. americanus* *A. duodenale* *A. lumbricoides*	Muscle depolorisation and flaccid paralysis
Praziquantel	CESTODES *T. saginata* *T. solium* *H. nana* TREMATODES *S. mansoni* *S. haematobium* *S. japonicum*	Stimulates motility of cestodes and impairs the function of their suckers
Hycanthone	TREMATODES *S. mansoni* *S. haematobium*	(a) Interferes with neuronal storage of 5-HT (b) Inhibits cholin- esterase Both lead to muscle paralysis

Diethylcarbamazine (DEC)

Diethylcarbamazine (banocide) is derived from piperazine (Fig. 11.12). The drug is used in the treatment of filiariasis caused by *Wuchereria bancrofti, Loa loa*, and *Onchocerca*. The drug removes all the microfilaria (the prelarval forms of the worm) from the blood and also kills the adult forms of *Loa loa*. The adult forms of onchocerca are not killed. Therefore treatment of onchocerciasis with the drug results in only temporary removal of microfilariae from the body. The surviving adult worms soon produce microfilariae and the disease returns.

The mechanism of action of diethylcarbamazine (DEC) is not known nor is the basis for its selective toxicity. The drug is inactive *in*

Fig. 11.12. Diethylcarbamazine.

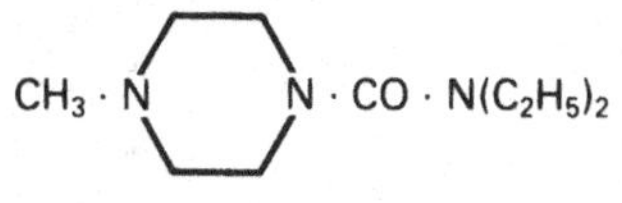

$CH_3 \cdot N$⬡$N \cdot CO \cdot N(C_2H_5)_2$

vitro suggesting that *in vivo* an active metabolite is formed. Alternatively DEC may aid the body's defences to remove the parasite. It is known that the drug causes the worms to migrate from tissue sites into the liver where they become trapped and phagocytosed. The worms are possibly dislodged from their sites by increased muscular contractions caused by the drug through its anticholinesterase activity. The drug may also cause surface antigens on the worm to be exposed to host's antibodies leading to the formation of antigen–antibody complexes and facilitating phagocytosis.

DEC is absorbed from the gastrointestinal tract and has a wide variety of untoward effects, including severe hypersensitivity reactions arising from the release of allergens from dead worms.

Praziquantel

Praziquantel (Fig. 11.13) is a prazinoquinoline derivative originally developed for the treatment of schistosomiasis. It is effective against a wide range of cestodes in which it stimulates motility and impairs functioning of their suckers.

In therapeutic doses (100 ng–1.0 µg/ml) the drug causes a powerful contraction of cestode muscle by increasing the permeability of muscle cell membranes to Ca^{2+}. The taenicidal effect of the drug *in vivo* arises from dislocation of the worm as a consequence of the violent muscle contraction. Praziquantel is also effective against all forms of schistosomiasis. It may also affect carbohydrate metabolism.

Hycanthone

Hycanthone is one of a series of thioxanthones which had their origin as miracil compounds in the late 1930s. The first useful miracil drug was lucanthone (miracil D). Hycanthone is the active

Fig. 11.13 Praziquantel.

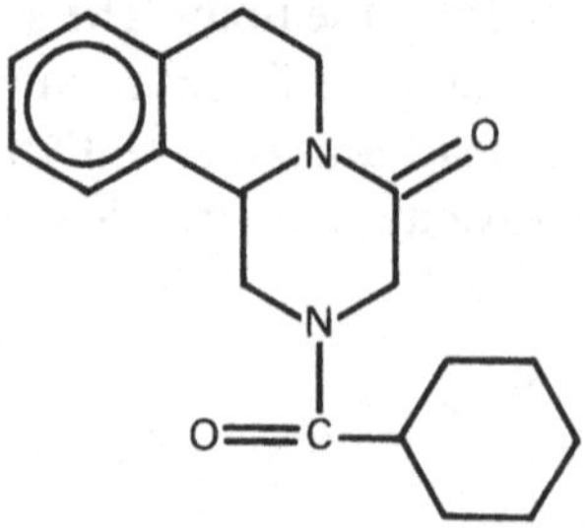

Praziquantel

hydroxylated metabolite of lucanthone. The drug is active against the adult forms of *S. haematobium* and *S. mansoni*, but ineffective against *S. japonicum*. The drug interferes with laying of eggs, induces separation of paired worms and induces a shift of worms from the mesenteric vasculature to the liver where they are subject to removal by enzyme action and phagocytosis.

After an intramuscular injection of the drug into mice infected with *S. mansoni*, the worms take up hycanthone from plasma against a concentration gradient. It is thought that hycanthone, and not a metabolite, is responsible for the antischistosomal action.

The mechanism of action is not fully understood. Bueding's studies suggest that 5-hydroxytryptamine (5-HT) and ACH are involved. In schistosomes, 5-HT and acetylcholine are putative neurotransmitters. The worms contain 5-HT (and can take it up), ACH, and acetyl-cholinesterase. There is evidence that hycanthone stimulates schistosome's uptake of 5-HT, but the 5-HT is taken up more into non-neuronal sites (low-affinity uptake) than into neuronal sites (high-affinity uptake) (compare with uptake₁ and uptake₂ in mammalian adrenergic systems). There is also evidence that hycanthone has anticholinergic activity in schistosomes. However this action is weak in mammalian smooth muscles suggesting that cholinergic receptors in schistosomes are pharmacologically diferent from those of higher animals. The interaction between this group of drugs and ACH and 5-HT has not been fully explored. Bueding's experiments on 5-HT were done more than 10 years ago. Since then a great deal more has become known about 5-HT receptors and their selective agonists and antagonists. The 5-HT and ACH involvement in the action of hycanthone may be usefully explored experimentally now.

Metrifonate

Metrifonate is an organophosphorus compound converted to a schistosomicidal metabolite *in vivo*. It is effective against *S. haematobium* infections. Metrifonate may be used in combination with oxaminiquine in mixed infections. The drug causes spastic paralysis of the worm through inhibition of cholinesterase.

Oxaminiquine

In therapeutic doses (50mg/kg) the drug causes a shift of worms from the mesentery to the liver. The worms became separated and egg production ceases. The worms die within 6 days of commence-ment of treatment. Oxaminiquine is effective against *A. mansoni* infections, weakly active against *S. haematobuim* but practically useless against *S. japonicum*. Not much is known of the mechanism of action of oxaminiquine. It is unusual among antischistosomal drugs in that it affects male worms more powerfully than females.

FURTHER READING

Barrett, J. (1981). *Biochemistry of Parasitic Helminths*. Macmillan Publishers Ltd., London & Basingstoke.
Chou, T. T., Bennett, J. L., Pert, C. & Bueding, E. (1973). Effect of hycanthone and two of its structural analogues on levels of and uptake of 5-hydroxytryptamine in *Schistosoma mansoni. J. Pharm. exp. Ther.* 186, 408–15.
Croll, N. A. & Matthews, B. E. (1977). *Biology of Nematodes*. John Wiley & Sons, New York, Toronto.
James, D. M. & Gilles, H. M. (1985). *Human Antiparasitic Drugs*. John Wiley & Sons, Chichester, New York.
Saz, H. J. & Bueding, E. (1966). Relationships between anthelmintic effects and biochemical and physiological mechanisms. *Pharmacol. Rev.*, 18, 871–94.
World Health Organisation (1954). *Report of the Expert Committee on Onchocerciasis*. Technical Report No. 87, WHO, Geneva.
World Health Organisation (1967). *Report of the Expert Committee on Filariasis*. Technical Report No. 359, WHO, Geneva.
World Health Organisation (1973). *Report of the Expert Committee on Schistosomiasis Control*. Technical Report No. 515, WHO, Geneva.

12

Anticancer and antiviral drugs

12.1   INTRODUCTION

Cancer (neoplastic disease) is malignant cell growth in which the restraints that normally regulate cell differentiation, cell proliferation and organ size are absent; the abnormal cell population which constitutes the cancer eventually invades and destroys surrounding tissues. This does not mean that the rate of growth of malignant tumour cells is necessarily faster than that of normal cells. The critical difference is that malignant tumour cells do not differentiate normally. The genes coding for normal differentiation are shut off, whereas the genes coding for proliferation are derepressed so that what are formed are abnormal cells.

There are several reasons why cancer is a most terrifying disease. The cause of most cancers is multifactorial and imprecisely understood. Treatment is unpredictable. Furthermore, surgical removal of the primary disease does not guarantee cure because by the time the primary tumour is large enough to be detected, the disease would usually have established itself at secondary sites (metastasis). Radiotherapy and anticancer drugs are highly toxic and in some cases are as likely to kill the patient as the disease. Advances are being made in the chemotherapy of cancer. These are due to increased understanding of the nature of tumour cell growth and improvements in the clinical integration of different treatment strategies – surgery, radiotherapy and drugs.

Cancer is a leading cause of death in Western industrialised societies where there is increasingly an awareness and avoidance of the sort of behaviour likely to cause cancer. This, coupled with the fact that there have been improvements in the technology for early detection and treatment, has resulted in decline in the incidence of certain cancers, e.g. stomach cancer (people are presumably eating less smoked foods contaminated with nitrosamines). This point is made to show that the incidence of cancers can be reduced when people are informed as to their most likely causes. What is disturbing, though, is that there continues to be increases in the last two decades in lung and colonic cancers (due to cigarette smoke and consumption of foods lacking in fibre) in industrialised societies where reliable statistics have been kept. This is in spite of vigorous anit-smoking campaigns that have resulted in a reduction in the average number of cigarette smokers in these societies.

12.2   CANCERS IN THE TROPICS
Until fairly recently, the impression that cancer was rare in the tropics was widespread. Cancer was previously unrecognised and unrecorded in the tropics; death from cancer in traditional societies was most likely attributed to malevolent forces. In recent times the major cancers seen in industralised western societies, e.g. cancers of breast, lungs, prostate, and the leukaemias, are also now seen in the tropics. As countries advance industrially and the quality of life of their citizens improves materially, cancer seems to take a leading role as a cause of death, ahead of poverty-related diseases. Lambo, a Deputy Director General of WHO illustrated this point by pointing to Singapore which by 1979 had 'moved rapidly from the status of a developing country in which cancer has moved just as rapidly to become the fore-most cause of death'. Not only that, certain cancers more frequently encountered in Africa have been identified. For example, the idiopathic pigment sarcoma of the skin (Kaposi's sarcoma) described by the Viennese physician Kaposi in 1872 is rare in Europe but has high incidence in Africa. Other tumours with high incidences in the tropics are: (a) liver cell carcinoma; (b) a group of tumours found among children in Africa called Burkitt's lymphoma (named after Dr Dennis Burkitt who first described the disease in Uganda); (c) Squamous cell carcinoma of the cervix and choriocarcinoma (see also Solanke, Osunkoya, Williams & Agboola, 1982). Burkitt's lymphoma is unique in many ways among all types of human cancers. It is the fastest growing human neoplasm with a tumour doubling time of days rather than months and a unique sensitivity to a number of chemotherapeutic agents e.g. cyclophosphamide, vincristine, methotrexate, and cytosine arabinoside. Thus it is curable in more than 50% of patients.

12.3 ENVIRONMENTAL FACTORS

Several environmental chemicals are thought to cause chromosome damage (mutagenesis) and to be responsible for human cancers. In the tropics, chemical constituents of some plants consumed as food or as medicine have been shown to be carcinogenic in experimental animals and are thought to contribute to the high incidence of hepatocellular carcinoma.

Aflatoxin

Livers of experimental animals dosed with aflatoxins show hepatic cell necrosis, proliferation of bile ducts and a high incidence of primary liver tumours. *A. flavus* is the major source of aflatoxins but other fungal strains, e.g. ochratoxin A is produced by *Aspergillus ochraceus* and aspertoxin from various other strains of *Aspergillus* and *Penicillium*.

Polycyclic aromatic hydrocarbons

Polycyclic hydrocarbons, e.g., benzanthracene, and benzopyrene, which are well known environmental contaminants (from motor vehicle exhausts, power plants and other industrial processes) appear to contaminate many tropical foods such as smoked-dried fish and meat and the popular suya (shish-kebabs) cooked over open fires.

Cigarette smoking

There is a strong correlation between cigarette smoking and the incidence of cancers of the larynx, pharynx, oesophagus, pancreas, and lungs, as well as cardiovascular diseases. Cancer risk is 10 times greater for smokers than for nonsmokers. Cigarette smoking is increasing in poorer third world countries because cigarette manufacturers advertise it as a symbol of progress and modernity to third world people, especially the young. Whereas the US and Europe have recorded declines in the percentage of adult cigarette smokers annually since 1965, cigarette manufacturers have been able to expand their operations in third world countries because in these countries, they face none of the stiff advertising and health warning requirements that governments in Europe and North America have imposed on them.

12.4 SELECTIVE TOXICITY IN CANCER CHEMOTHERAPY

As in infectious diseases, the aim in cancer chemotherapy is that the drug should kill the malignant tumour cells at doses that do not harm normal cells. Selective toxicity is more difficult to achieve here than in bacterial or parasitic infections because in cancer the disease-causing cells share a great many characteristics with normal cells. Thus most anticancer drugs are also toxic to normal tissues with rapid rates of cell turnover. A more realistic objective is that the drug should kill most of the tumour but should allow enough of the cells of the patient's critical tissues to survive the effect of the drug so that complete recovery can occur.

In a malignant tumour, not all the cells are dividing. The *growth fraction* is the proportion of cells in a tumour mass that is actually dividing. The higher the growth fraction, the greater is the sensitivity of the tumour to chemotherapeutic agents. Anticancer drugs are most effective in lymphomas, e.g. Burkitt's lymphoma and leukaemias. Common malignant tumours such as those of breast, lung, colon, and rectum, are solid tumours with low growth fractions and are less sensitive to drugs.

Another factor that affects the sensitivity of the tumour cells to drugs is the stage of growth of these cells. Tumour cell growth is described by the standard Gompertzian curve – the tumour size increases logarithmically (exponentially) with time until a plateau is reached (Fig. 12.1). The tumour is sensitive to drugs in the logarithmic but not in the plateau phase; hence one should initiate therapy when the tumour is in the proliferative phase. This underlines the importance of early detection.

12.5   TOXICITY OF ANTICANCER DRUGS

Each group of drugs has its peculiar type of toxic effects which should be noted. A general point to note is that several normal tissues, e.g. hair follicles, bone marrow, and gastrointestinal tract, have high growth fractions, e.g. bone marrow has a growth fraction of 30% or more. Thus most drugs are toxic to bone marrow at doses at which they kill cancer cells. Hence typical undesirable effects of anticancer drugs are the following.

> Bone marrow depression leading to leucopoenia, lymphocyto-
> poenia, thrombocytopoenia, immunosuppression, infection,
> haemorrhage, and anaemia.
> Gastrointestinal tract effects such as ulceration, diarrhoea.
> Effects on the gonads are menstrual irregularities, infertility,
> sterility, and impaired spermatogenesis.
> Hyperuricaemia; rapid destruction of tumour cells can cause

release of nucleic acids and deposition of uric acid in the kidney leading to renal damage. If this is the case allopurinol should be given.

Most anticancer drugs have a therapeutic index approaching unity. Long-term dangers are carcinogenicity, mutagenicity and teratogenicity.

Toxicity can be minimised by the following.

Use of *intermittent high dose* therapy in which the patient's bone marrow is allowed to recover from the effects of the drug between courses of treatment,

Protecting normal cells from the cytotoxic effects of the anticancer drug, e.g. by the use of citrovorum factor (folinic acid) after high doses of methotrexate (the socalled citrovorum rescue).

Fig. 12.1. Diargammatic representation of Gompertzian Curve of tumour growth. Note that initially the time to double the tumour size (doubling time) is short (dt_1) but as the growth approaches its plateau, the doubling time increases (dt_2, dt_3).

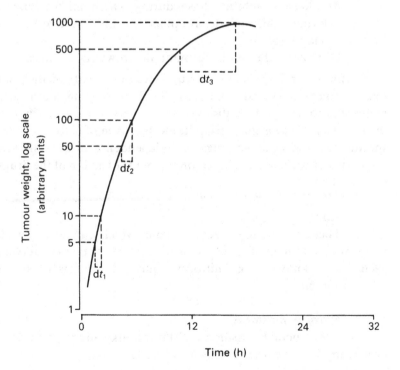

Combination of drugs with different mechanisms of action,
e.g. VAMP (i.e. vincristine, amethopterin, 6-mercaptopurine,
plus prednisolone) in the treatment of acute leukaemia,

Using the drugs as adjuvant to surgery and radiotherapy. After
removing a large tumour by surgery or irradiation, the
tumour cells left behind may be stimulated into logarithmic
growth; metastases may similarly have growth fractions and
doubling times resembling primary tumours in logarithmic
growth. Hence in adjuvant therapy lower and safer doses of
anticancer drugs can be used.

12.6   ANTICANCER DRUGS

Anticancer drugs may be classified in terms of the phase of the
cell cycle on which the drug acts. Cell cycle phases are:

G_1 phase – active growth of cell.

S phase – during which there is active synthesis of DNA/RNA
and proteins.

G_2 phase – premitotic phase, growth of cell and some protein
synthesis takes place.

M phase – mitotic phase during which microtubules are
formed; this includes prophase, metaphase, anaphase, and
telophase.

G_0 phase – the cell is dormant, no growth takes place.

Some anticancer drugs act to interrupt development at specific phases,
e.g. actinomycin D and asparaginase (G_1 phase); methotrexate, 6-
mercaptopurine, and antinomycin D (S phase); vincristine
(metaphase). There is an overlap in the spectrum of activity of phase-
specific drugs while some drugs act independently of the cell cycle.

Another classification is based on the mode of action of the drugs as
described below.

Alkylating agents

These are highly reactive agents which can form covalent
bonds with a number of cellular constituents. Many types of alkylating
agents are known, e.g. nitrogen mustards, nitrosoureas, and
alkylsulphonates.

Nitrogen mustards

The structures of some well known alkylating agents derived
from nitrogen mustard are shown in Fig. 12.2.

Mechanism of action

At neutral pH, one of the chlorethyl side chains undergoes cyclisation, releasing a chloride ion to form a three-member ringed structure called *immonium ion*. This highly reactive ion can attack and form covalent bonds with nucleophilic groups such as amino, carboxylic and sulphydryl-moieties of proteins and nucleic acids. In bifunctional alkylating agents such as the nitrogen mustards, the two side chains independently cyclicise and interact with separate moieties of nucleic acids and can cross-link DNA strands. The cytotoxicity of the nitrogen mustards is due to inhibition of DNA replication (see Fig. 12.3).

The experimental evidence which shows that alkylating agents interact with nucleic acids is interesting. If a solution of normal double-

Fig. 12.2. Molecular structures of some nitrogen mustards.

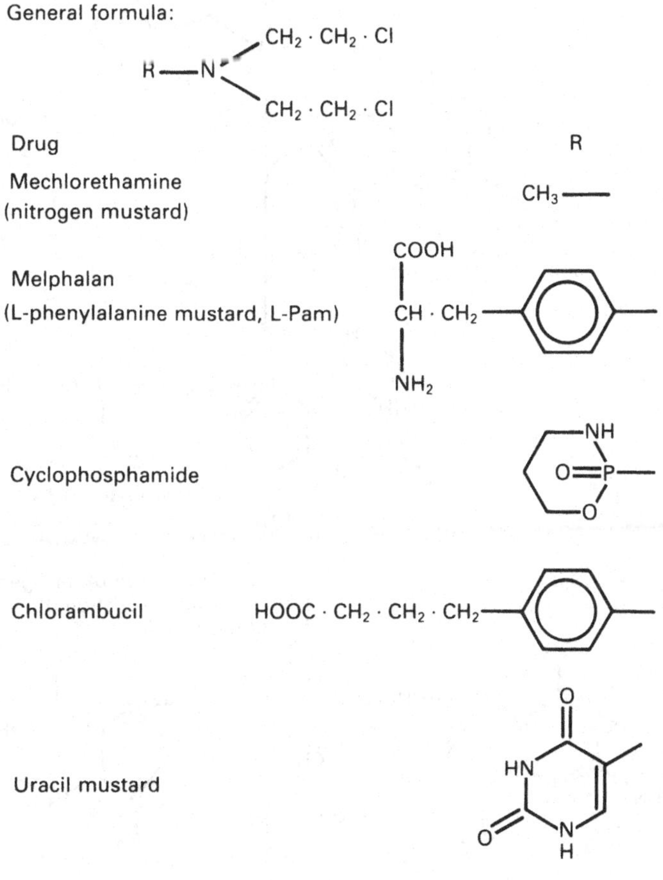

stranded DNA is made alkaline, denaturation of the DNA occurs and the molecule separates into single strands. On neutralisation, strands with appropriate hydrogen bonding sequence come together to form double strands (renaturation). Renaturation is only partial because the coming together of suitable strands is random. If the solution has been

Fig. 12.3. Mechanism of alkylation of nucleic acid by nitrogen mustard.

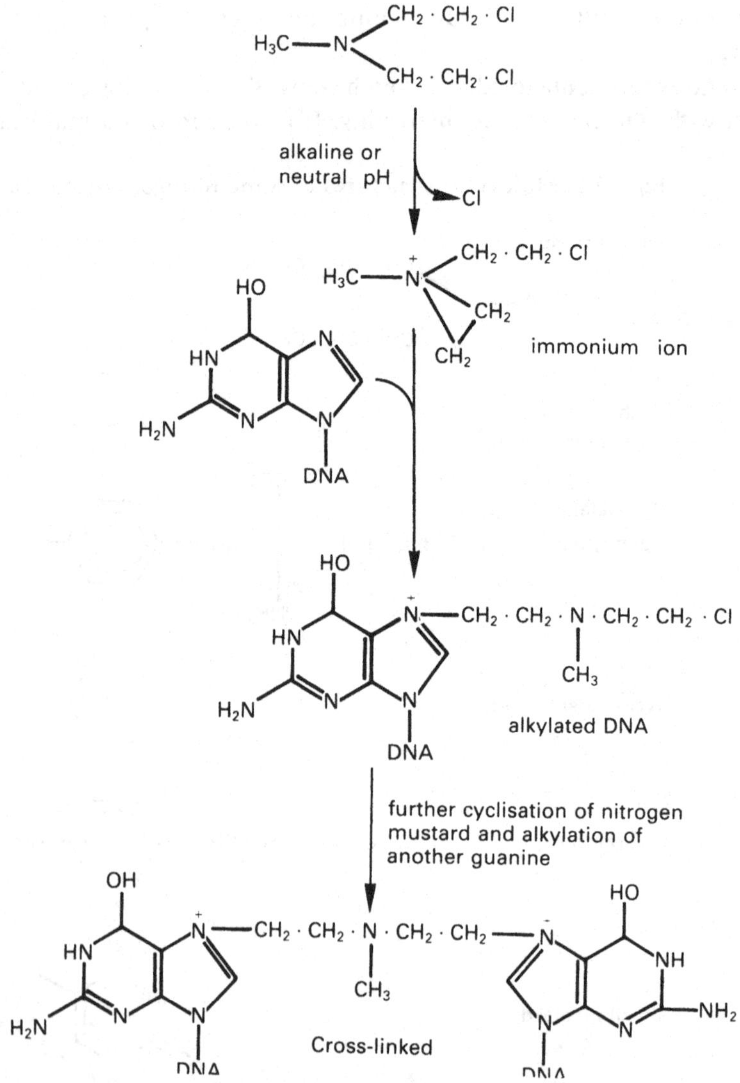

treated with an alkylating agent before alkalinisation, denaturation also occurs, but on neutralisation, renaturation is virtually complete. This is because, even though hydrogen bonding is disrupted by alkalinisation, the pairs of strands with appropriate hydrogen bonding sequence are still held together (cross-linked) by the alkylating agent. On neutralisation, hydrogen bonding (zipping up) can now take place (see Fig. 12.4).

By cross-linking DNA, alkylating agents interfere with DNA and protein synthesis. Proliferating and resting cells are affected but the drugs are most cytotoxic to rapidly dividing cells.

Phenylalanine mustard (melphalan) was developed on the rationale that since phenylalanine is actively taken up by melanin-containing tissues, the drug should be selectively toxic to melanomas. Nitrogen mustards linked to pyrimidines, e.g. uracil mustard and phenylbutyric acid (chlorambucil) have been developed on similar reasoning.

Fig. 12.4. Alkaline denaturation of normal DNA (A) and alkylated DNA (B). On neutralisation, renaturation of alkylated DNA is complete whereas that of normal DNA is only partial.

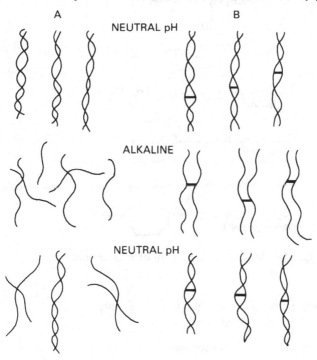

Nitrosoureas

(Fig. 12.5) alkylate as well as carbamylate proteins and nucleic acids thereby inhibiting DNA and protein synthesis. They are converted in the liver by cytochrome p-450 to highly lipophilic alkylating products.

Busulphan

(Fig. 12.6) is an alkyl sulphonate. *In vivo*, the alkyl oxygen bonds split allowing alkylation of a variety of cellular constituents such as DNA guanines, to take place. Alkylation of DNA is crucial to the cytotoxicity of all aklylating agents. That is why cross-sensitivity and cross-resistance to these drugs can occur. Resistance to alkylating agents can be due to decreased uptake of drug or increased ability of tumour cells to repair drug-induced DNA injury. In general, resistant cells take up less drug than sensitive cells although the difference is not

Fig. 12.5. Molecular structures of some nitrosoureas.

General formula

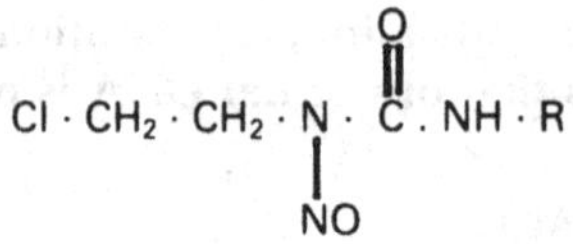

$$Cl \cdot CH_2 \cdot CH_2 \cdot N \cdot \overset{\overset{\displaystyle O}{\|}}{C} \cdot NH \cdot R$$
$$\underset{NO}{|}$$

Carmustine, R = - $CH_2 \cdot$ $CH_2 \cdot Cl$
(BCNU)

Lomustine, R =
(CCNU)

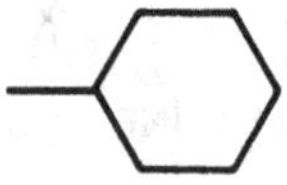

Semustine, R =   —CH_3
(MethylCCNU)

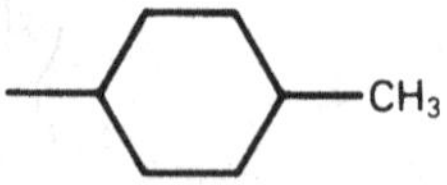

Fig. 12.6. Molecular structure of busulphan.

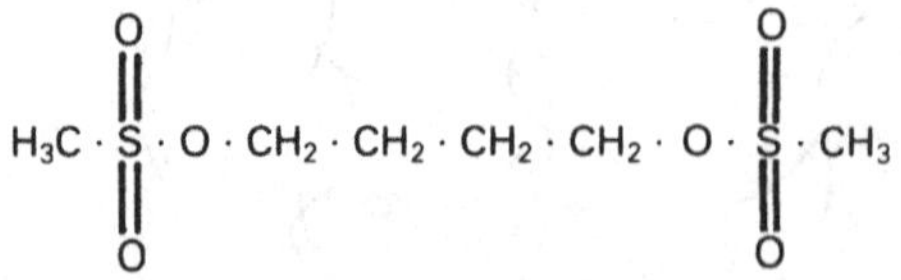

$$H_3C \cdot \overset{\overset{\displaystyle O}{\|}}{\underset{\underset{\displaystyle O}{\|}}{S}} \cdot O \cdot CH_2 \cdot CH_2 \cdot CH_2 \cdot CH_2 \cdot O \cdot \overset{\overset{\displaystyle O}{\|}}{\underset{\underset{\displaystyle O}{\|}}{S}} \cdot CH_3$$

Busulphan

enough to account for resistance. Nitrogen mustard is actively transported into tumour cells. The mechanism of reduced uptake in resistant cells is not known, but it could be that in high doses, the drug blocks its own uptake by inhibiting the uptake pump.

Tumour cells can excise alkylated bases and repair damaged DNA. The repair process is initiated by *endonucleases*, i.e. enzymes which can recognise alkylation-induced injury to DNA as mistakes and then 'nick' the DNA at the damaged site, subsequently synthesising a new segment to replace the excised segment. A *ligase* enzyme then links the newly synthesised segment covalently to the existing strand to form the original DNA. Resistant tumour cells are able to repair drug-induced injury more readily than sensitive cells.

Drug administration

The important issue here is that many alkylating agents are potent vesicants – highly irritant on contact with the skin. Therefore, if the drug can be absorbed from the gastrointestinal tract it must be given orally. If not it must be given intravenously taking care to avoid contact with the skin. Busulphan and chlorambucil are active orally.

Metabolism

Most of the drugs are inactivated by liver enzymes. Some are converted to active products by the mixed function oxidase system of the liver. For example, cyclophosphamide is converted to the cytotoxic products phosphoramide mustard and acrolein by liver enzymes.

Uses

Aklylating agents have a broad spectrum of antitumour activity. They are used in the treatment of Hodgkin's lymphoma, carcinomas of the breast, ovary and lung, and leukaemias. The most commonly used alkylating agent is cyclophosphamide administered orally or by i.v. injection in Hodgkin's disease, Burkitt's lymphoma, sarcomas, and a variety of solid tumours. Cyclophosphamide is also used to treat chronic rheumatoid arthritis. It is immunosuppressive and therefore used in transplant surgery to prevent rejection. Nitrosoureas are active after oral administration, are lipophilic, penetrate the blood–brain barrier and are used to treat tumours of the CNS.

Antimetabolites

These prevent the formation of essential metabolites which the cell needs to synthesise nucleic acids and proteins.

(a) Folic acid analogues

These act by inhibiting the enzyme dihydrofolate reductase; examples are methotrexate (Fig. 12.7) and aminopterin. The mechanism of this action is discussed in detail on page 218. Essentially, dihydrofolic acid (FH_2) must be reduced to tetrahydrofolic (FH_4) before the cell can use it to make thymidine, purines, glycine, etc.; methotrexate blocks dihydrofolate reductase activity and so folate is trapped in its unusable form.

The covalent binding of methotrexate to enzyme is virtually irreversible. The inhibition of thymidine synthesis is the critical factor in cell death. Methotrexate is most active against rapidly growing tumours and cells in S phase. Consequently, it is highly toxic to bone marrow and gastrointestinal tract. The mechanism of resistance to methotraxate includes:

> Production by the tumour cells of altered dihydrofolate reductase enzyme with decreased affinity for the drug (see figure 13.6).
>
> Production of an increased amount of dihydrofolate reductase enzyme.
>
> Decrease drug transport into the cells; methotrexate is specifically taken up into sensitive tumour cells by a folinic acid carrier mechanism.

Uses

Methotrexate is administered orally, intravenously or intrathecally. The drug does not enter the CNS unless directly administered. High doses in intermittent schedule of administration (pulse therapy) should be used to enhance selective toxicity and folinic acid (citrovorum) given to prevent damage to normal cells. Methotrexate is

Fig. 12.7. Molecular structure of methotrexate.

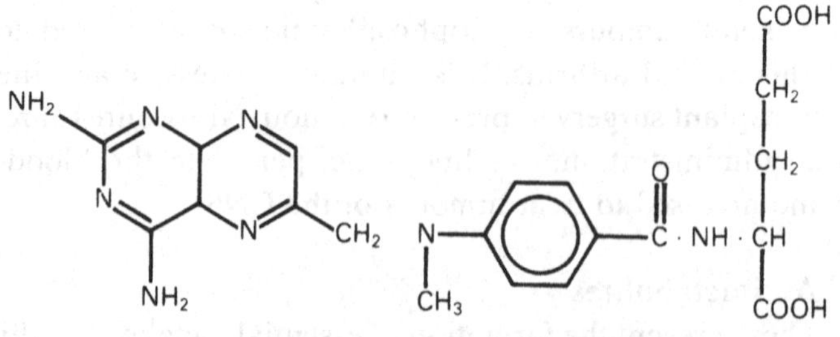

Methotrexate

useful in gestational choriocarcinomas, leukaemias, sarcomas, and Burkitt's lhymphoma. It is also used in the treatment of a number of non-neoplastic diseases, eg. psoriatic arthritis, systemic lupus erythematosus, and chronic rheumatoid arthritis.

(b) The purine analogues

These inhibit purine synthesis in tumour cells. DNA synthesis is blocked. Examples are 6-mercaptopurine, 6-thioguanine used in the treatment of acute leukaemia, azathioprine (immunosuppressant), and allopurinol (used in the treatment of gout).

6-Mercaptopurine

(6-MP) (Fig. 12.8) is converted by a hypoxanthine-guanine phosphoribosyl-transferase enzyme to 6-mercaptopurine-ribose-phosphate (6MPRP) which inhibits purine synthesis in tumour cells by a negative feedback inhibition of enzymes in the purine biosynthetic pathway. 6-MP cytotoxicity may also involve other actions and so may its metabolites

6-thioguanine

(6-TG) is also converted to the nucleotide 6-thioguanine-ribose-phosphate (6-TGRP) which blocks the conversion of inosinic to guanylic acid. Resistance to 6-MP and 6-TG is due to inability of the cells to commit lethal suicide, i.e. they lack the enzyme hypoxanthine guanine phosphoribosyltransferase, so that the parent compounds are not converted to cytotoxic products.

(c) Pyrimidine analogues, e.g. 5-fluorouracil (FU)

FU (see Fig. 12.9) is used in the treatment of several solid tumours, e.g. breast cancer usually in combination with cyclophosphamide and methotrexate. FU is converted to 5-fluoro-2-doxyuridine-

Fig. 12.8. Molecular structures of purine analogues.

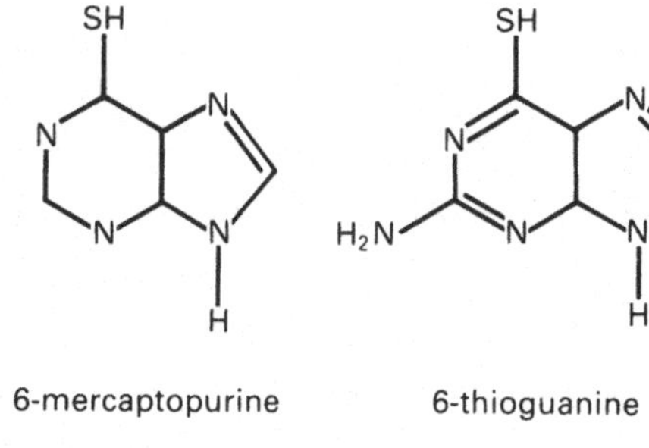

6-mercaptopurine   6-thioguanine

5'-monophosphate (FDUMP) which is the cytotoxic agent. The conversion is catalysed by pyrimidine phosphoribosyltransferase. Resistance to FU is probably due to failure in conversion of FU to FDUMP. Cytotoxicity is due to inhibition of thymidylate and DNA synthesis. Higher uptake by, and greater conversion of FU to FDUMP, in tumour cells than normal cells account for relative selective toxicity.

Natural products
(a) Antibiotics
A number of antibiotics are used in the treatment of cancer. They all directly or indirectly alter DNA function. *Actinomycin D,* and *adriamycin* bind noncovalently to DNA and are called intercalating agents. *Mithramycin* binds to DNA but does not intercalate and bleomycin causes DNA strand cleavage. Actinomycin D is used in the treatment of a wide range of cancers including several solid childhood tumours, Wilm's tumour, Kaposi's sarcoma and Burkitt's lymphoma, often in combination with radiotherapy. *Adriamycin* and *daunorubicin* are used for the treatment of acute leukaemias.

Actinomycin D (dactinomycin)
(Fig. 12.10) binds to double-stranded DNA and blocks DNA-directed functions, e.g. prevents the synthesis of RNA. The drug is cytotoxic to cells in any phase of the cell cycle and affects cells in the logarithmic as well as those in the plateau phase of growth. Resistance is associated with impaired entry of the drug into the cell due to change in cell membrane composition. *Amphotericin B* (page 207), a polyene antibiotic that can increase the permeability of mammalian cell membranes to ions, increases the uptake of dactinomycin and its anticancer activity in resistant tumours. Dactinomycin can also be delivered to resistant cells in liposomes (page 329).

Fig. 12.9. Molecular structure of 5-fluorouracil.

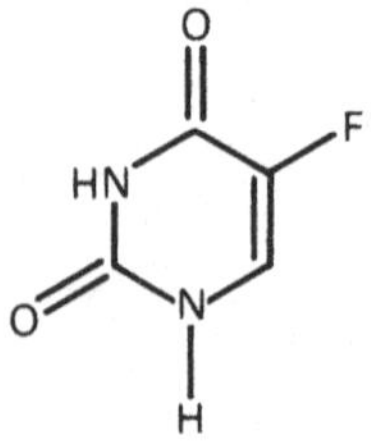

The drug is active orally and has the usual range of toxicities. Bone marrow depression and consequent fall in leucocyte and platelet counts give rise to ulceration of oral and gastrointestinal tract mucosa, and alopecia. It is also immunosuppressive, and in animal experiments, carcinogenic.

Anthracycline antibiotics

Examples are adriamycin, daunorubicin (see Fig. 12.11), and doxorubicin. Daunorubicin is used in the treatment of acute leukaemias. Adriamycin has a very broad spectrum of anticancer activity, being useful in a wide range of haematological malignancies and solid tumours. These antibiotics also have a wide range of toxicities. They cause bone marrow depression and consequently leucopoenia, thrombocytopoenia, and anaemia. In addition they cause acute cardiotoxicity and delayed progressive cardiomyopathy. In animal experiments they are also mutagenic and carcinogenic due to chromosome damage.

Intercalation of DNA

Both adriamycin and daunorubicin bind to DNA. Normally, the deoxyribose phosphate backbone of the DNA double helix is twisted (right-handed supercoiled) round the stacked bases. When an intercalating drug, e.g. adriamycin, becomes inserted between the base pairs, an uncoiling of the double helix occurs. Uncoiled DNA sedi-

Fig. 12.10. Molecular structure of actinomycin D (dactinomycin). Thr = threonine; Val = valine; Pro = proline; Sar = sarcosine; Meval = N-methylvaline.

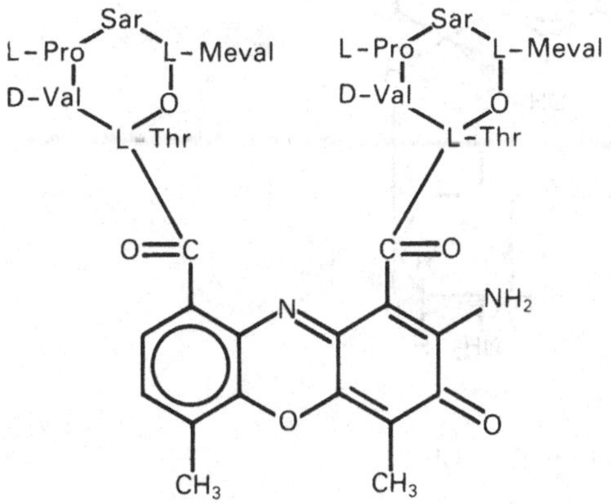

ments at a different rate from supercoiled DNA. Intercalation can therefore be estimated by measuring the sedimentation coefficient of normal DNA after interaction with an intercalating drug. An intercalated DNA is unable to function as a template in nucleic acid and protein synthesis. The drugs are cytotoxic to tumours in logarithmic and plateau phases, S-phase cells being more sensitive than cells in the G phase. Other antibiotics used in cancer chemotherapy are: mitomycin (alkylation and cross-linking of DNA); bleomycin (catalyses the degradation of DNA; useful in the treatment of squamous cell carcinoma of skin and genitalia, i.e. vagina and penis) and rarely causes bone marrow depression, therefore useful in combination with other drugs.

Alkaloids

The most important alkaloids used in the treatment of cancer are those obtained from the rose periwinkle plant *C. roseus (Vinca rosea)*. These alkaloids are mitotic inhibitors (or spindle poisons). The drugs interfere with the formation of microtubules; the latter are tube-like organelles found in all mammalian cells. Microtubules play an important role in the movement of cells relative to one another and in the movement of cell constituents and are referred to as *cytoskeleton*. Cell mitosis depends on microtubule function. The cytotoxicity of

Fig. 12.11. Molecular structures of anthracycline antibiotics.

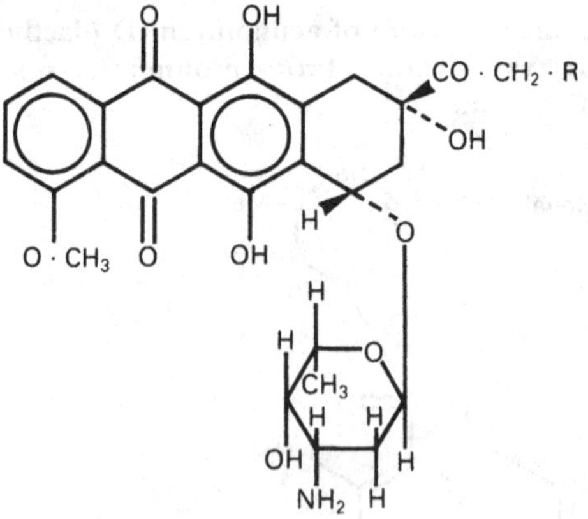

Adriamycin, R = -OH

Daunorubicin, R = -H
(daunomycin)

Vinca alkaloids comes from their ability to arrest cell mitosis specifically in metaphase. The mechanism of action of the *Vinca* alkaloids (also of colchicine and podophyllotoxin) is thought to be as follows: Microtubules are polymers made up of large protein molecules called tubulin (molecular weight, 120000). Tubulin is the specific receptor for *Vinca* alkaloids. Normally, the microtubules of the mitotic apparatus are in equilibrium with a pool of soluble tubulin in the cytoplasm; this equilibrium is maintained by continuous disassembly of microtubules and polymerisation of tubulin molecules. By binding to tubulin molecules to form drug–tubulin complexes, *Vinca* alkaloids prevent polymerisation and cause disassembly of microtubules. *Vinca* alkaloids can also inhibit the transport of aminoacids and the synthesis of nucleic acids. Selective toxicity is due to preferential concentration of the alkaloids in tumour cells.

The drugs are highly irritant to skin and tissues, and are given by the intravenous route. Care should be taken to prevent extravasation and contact with the skin. The drugs are highly bound to tissues, hence have very large volumes of distribution; they do not enter the CNS.

Vinca alkaloids are used in the treatment of Hodgkin's disease, lymphocytic leukaemias, and Burkitt's lymphoma, and in combination with dactinomycin or cyclophosphamide in the treatment of paediatric solid tumours.

Vincristine is thought to depress bone marrow less (marrow-sparing) compared to other anticancer drugs, but it is also neurotoxic due to its binding to neurotubulin and causing dissolution of neurotubles.

(c) Enzymes
L-asparaginase (L-asparagine amidohydrolase)
This is the only enzyme preparation used in the treatment of cancer. The enzyme catalyses the hydrolysis of the aminoacid asparagine to aspartic acid and ammonia. Most normal cells synthesise sufficient L-asparagine for their metabolic needs. Certain neoplastic tissues such as lymphoblastic leukaemic cells in children require an exogenous source of the amino acid. L-asparaginase, by hydrolysing it, deprives the malignant cells of the asparagine available in extracellular fluid, resulting in cell death.

In contrast to other anticancer drugs L-asparaginase has minimal effects on the bone marrow, and so does not damage oral or gastro-intestinal mucosa or the hair follicles; but asparaginase causes other severe toxicities on the liver, kidneys, pancreas, and CNS, and affects the clotting mechanism of blood. It is probable that the various toxic effects result from inhibition of protein synthesis in the different organs. Since L-asparaginase is a large molecular weight protein, it is antigenic (most asparaginase enzymes are obtained from *E. coli*) and hypersensitivity reactions ranging from allergy to anaphylactic reactions are common.

The anticancer spectrum of activity of L-asparaginase is narrow, it being used mostly in the treatment of acute lymphoblastic leukaemia.

Steroid hormones

The rationale for the use of steroid hormones or hormone antagonists in the treatment of some cancers is that the growth of these cancers, e.g. prostatic cancer and breast cancer, is stimulated by certain hormones. The aim in steroid hormone therapy is to remove the hormonal stimulus which normally promotes the growth of hormone-sensitive tumours.

Cancer of the prostate gland

Androgens, e.g. testosterone, maintain normal prostate size and function. Oestrogens antagonise this action. The mechanism is not clearly understood, but involves inhibition of the formation of interstitial cell stimulating hormone (ICSH) by the adenohypophysis. ICSH promotes the synthesis of androgens by the Leydig cells of the testis. Oestrogens may also have a direct action on prostatic tumour growth. Diethylstilboestrol is used in the treatment of prostatic cancer.

Breast cancer

Diethylstilboestrol was also formerly used in the treatment of breast cancer. Oestrogens have the paradoxical effect of causing regression of breast cancer rather than promoting its growth. Prolonged use of diethylstilboestrol causes uterine bleeding and cardiovascular toxicities. In theory, androgens should be useful in the treatment of breast cancer, since the male sex hormones reduce the oestrogen levels through inhibition of gonadotrophins. The major disadvantage of testosterone in the treatment of breast cancer is hirtuism, deepening of the voice, and increase in muscle mass, i.e. masculinisation.

Antioestrogens

Tamoxifen (Fig. 12.12) antagonises oestradiol by binding to estrogen receptors. Possibly by acting as an oestrogen agonist, tamoxifen causes a down regulation of oestrogen receptors in the tumour, so that the hormone does not stimulate tumour growth.

Side effects are numerous, e.g. hypercalcaemia, retinopathy, and corneal damage; some are due to its oestrogenic agonist activity. Another antioestrogen is *nafoxidine*. These drugs are used to treat breast cancer in post-menopausal women.

Oestrogen activity can also be reduced by drugs which block the enzyme aromatase. The main source of estrogens in pre-menopausal women is the ovaries, while in post-menopausal women oestrogens are derived from aromatisation of androgens in peripheral tissues. Aromatisation (i.e. the conversion of the 'A' ring of an androgen to the unsaturated or aromatised 'A' ring of an oestrogen) is catalysed by the enzyme *oestrogen synthetase* or *aromatase* (see Fig. 12.13). This reaction takes place in several peripheral tissues including liver, muscle, and breast tumour itself. The aromatase enzyme is blocked by several steroidal and non-steroidal (e.g. aminoglutethimide) compounds. These compounds also inhibit other steroid hydroxylase enzymes, thereby causing chemical adrenalectomy. Hence aminoglutethimide is given in combination with hydrocortisone. This treatment produces remission of tumour in about 50% of post-menopausal women where there is evidence that the cancer is supported by oestrogen (oestrogen receptor positive). *Androgens*, e.g. testosterone propionate, fluoxy-mesterone, and testolactone are used in the treatment of advanced breast cancer in women in menopause. They cause hypercalcaemia, masculinisation, hirtuism, and increased libido. Testolactone lacks these androgenic activities. *Glucocorticoids* act on a wide range of tissues and organs, unlike the sex hormones which are selective to a group of sex-related target organs. Glucocorticoids (e.g. prednisolone) are used in the treatment of acute lymphoblastic leukaemias of child-hood in combination with other antineoplastic drugs. Prednisolone

Fig. 12.12. Molecular structure of tamoxifen.

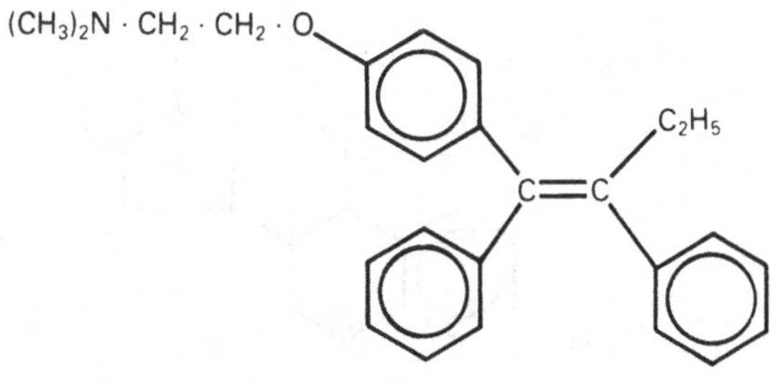

also produces remission in chronic lymphoblastic leukaemia, Hodgkin's disease, and lymphocytic lymphomas. The mechanism of action has been extensively studied but is not unequivocally understood. Steroids are highly lipophilic and readily enter the cytosol of cells. In the cytosol the steroid binds to an intracellular receptor protein. The potency of the glucocorticoid is directly proportional to the affinity of the drug for this receptor protein. The steroid receptor complex in turn binds to an acceptor site, probably DNA, in the cell nuclens. This leads to the formation of specific mRNA's in the cell and hence the synthesis of new proteins which are toxic to the tumour cell. Beware of the characteristic side effects of steroid therapy.

12.7   ANTIVIRAL DRUGS

Introduction

Viruses are submicroscopic agents that infect plants and animals, usually manifesting their presence by causing diseases. Viruses are unable to multiply outside the host's tissues. The mature virus (called a virion) consists of nucleic acids enclosed within a protein-glycoprotein or lipoprotein coat. The nucleic acid is either DNA or

Fig. 12.13. Formation of oestrogen from androgen (aromatisation) under the influence of aromatase.

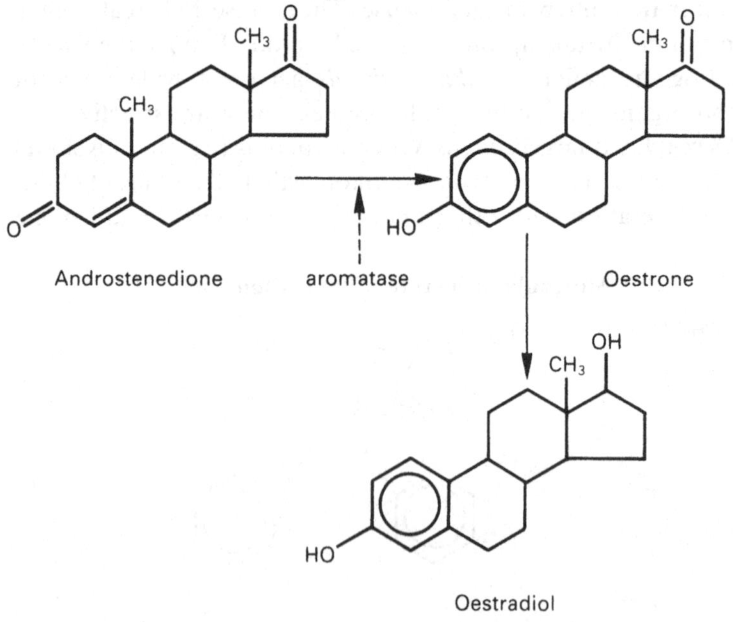

Androstenedione   aromatase   Oestrone

Oestradiol

RNA in animal viruses, whereas it is RNA in plant viruses. Infectivity resides in the nucleic acid component. The nucleic acid is released from the virion into the infected cell where it initiates the synthesis of more virions. Some virions contain or induce the synthesis of enzymes which aid their penetration of host cells.

Viruses are of great medical and agricultural importance causing diseases such as poliomyelitis, smallpox, measles, yellow fever, acquired immune deficiency syndrome (AIDS), common cold, and various diseases of food and cash crops, foot and mouth diseases of cattle, etc. The composition of the lipoprotein coat is unique to each virus and can be used to characterise it, as well as to induce in the host the formation of specific antibodies. This latter is the basis of vaccines which are available for protection against many viral diseases. Immunistion has virtually eradicated smallpox and diseases like poliomyelitis, yellow fever, and measles are now rare due to the availability of effective immunisation. Some viral diseases are not controlled by immunisation. This is why there is the need for effective antiviral drugs.

The search for drugs which can be used to treat viral diseases has been intense and prolonged. Yet very few drugs have been found which have wide effective clinical applications. The few drugs that are clinically useful have narrow spectrum of activity and limited to only one or two specific viruses. The problem is that, in contrast to most other infectious agents (bacteria, fungi, protozoa, etc.), viruses are obligative intracellular parasites which require the metabolic processes of the invaded cell for the virus to replicate. Selective toxicity against the virus is thus a difficult goal in the development of antiviral agents. Agents that may inhibit the replication of viruses are also likely to cause injury in the host cells invaded by the virus. Another problem is that viruses do not have complicated and elaborate biochemical and physiological processes different from those of host cells which can be exploited in drug development.

Antiviral drugs and their sites of action
Infection of a host cell by a virus involves the following.

(a) Specific binding of the virus with components of the host cell membrane.

(b) Entry of the virus into the host cell.

(c) Uncoating of the virus to expose its nucleic acids.

(d) Transcription, that is synthesis of RNA made up of a particular sequence of nucleotides using the viral DNA as template.

In the case of retroviruses, e.g. human immunodeficiency virus (HIV), a *reverse transcriptase* enzyme catalyses the production of DNA copies of the viral RNA which are then used to replicate the virus.

(e) Virus particles are assembled and released through the plasma membrane.

In theory, all of these steps can be targets for antiviral drug action. In practice, most of the useful antiviral drugs affect replication. Examples of useful antiviral drugs are given below.

Idoxuridine

This is a halogenated pyrimidine with structural resemblance to thymidine which is a component of DNA. Idoxuridine is phosphorylated within host cells after which the triphosphate derivative is incorporated into both viral and mammalian DNA. Such DNA is susceptible to breakage and may give rise to the synthesis of altered viral proteins due to faulty transcription (see page 209). The activity of idoxuridine is limited to DNA viruses, primarily the herpes virus group. The principal use of idoxuridine is in the treatment of herpes simplex keratitis. The drug is administered in drops into the conjunctiva using an 0.1% solution. Infections caused by other types of herpes simplex do not respond well.

Amantadine

is a synthetic antiviral agent with an unusual structure. It is a tricyclic amine. The drug inhibits replication of influenza type A virus. Host cells are not inhibited. The replication of most strains of influenza type A virus is inhibited by a concentration of less than 1 μg ml^{-1} of amantadine, which is achieved by the usual therapeutic dose of 150–200 mg per day. Some studies suggest that amantadine is effective only if treatment is initiated early in an attack of 'flu. The drug can also be used as a prophylactic in an epidemic when people who are in contact with sufferers have yet to show signs of infection. Amantadine is a useful drug in the treatment of Parkinsonism. It is proposed that the drug releases dopamine from dopaminergic nerves in the nigrostriatum of patients with the disease.

Vidarabine (adenine arabinoside)

is an analogue of adenosine. The compound is phosphorylated within the cell and acts by inhibiting viral DNA polymerase. Mammalian DNA synthesis is inhibited less. Vidarabine is metabolised to hypoxanthine arabinoside; although less active, this metabolite synergises with the parent compound to inhibit the replication of large DNA viruses, e.g. that causing herpes simplex encephalitis. The drug can also be used to treat herpes zoster infections and topically in herpes simplex keratoconjunctivitis.

Human interferon

The interferons are an interelated group of glycoproteins liberated by cells infected by a virus. They act to make neighbouring cells less susceptible to virus infection. Interferon is thus an important part of the body's defence mechanism against viral infection. Interferons are in general, virus-specific. The interferon induced by one virus cannot usually be used to protect against infection by a different virus. However effective interferons induced by DNA or RNA virus can give protection against a wide variety of DNA or RNA viruses. The mechanism of action seems to be interference with viral replication in host cells.

The problem is how to make sufficient amount of interferons available for use. One approach is the use of tissue culture. This is expensive. Another approach uses genetic engineering to cause bacterial cells, e.g. *E. coli*, to make human interferon. This is less expensive. Another approach is to use interferon inducers such as double-stranded RNA. Clinical trials have shown interferons to be effective in controlling infections caused by herpes zoster, rabies virus, and hepatitis B virus, especially in combination with vidarabine.

Acquired immune deficiency syndrome (AIDS)

This disease has become an important health problem around the world. AIDS is sexually transmitted (both heterosexually and homosexually), by contaminated blood transfusion and by injection of drugs using contaminated needles. AIDS is caused by the retrovirus, human immune deficiency virus (HIV). The virus causes a progressive and severe immune deficiency resulting in death due to opportunistic infections and certain malignancies (especially Kaposi's sarcoma and certain lymphomas). HIV preferentially infects and destroys helper/inducer phenotype T-cells expressing CD4 antigen making it impossible for the victim to mount immunological defence against infections.

The approaches to the treatment of AIDS and related syndromes include: (a) therapy for opportunistic infections and malignancies; (b) destruction or inhibition of replication of the HIV virus; and (c) immune reconstitution or immunopotentiation.

Zidovudine (formerly known as Azidodeoxythymidine, AZT)
is a thymidine analogue which was the first antiviral agent to
be licensed for the treatment of AIDS. Zidovudine is converted to a
triphosphate by cellular enzymes. This triphosphate form binds to
retroviral reverse transcriptase leading to inhibition of viral
replication. Cellular DNA polymerase is about 100 times less susceptible
to inhibition by zidovudine. This difference provides an advantage of
relatively low host cytotoxicity. In clinical trials some AIDS patients
treated with zidovudine show significant recovery of immune competence and clinical improvement. The drug does not cure AIDS and
since it only suppresses viral replication, treatment must be maintained or else the disease re-establishes itself. The drug is well
absorbed from the gastrointestinal tract and can enter the CNS. This is
a useful property since HIV can infect the CNS.

Other antiviral drugs used in the treatment of AIDS: dideoxycytidine

This is an antiviral drug that inhibits reverse transcriptase
enzyme and so prevents viral replication. It has been developed by the
National Cancer Institute in America and is undergoing clinical trials.
It is claimed that dideoxycytidine has good oral bioavailability, good
kidney clearance, and appears to disturb normal cellular metabolism
less than zidovudine. It may cause less side effects, especially bone
marrow suppression, than zidovudine.

Suramin,

the antitrypanosomal drug (page 248) has been found to
inhibit HIV replication *in vitro* and has been tried with limited success
in the treatment of AIDS patients.

Antimoniotungstate (HPA-23)

is another reverse transcriptase inhibitor which has been
clinically investigated in AIDS with some success. The side effects
include thromibocytopoenia and hepatitis.

None of these drugs eradicate the AIDS virus. Even when effective
and safe, the drugs can only suppress the infection, and on cessation of
treatment the infection is re-established. An alternative approach to a
direct attack on HIV reverse transcriptase is immunorestorative therapy.
The aim of this is to improve the immune competence of the AIDS
patient since the major problem in this disease is that the victim's
immune system is severely damaged by HIV. Immune restoration may

involve transplantation of cross-matched bone marrow or bone marrow from an identical twin. Lymphocyte transfusion has also been tried. These measures are unlikely to be successful because HIV will infect the newly transfused cells.

Immunorestorative therapy can also be achieved by the use of biologically active molecules such as: *thymic hormones* which induce maturation and differentiation of lymphocytes; *interleukin 2*, a low molecular weight glycoprotein which aids differentiation, maturation and growth of T cells; and *recombinant d-A interferon* which, *in vitro*, inhibits HIV replication. The problem with the use of measures such as interleukin 2 is that, by activating T cells *in vivo* they could provide more substrate for HIV, i.e. more cells in which the virus can replicate. It is unlikely that any of the presently available antiviral agents and immunorestorative strategies alone will cure patients with AIDS or AIDS-related diseases. Therefore a combination of approaches will probably be the best strategy in the treatment of this deadly disease. The ideal antiviral drug should be virucidal or if virustatic, it should be active orally and free of side effects since it would have to be taken for prolonged periods. Such an antiviral drug should be used in combination with a potent and safe immunopotentiator.

FURTHER READING

Solanke, T. F., Osunkoya, B. O., Williams, C.K.O., & Agboola, O. O., eds. (1982). *Cancer in Nigeria*. Ibadan University Press, Ibadan.

Pratt, W. B. & Ruddon, R. W. (1979). *The Anticancer Drugs*. Oxford University Press, New York, Oxford.

Chabner, B. A. & Pinedo, H. M., eds. (1986). *The Cancer Pharmacology Annual*. Elsevier Science Publishers, Amsterdam, New York.

Gupta, S. (1986). Therapy of AIDS and AIDS related syndromes. *TIPS* 7, 393–7.

13

Drug resistance

13.1 INTRODUCTION

Drug resistance is said to exist when an organism acquires the ability to survive concentrations of a drug several times higher than those which would normally kill it or inhibit its growth. Resistant microbes can transfer this acquired property to their offspring when the microbes divide. Furthermore, mechanisms exist by which the resistance machinery can pass from resistant to sensitive organisms of the same or even different strains. This means that once resistance is established among a population of micro-organisms, it can spread by infecting sensitive bacteria; this is a serious threat to the continued usefulness of chemotherapeutic agents.

Among the factors which favour the emergence of resistant organisms is inappropriate use of antimicrobial drugs. In industrialised nations, extensive use of antibiotics in animal husbandry has been named as a major cause of the spread of resistance. In the tropics where there is extensive self-medication and where antibiotics can be sold without licence and purchased without prescription, large reservoirs of resistance are building up. The recent emergence of a penicillinase-producing strain of *Neisseria gonococcus* (PPNG) which is resistant to benzylpenicillin in West Africa and South East Asia has been attributed to the inappropriate use of the penicillins.

In one survey, it was found that more than 76% of *E. coli* isolates from the Philippines, Korea, Taiwan and Indonesia were resistant to one or more antibiotics and 44% to four or more (Echeverria *et al.*, 1978). The same survey found that in the Phillipines (where antibiotics are available without prescription) 98% of children admitted into hospital for gastroenteritis had been treated with antibiotic before admission. Third world countries thus find themselves in a situation where

296

they spend scarce resources buying antimicrobial agents which may be in effect therapeutically useless.

The aim in this chapter is to emphasise the importance of this problem. It should be read with Chapter 5 since an understanding of the mechanisms by which micro-organisms develop resistance to antibiotics has proved helpful in unravelling how some of these drugs work.

13.2 HOW MICRO-ORGANISMS DEVELOP RESISTANCE TO ANTIMICROBIAL AGENTS

1. Mutation

One mechanism by which micro-organisms develop resistance to antimicrobial agents is spontaneous mutation, that is, a change in the structure of the nuclear DNA. This enables the organism, for example, to produce enzymes which destroy the antimicrobial agent or to produce binding sites (receptors) with lowered affinity for the antimicrobial agent. Any population of micro-organisms which is overall sensitive to a given antimicrobial agent may contain a small number of mutant organisms which are resistant to the antimicrobial agent. When the population is exposed to the agent, the sensitive members are killed, but the mutants survive (Fig. 13.1). Usually these mutants are eliminated by the body's immune system; but if they are protected in mucous membranes, or lung cavities, they may grow and give rise to a new generation of organisms which are totally resistant to the antimicrobial agent. This process whereby resistant mutants are selected out by antimicrobial agents is known as *drug selection pressure*.

The change from sensitivity to resistance can occur by a single step mutation such as is seen with streptomycin where total resistance of *Mycobacterium tuberculosis* can occur after one exposure to the antibiotic. Resistance can also result from stepwise selection of mutants with

Fig. 13.1. Emergence of resistance under drug pressure; ○, Sensitive strain; ●, resistant mutants.

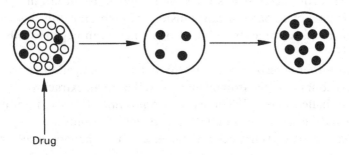

Drug

increasing resistance to successively increasing doses of the antimicrobial agent. Another way by which resistant mutants can emerge is by exposure of sensitive organisms to sublethal doses of the agent.

2. Transduction

Sensitive organisms can also acquire resistance by the process known as *phage transduction*. When a bacterial virus (bacteriophage or phage) infects a bacterial cell, the DNA of the phage and that of the bacterium become integrated. During phage replication, pieces of the bacterial DNA become incorporated in the phage DNA. If the bacterium happens to be carrying a drug-resistance determinant in its chromosome, these determinants become incorporated in the phage. When the bacterial cell eventually lyses, it releases multiple copies of resistance-carrying phages. When these now infect drug-sensitive bacteria, the latter become resistant. Resistance plasmids (*vide infra*) can also be transferred from one bacterium to another of the same species by phage transduction. The spread of drug resistant *Staphylococcus aureus* in hospitals is believed to be due to phage transduction of resistance plasmids. This Gram-positive organism can harbour plasmids which confer resistance simultaneously to several important antibiotics such as penicillin, chloramphenicol, and erythromycin.

3. Transmission of resistance factors (R-factors) by conjugation

The discovery that cellular conjugation in Gram-negative bacteria is responsible for the spread of drug resistance was made during epidemics of bacillary dysentery in Japan. It was found that strains of *Shigella* isolated from patients suffering from dysentery were resistant to a large number of drugs including sulphonamides, streptomycin, chloramphenicol, and tetracyclines. Also, resistant and sensitive strains of the same organism could be isolated from the same patients. Moreover, patients harbouring multi-resistant *Shigella* also harboured multi-resistant *E.coli*. It was then found that resistant Gram-negative organisms such as *Shigella* can transfer resistance, not only to sensitive organisms of the same strain but also to other Gran-negative cells such as *E.coli*.

The transfer of resistance occurs through cell conjugation. In bacteria, DNA is contained in chromosomes as well as in an extrachromosomal element called plasmid. The extrachromosomal DNA is responsible for most drug resistance in micro-organisms. Plasmids are not present in all strains of a given species of bacterium. They are not necessary for the normal function of the cell, but like nuclear chromosomes, plasmids are genetic elements. They can confer on the organisms distinct hereditary characteristics including drug resistance. The complexes of genes on a plasmid responsible for drug resistance are called R-factors. R-factors consist of genes called R-Determinants (RDS) that carry the code for resistance to different antimicrobial agents and those that promote the transfer of resistance from one micro-organism to another; the latter are called Resistance Transfer Factors (RTFs) (Fig. 13.2). One R-factor can have several genes, each responsible for resistance to a different antimicrobial agent. By the process of cell conjugation a resistant Gram-negative bacterium can confer resistance properties on a previously drug sensitive strain. Even more problematic, from the therapeutic point of view, is the fact that nonpathogenic coliform organisms which are normal inhabitants of the alimentary canal can become carriers of resistance plasmids which they can transfer to sensitive pathogens. Readers who wish to explore the details of the fascinating subject of resistance plasmids may do so in the reviews listed at the end of this chapter.

13.3 RESISTANCE TO SPECIFIC ANTIMICROBIAL AGENTS

To acquire resistance to antimicrobial agent microbes may produce:

Fig. 13.2. Bacterial resistance factors. (a) Bacterial cell: fl, flagellum; pl, R-factor carrying plasmid; N, nucleus; pi, pilus. (b) A complete R-factor: RTF, resistance transfer factor, RD₁, ₂, ₃, ₄, resistance determinants to various antibiotics.

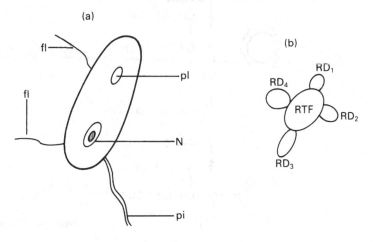

An enzyme which inactivates the drug;

An altered binding site (receptor) with reduced affinity for the
   drug;

An altered carrier with reduced uptake for the drug;

An alternative enzyme to the one inhibited by the drug;

Increased amounts of the enzyme inhibited by the drug; or

An increased amount of a metabolite for which the drug is a
   competitive antagonist.

Sometimes more than one mechanism can operate against a given
antimicrobial agent.

13.4   PRODUCTION OF AN ENZYME WHICH INACTIVATES AN ANTIBIOTIC

(a) Chloramphenicol

Resistance to chloramphenicol has been observed in both
Gram-positive and Gram-negative bacteria such as *E. coli, S. aureus,*

Fig. 13.3. Inactivation of chloramphenicol by a specific acetyltransferase produced by bacteria in response ot drug pressure.

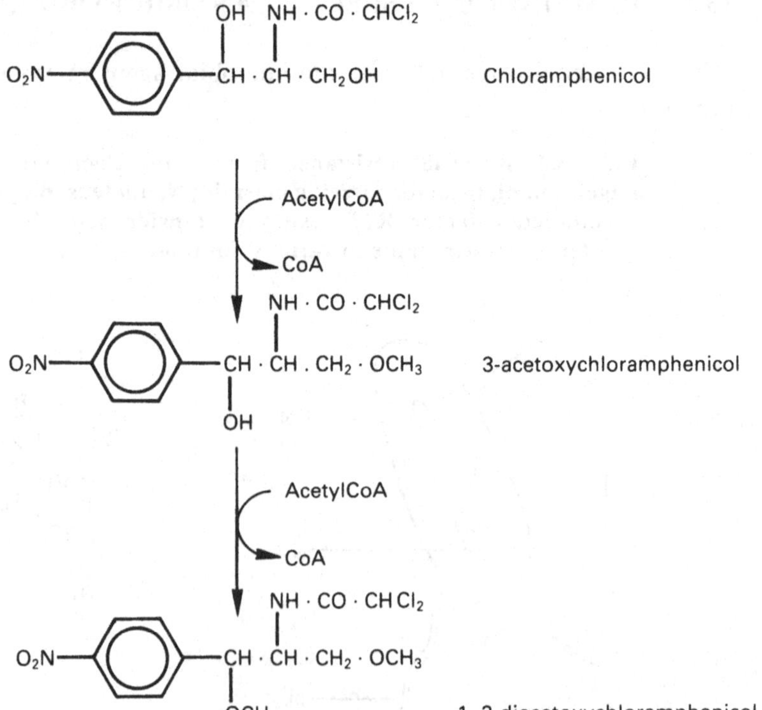

Pseudomonas and *Salmonella typhi*. Resistance is due to the production of an enzyme, chloramphenicol acetyltransferase, which destroys the antibiotic property of the drug (Fig. 13.3.).

The enzyme is produced by R-factor carrying bacteria and induced by chloramphenicol. How can a drug which is a potent inhibitor of protein synthesis induce the production of an enzyme? It seems that initially, inhibition of protein synthesis and induction of chloramphenicol acetyltransferase are in competition. Subsequently, the concentration of chloramphenicol falls below the level at which it can inhibit protein synthesis and then enzyme production rises rapidly.

(b) Aminoglycosides

Resistance to the aminoglycosides can be caused by three types of inactivating enzymes which bring about:

Phosphorylation;

Acetylation; and

Adenylation

Phosphorylation and adenylation occur on -OH groups and acetylation on $-NH_2$ groups. The enzyme responsible for the catalysis of the reactions are of different forms. Thus streptomycin is a substrate for O-nucleotidyltransferase (adenylation) and O-phosphotransferase (phosphorylation) but not N-acetyl-transferase (acetylation); whereas kanamycin is acetylated and adenylated.

The enzymes are produced by both Gram-negative and Gram-positive bacteria as a result of chromosomal mutation or acquisition of genes carried on plasmids. The modified drug is inactive, that is, it fails to bind to the receptor protein on 30s ribosome and blocks permeation into the bacterial cell thereby preventing its own access and the access of active molecules to the active site.

(c) Penicillins and cephalosporins

Resistance to penicillin is due to the production by resistant organisms of the inactivating enzyme usually called *penicillinase*. However, because the target for these enzymes is the β-lactum ring of the penicillin molecule (Fig. 13.4) and because the cephalosporins which possess a β-lactam ring are also substrates for these enzymes, the more embracing term β-*lactamase* is preferred. Particular β-lactamases may exhibit a preference for either cephalosporin or penicillin as substrate. Therefore, cross-resistance between these groups of drugs may not be complete.

The code for the structure and production of β-lactamase is carried by plasmid genes in R-factors. Gram-positive and Gram-negative bacteria can produce inactivating β-lactamases. The production of β-lactamase is induced by exposure of the bacterium to a β-lactam drug. All the penicillins can act as inducers to the enzyme. By far the most widely distributed β-lactamase is that produced by *S. aureus* known as the TEM-1 enzyme which can destroy a wide range of pencillin and cephalosporin drugs.

A great deal is known about β-lactamases. The enzyme is made inside the cell and transported through the cell membrane to the external surface. In Gram-positive bacteria which produce very large amounts of β-lactamase (for example, when fully induced, *S. aureus* production of β-lactamase is up to 3% of its total protein synthesis) most of the enzyme is released into the external *milieu*. On the other hand, Gram-negative organisms usually produce smaller amounts of enzyme which remain associated with the outer portion of the cytoplasmic membrane and destroy the β-lactam as it tries to enter the cell. β-lactamase-sensitive antibiotics are completely ineffective against β-lactamase-producing bacteria as the latter produce enough enzyme to destroy almost any amount of antibiotic administered.

As has been pointed out, the resistance determinant can be transferred from one strain of bacterium to another of the same or even a

Fig. 13.4. Inactivation by hydrolysis of (a) penicillin, and (b) cephalosporin, by beta-lactamase produced by bacteria in response to drug pressure.

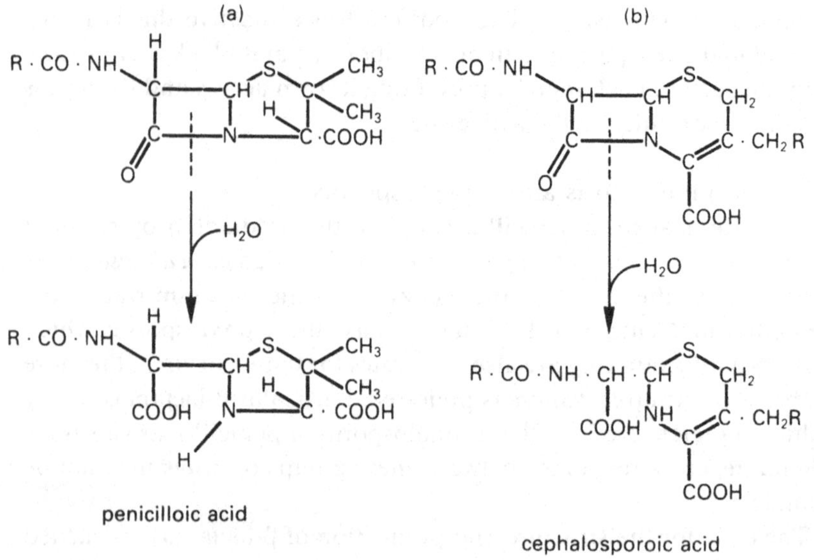

(a)

penicilloic acid

(b)

cephalosporoic acid

different species. Thus it is sometimes found that organisms cultured from the site of an infection not responding to pencillin, are sensitive to penicillin *in vitro*. This has been seen with streptococcal infections. The reasons for this is that *in vivo*, the organisms may be protected from the antibiotic by β-lactamase produced by other nonpathogenic organisms such as *E. coli*.

β-Lactamase-resistant penicillins

In β-lactamase-sensitive penicillins, the antibiotic has a higher affinity for the β-lactamase enzyme than for the cell wall-building enzyme, peptidoglycan transpeptidase. To overcome the problem of β-lactamase resistance derivatives of β-lactam antibiotics with greater affinity for transpeptidase than for β-lactamase can be made. Different substitutions on the side chain of penicillin G give rise to compounds with different susceptibilities for the β-lactamase enzyme. For example, methicillin has 10000 times lower affinity than penicillin G for β-lactamase, and a greater affinity for peptidoglycan transpeptidase than for β-lactamase. Methicillin is therefore resistant to β-lactamase.

Methicillin is useful in the treatment of β-lactamase-producing resistant bacteria. Unfortunately, its intrinsic antibiotic activity is much lower than that of benzylpenicillin. Moreover, the drug is ineffective against Gram-negative organisms as it is unable to penetrate the outer membrane of these organisms, and even more disturbing are reports of organisms resistant to methicillin by mechanisms not involving β-lactamase production. Resistance to methicillin and other β-lactamase-resistant antibiotics is not yet widespread, but its occurrence points to the extraordinary capacity of bacteria to adapt.

13.5   INHIBITORS OF β-LACTAMASE

Another way to overcome the problem of β-lactamase restistance is to inhibit the enzymes with a drug which has high binding affinity for, but is not hydrolysed by, the enzyme. Clavulanic acid (Fig. 13.5) is such a drug. This naturally occurring antibiotic is a weak

Fig. 13.5. Clavulanic acid.

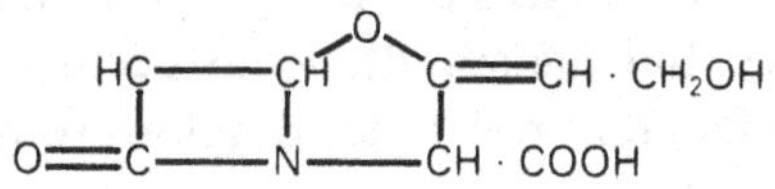

inhibitor of peptidoglycan transpeptidase but is a potent inhibitor of β-lactamase in Gram-negative and Gram-positive bacteria. Clavulanic acid contains a β-lactam ring; the drug binds covalently to the active site of β-lactamase, thereby causing an irreversible inactivation of the enzyme. Clavulanic acid, therefore, enhances the antibiotic activity of β-lactamase-sensitive antibiotics. Formulations containing clavulanic acid and β-lactam antibiotics (e.g. augmentin) are currently in clinical use. Thienamycin is an interesting β-lactam antibiotic which can inhibit both β-lactamase and peptidoglycan transpeptidase. It is still under investigation (see also Table 13.1).

13.6   PRODUCTION OF AN ALTERED BINDING SITE WITH REDUCED AFFINITY FOR THE ANTIMICROBIAL AGENT

For an antimicrobial agent to inhibit a biochemical pathway in the micro-organism it must bind to a specific receptor in the enzyme to be inhibited. Micro-organisms are known which adapt to such situations by producing an enzyme with reduced affinity for the antimicrobial agent but not for the natural substrate. This suggests that the antibiotic binds to a separate site on the enzyme to produce an allosteric enzyme inhibition (see Fig. 13.6).

The best known examples of this mechanism are in resistance to

  (a) streptomycin:
  (b) erythromycin; and
  (c) rifampicin.

(a) Streptomycin

This type of resistance occurs to streptomycin by mutation, that is, a change in the chromosomal gene which results in the formation of 30S ribosomal subunits with reduced affinity for streptomycin. The change in ribosomal structure has been traced to the S12 protein fraction of the 30S ribosomal subunit (the protein is referred to as S12 to indicate its mobility on gel electrophoresis). The altered ribosome can effectively direct protein synthesis. It must therefore be that the binding of aminoacyl-tRNA to the ribosome is not affected by the change. This type of resistance is much less clinically significant than the plasmid-mediated resistance, but the simultaneous occurrence of both types may account for the fact that resistance develops so readily to streptomycin.

Table 13.1 *Clinical usefulness of drugs with varying affinities for β-lactamase and peptidoglycan transpeptidase enzymes*

Drug	Affinity for		Remark
	β-lactamase	Peptidoglycan transpeptidase	
Penicillin G ⎫ Cephalosporin ⎰	High	High	Ineffective against β-lactamase-producing bacteria
Methicillin	Low	High	β-lactamase resistant
Clavulanic acid	High	Low	Enhances the activities of β-lactamase-sensitive antibiotics
Thienamycin	High	High	Effective against β-lactamase-producing bacteria

(b) Erythromycin

Erythromycin inhibits protein synthesis by binding to 50S ribosomal subunits and preventing peptidyl-tRNA from translocating, thereby preventing chain elongation (page 210). Micro-organisms resistant to erythromycin are mutants which produce an altered form of 50S subunit in which the erythromycin receptor has a reduced binding affinity for the antibiotic. The mutant receptor protein can bind peptidyl-tRNA and so translocation and peptide enlongation can take place. The resistant organisms can thus grow in the presence of the antibiotic.

(c) Rifampicin

Rifampicin provides another example. This antibiotic inhibits protein synthesis by blocking RNA polymerase (page 216). In resistant mutants, the polymerase enzyme has a reduced affinity for the antibiotic. In some cases the enzyme fails totally to bind the drug. The binding of the enzyme to the natural substrate is not affected.

13.7 REDUCED UPTAKE OF THE ANTIMICROBIAL AGENT

Penetration into the intracellular compartment of the micro-organism by the antimicrobial agent is a critically important step in the action of the drug. This is so because virtually all antimicrobial agents act on processes taking place inside the cell. Therefore an obvious mechanism by which organisms can protect themselves from injury is to reduce the amount of antimicrobial agent entering them. There are several examples of this type of resistance discussed below.

(a) Aminoglycosides

In resistant bacteria, aminoglycosides are phosphorylated, adenylated or acetylated to inactive products by a variety of inactivating enzymes. These products inhibit the permease which normally facilitates the accumulation of the antibiotic in the micro-organism. The result is that not only do the inactivated products not enter the cell, but they also prevent the entry of any aminoglycoside molecules that have escaped inactivation.

Fig. 13.6. A mechanism of resistance.
(A) Substrate (S) binds to substrate binding site (Sbs) on enzyme to complete an essential biochemical step.
(B) An inhibitor antimicrobial agent (I) binds to an allosteric site on the enzyme (Ibs) and thereby alters Sbs so that substrate cannot bind.
(C) A resistant microorganism makes an enzyme in which Ibs has reduced affinity for the inhibitor therefore S can bind normally to Sbs even in the presence of inhibitor. The essential biochemical step is completed.

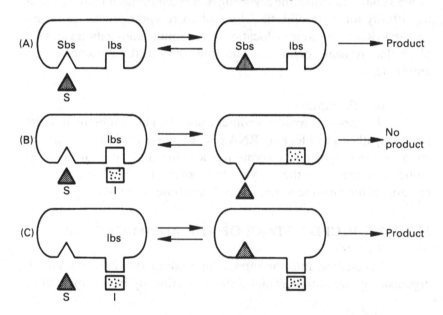

(b) Loss of intracellular binding site

Reduced drug uptake can also occur if covalent binding to intracellular structures is abolished. For example, streptomycin normally binds covalently to 30S ribosome in sensitive cells. However, resistant mutants produce a form of 30S ribosome that fails to bind streptomycin. Therefore streptomycin leaves the cell as quickly as it enters. Measurement of intracellular streptomycin would thus show reduced uptake even though the cell membrane transport of streptomycin is not altered. A similar mechanism also operates in *Plasmodium falciparum* resistance to chloroquine.

(c) Reduced membrane permeability

A well known example of this is in resistance to tetracycline. The tetracyclines inhibit bacterial cell growth by blocking protein synthesis. Entry of the antibiotic into the cell is by a facilitated transport requiring metabolic energy. In resistant organisms, tetracycline induces the production of another protein that blocks the activity of the tetracycline specific carrier protein, thereby reducing the amount of tetracycline reaching the protein-synthesising site.

13.8 PRODUCTION OF AN ALTERNATIVE ENZYME TO THE ONE INHIBITED BY THE ANTIMICROBIAL AGENT

Many antimicrobial agents interfere with microbial cell function by blocking specific enzyme systems. Resistant micro-organisms survive the toxic effect of such agents by switching on an alternative enzyme to the one that is blocked. This mechanism has been encountered in organisms resistant to sulphonamides and diaminopyrimidines.

(a) Sulphonamides

Sulphonamides block the enzyme dihydropteroate synthetase and prevent PABA utilisation in folic acid synthesis. The production of this enzyme in sensitive organisms is directed by chromosomal genes whereas resistance to sulphonamides is carried on R-factors. The R-factor genes direct the formation of a type of the enzyme which is at least 1000 times less sensitive to inhibition by sulphonamides than the chromosomal enzyme. Therefore resistant organisms are able to utilise PABA for folic acid synthesis in the presence of high concentrations of sulphonamides (Fig. 13.7).

(b) Diaminopyrimidines

Resistance to diaminopyrimidines such as trimethoprim and pyrimethamine occur by a similar mechanism. The target enzyme for these drugs in the chromosomal dihydrofolate reductase. R-factor-determined enzymes are insensitive to trimethoprim. Therefore, resistant organisms including bacteria and malaria parasites are able to produce tetrahydrofolate in the presence of high concentrations of trimethoprim or pyrimethamine.

The sulphonamide, sulphamethoxazole, is often combined with trimethoprim on the principle that sequential blockade of tetrahydrofolate production in micro-organisms would prevent the emergence of resistance. However, bacteria and *P. falciparum* are now emerging that harbour R-factors with resistance markers for both sulphonamides and trimethoprim.

Fig. 13.7. A mechanism of resistance to sulphonamides.
(a) **In sensitive organisms sulphonamides (△) prevent the chromosomal enzyme (CE)-directed utilisation of PABA (△) in the synthesis of folic acid.**
(b) **In resistant organisms, R-factor genes make a new enzyme (NE) which can utilise PABA for folic acid synthesis, but is not blocked by sulphonamides.**

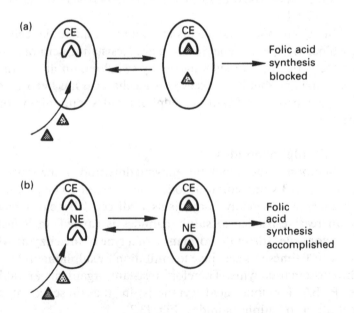

13.9 PRODUCTION OF INCREASED AMOUNTS OF THE ENZYME INHIBITED BY THE ANTIMICROBIAL AGENT

Trimethoprim

Where an antimicrobial agent interferes with an enzyme in the micro-organism, the agent and a natural substrate compete for the active site on the enzyme. If an organism can achieve an increased synthesis of the target enzyme, it can overcome the effect of the agent by providing excess enzyme for the natural substrate. Many examples of this form of resistance are known. Resistance to trimethoprim and amethopterin, both inhibitors, of dihydrofolate reductase, is associated with increased levels of the enzyme which may be several hundred-fold greater than in sensitive cells.

13.10 DRUG RESISTANCE IN MALARIA

Introduction

Drug resistance in malaria is defined by the World Health Organisation as the 'ability of a parasite strain to survive and/or multiply despite the administration and absorption of a drug given in doses equal to or higher than those usually recommnded but within the limits of tolerance of the subject'. For drug resistance to be evoked as the reason for therapeutic failure, it must be ascertained that the resistant parasite has been exposed, during therapy, to plasma concentrations of the drug equal to or higher than those which normally kill sensitive parasites. Thus therapeutic failures arising from inadequate dosage, inadequate absorption, or failure of host tissues to form active metabolites from pro-drugs, are not cases of resistance. Drug resistance must also be distinguished from inherent insusceptibility of the malaria parasite to a given drug. Thus the sulphonamides are normally less effective against forms of malaria other than *P. falciparum*, and chloroquine is more effective in *P. falciparum* than in *P. malariae* infections.

The problem of drug resistance embraces all human species of malaria parasites and all groups of drugs used in their treatment. However, the most crucial practical problem relates to resistance of *P. falciparum* to 4-aminoquinolines and specifically to chloroquine. This is so because, of all the species of human malaria parasites, the infection caused by *P. falciparum* is the most lethal, and chloroquine is by far the most effective drug in the treatment of an acute falciparum malaria attack. None of the other available drugs, alone or in combination, has the therapeutic efficacy of chloroquine. Furthermore, the

widespread and high level resistance to 4-aminoquinolines seen with
P. falciparum is not encountered in *P. malariae, P. vivax* or *P. ovale.*

P. falciparum is at present the only species of human malaria parasite to develop resistance to chloroquine. It is also the case that where
high level resistance to chloroquine is prevalent, resistance to other
antimalarial drugs is frequently encountered.

13.11   GRADATION OF RESISTANCE

Drug resistance is suspected when infected patients fail to
respond to therapy in the usual way. Different degrees of resistance are
recognised. In mild forms of resistance, the asexual erythrocytic parasites survive the effect of the drug in numbers insufficient for detection;
clinical symptoms of the disease subside. However, when the drug
therapy is stopped, the surviving parasites resume development and
recrudescence ensues. In high level resistance, the asexual parasites continue to multiply in the presence of the drug. The WHO has
recommended the gradation of responses set out in Table 13.2.

13.12   MODELS FOR THE STUDY OF DRUG RESPONSE IN MALARIA

Drug response can be studied in the field on patients naturally
infected by *P. falciparum* malaria, in experimental animal models, or *in
vitro* according to the methods developed by Trager & Jensen (1976).
Experimental animal models include *P. burghei burghei* in rodents, *P.
cynomolgi* and *P. knowlesi* in rhesus monkeys (*Macaca mulata*) and *P.
vivax* and *P. falciparum* in owl monkeys (*Aotus trivirgatus*). The basis of
the *in vitro* tests is that maturation of the ring forms of *P. falciparum*
parasites into mature schizonts, containing two or more nuclei, is
inhibited by chloroquine and DHFR inhibitors (see page 221).

13.13   GEOGRAPHICAL DISTRIBUTION OF
P. FALCIPARUM RESISTANCE

High to moderate level resistance is now a well established
problem in several countries of South East Asia, e.g. Bangladesh,
Burma, Kampuchea, Malaysia, Papua New Guinea, The Philippines,
Southern China, North East India, Thailand, and Vietnam. It is said
that the entire malarial pool in Thailand is resistant to 4-amino-
quinolines. In South America, *P. falciparum* resistance has been found
in parts of Brazil, Colombia, French Guiana, Guyana, Surinam,
Bolivia, Ecuador, and Venezuela. In Africa where resistance was

Table 13.2 *WHO grading of resistance of asexual parasites (P. falciparum) to schizonticidal drugs*

Response	Recommended symbol	Evidence
Sensitivity	S	Clearance of asexual parasitaemia within 7 days of the first day of treatment without recrudescence
Resistance	RI	Clearance of asexual parasitaemia as in sensitivity, followed by recrudescence
	RII	Marked reduction of asexual parasitaemia, but not clearance
	RIII	No marked reduction of asexual parasitaemia

unknown until 1979, *P. falciparum* resistance of the RI grade has been reported in Kenya, Tanzania, Uganda and Madagascar. The reservoir of drug resistance in malaria is thus very large and increasing and threatening.

13.14 HOW DRUG RESISTANCE IN MALARIA DEVELOPS
Some major factors predisposing to the initiation of drug resistance in malaria are discussed below.

(a) The widespread use of chloroquine, especially for prophylaxis, might exert selection pressure allowing pre-existing resistant parasite mutants to survive. The therapeutic use of 4-aminoquinolines for the exclusive purpose of treating acute infections exerts little selection pressure. Chloroquine resistance usually occurs on a large scale, in places where the drug has been freely used for prophylactic purposes.

(b) Transmission of resistant mutants from endemic areas to areas where mosquitoes able to establish a resistant strain exist. Most species of anopheline mosquito can serve as vector for any strain of resistant *P. falciparum*.

(c) When sporozoites of a resistant strain of *P. falciparum* are injected into man, gametocytes developing from them can mate with gametocytes from a sensitive strain present at the same time and so produce a hybrid-resistant strain. In the absence of hybridisation, the resistant parasite can survive several transmissions in the mosquito and outlive sensitive strains. Thus once a resistant strain is introduced into a population, it eventually establishes itself. This is in contrast to bacterial resistance in which the organisms usually revert to sensitive forms when drug selection pressure is removed.

13.15 BIOCHEMICAL BASIS OF DRUG RESISTANCE IN MALARIA

Chloroquine resistance in *P. falciparum* is believed to be due to loss of high affinity binding sites in the resistant parasite. The evidence for this view is that the selective concentration of chloroquine by erythrocytes invaded by sensitive falciparum parasites is lost in infections by resistant parasites. In resistant cells there appear to be decreases in the number and binding affinity of chloroquine receptors (e.g. ferriprotoporphyrin, see page 239) in the malaria parasite.

Resistance to the 4-aminoquinolines (chloroquine and amodiaquine), the DHFR inhibitors (proguanil and pyrimethamine) and the sulphonamides, is the result of spontaneous mutation of nuclear genes (page 297). Chloroquine resistance develops after many years of exposure to the drug, whereas resistance to DHFR inhibitors can occur after a brief exposure of the parasite. Peters has suggested an explanation of this difference based on comparison of concentration/effect curves for chloroquine and DHFR inhibitors. It is pointed out that the curve for chloroquine is much steeper than the curve for proguanil. Consequently, for a relatively small increase in chloroquine concentration, its activity can be increased by a large amount. On the other hand, with proguanil, a large increase in concentration produces only a relatively small increase in activity. Furthermore, the action of proguanil and other DHFR inhibitors is *plasmodistatic* whereas the 4-aminoquinolines are *plasmodicidal*. Thus with the usual doses of both drugs, mutants resistant to proguanil have a higher chance of surviving therapy than chloroquine-resistant mutants. So it will take longer for any pre-existing chloroquine-resistant mutants to emerge than those resistant to proguanil.

13.16 DRUG TREATMENT OF *P. FALCIPARUM* MALARIA RESISTANT TO 4-AMINOQUINOLINES

The established drugs employed in the treatment of resistant *P. falciparum* are quinine, alone or in combination with pyrimethamine, dapsone, or other long-acting sulphonamide. In the hard-core areas of Indochina, quinine combined with tetracyclines has been found effective. Other drug combinations which have been found successful are: sulphadoxine + pyrimethamine (Fansidar); sulphalene + pyrimethamine; and sulphalene + trimethoprim.

The incidence of resistance encountered in the use of established antimalarial drugs has focused attention on the possibility of antibiotics being used in the treatment of malaria. Recent studies have shown that in concentrations normally achieved in antibacterial therapy, erythromycin, chloramphenicol, clindamycin, rifampicin, and tetracycline have antiparasitic effects.

Studies with antibiotics in the treatment of malaria are important for two reasons; the pharmacological profile of the drugs is already established, and as the mode of action of these drugs is reasonably clearly understood, their study should help to unravel further the complicated biochemistry of the malaria parasite.

FURTHER READING

Echeverria, P., Verhaert, L., Vlyangco, Romolarini, S., Ho, M. T., Orskov, F. & Orskov, I. (1978). Antimicrobial resistance and enterotoxin production among isolates of *Escherichia coli* in the Far East. *Lancet*, **2**, 589–92.

Franklin, T. J. & Snow, G. A. (1981). *Biochemistry of Antimicrobial Action*, 3rd edn. Chapman and Hall Ltd., London & New York.

Peters, W. (1969). Drug resistance in malaria – a perspective. *Trans. R. Soc. Trop. Med. Hyg.* **63**, 25–38.

Rolinson, G. N. (1971). Bacterial resistance to penicillins and cephalosporins. *Proc. R. Soc. Lond.* B **179**, 403.

Trager, W. & Jensen, J.B. (1976), Human malaria parasites in continuous culture. *Science*, **193**, 673.

14

Strategies for the development of new drugs

14.1 INTRODUCTION

Most of the drugs now used in the treatment of tropical diseases were introduced at a time when relatively little was known of the molecular and biochemical processes occurring in the causative agents. Drug development was empirical, based on testing a whole range of structurally related compounds to see which was most useful. In the last 10 years it has been possible to adopt rational approaches to drug development. These are based on improved knowledge of the biochemistry and other features of the disease-causing agents. Some of these new strategies are described in this chapter. Although useful drugs have not emerged from these approaches, this chapter is worth reading because the scientific principles on which they are based are interesting and will almost certainly form the background to the usage of a new generation of drugs in the tropics. The chapter opens with sickle-cell disease. The attempts so far made to develop anti-sickling drugs are discussed in some detail for two reasons. Firstly, the drug therapy for this important tropical disease is not dealt with elsewhere in this book, there being no specifically effective anti-sickling drugs in use. Secondly, a student of pharmacology in the tropics should know what sort of research is being done to find an effective anti-sickling drug and hopefully be inspired to go on to participate in this challenging endeavour.

14.2 SICKLE CELL DISEASE

The American physician, Herrick, first noted the presence of sickled red cells in the blood of a West Indian medical student suffering from anaemia in 1904. Herrick (1910) subsequently linked the occurrence of these peculiarly shaped elongated red blood corpuscles with the severe anaemia now known as sickle cell disease. In the 80 years since Herrick's first observation, much has been learnt about the nature of sickle cell disease. The disease is autosomally inherited. The gene has a high frequency among people of African descent and among people living in regions where falciparum malaria is or has been endemic. The disease is responsible for high rates of mortality especially in infants. In parts of Nigeria, the incidence of sickle cell trait (see below) is as high as 30% of the population. Many children born with sickle cell anaemia die before the age of five. *Abiku*, celebrated in poetry by Wole Soyinka and J. P. Clark are almost certainly sickle cell deaths (see page 18).

There is as yet no effective drug therapy for the disease. However, knowledge of the sickling process is advancing, and several attempts at drug development have been made. In the following pages, essential features of the sickling phenomen are presented together with some of the ideas on drug development.

Haemoglobin-A and haemoglobin-S

The normal human haemoglobin molecule consists of two separate moieties – haem and globin. Globin is a tetrameric protein and accounts for 97% of the mass of the haemoglobin molecule. The globin tetramer consists of 4 polypeptide chains – 2 alpha and 2 beta chains. The alpha and beta chains differ in respect of 10 amino acids. The haem moiety accounts for 3% of the mass of the haemoglobin molecule. In each haemoglobin molecule, there are four haem moieties each linked to one of the polypeptide chains of globin.

In 1949, Linus Pauling showed that the haemoglobin molecule from people who suffered from sickle cell anaemia was abnormal in its electrophoretic mobility. He termed the sickle cell haemoglobin, *Haemoglobin-S (Hb-S)* and the normal haemoglobin, *Haemoglobin-A (Hb-A)*. In electrophoresis, the velocity (V) of migration of a protein molecule in an electric field is described by

$$V = \frac{EZ}{f}$$

where E = strength of electric field; Z = net electric charge on the protein; and f =frictional resistance coefficient of the protein molecule.

The frictional resistance coefficient is a function of the size and shape of the molecule. Another property of protein molecules is the *isoelectric point*. This is defined as the pH at which there is no net charge on the protein molecule. At this pH the electrophoretic mobility is zero. Below the isoelectric pH, the molecule is positively charged: above the isoelectric pH, it is negatively charged. Thus proteins carrying different numbers of charged groups in their molecules have different isoelectric points.

The isoelectric pH difference between Hb-S and Hb-A is the same whether the haemoglobin is oxygenated or deoxygenated. The difference is due to the number of ionisable groups in the two kinds of haemoglobin molecules. Hb-S has two less negative charges per molecule than Hb-A. Figure 14.1 is a diagrammatic representation of the electrophoretic pattern of Hb-A, Hb-S and Hb-AS on starch gel.

Pauling's work thus demonstrated that sickle cell anaemia is a disease caused by an alteration in the structure of haemoglobin molecules, hence the term 'molecular disease' was used to describe sickle cell anaemia. In 1957 Ingram used the technique of finger-printing to show that Hb-S differs from Hb-A by a single aminoacid. The technique of finger-printing involves tryptic digestion of a protein molecule to yield small molecular weight peptides, and separation of the peptides by a two-dimensional procedure – electrophoresis in a horizontal direction and paper chromatography in a vertical direction. It was shown that Hb-S contains the aminoacid *valine* instead of *glutamic acid* at position 6 of the beta chain as shown below:

    Hb-A :   Val – His – Leu – Thr – Pro – Glu – Glu – Lys
    Hb-S :   Val – His – Leu – Thr – Pro – Val – Glu – Lys
beta chain :   1   2   3   4   5   6   7   8

The side chain of valine is non-polar whereas that of glutamate is highly polar. This alteration greatly reduces the solubility of deoxygenated Hb-S.

Inheritance of haemoglobin-S

An individual who inherits sickle cell genes from both parents is a sickle cell homozygote (Hb-SS) and suffers from sickle cell disease. Most of the haemoglobin in his red cells is Hb-S. An individual who inherits a sickle cell gene from one parent and a normal haemoglobin gene from the other parent is a heterozygote (Hb-AS): 25–40% of the haemoglobin in a heterozygote is Hb-S and the rest is Hb-A. This amount of Hb-S is not enough to cause sickling under normal circumstances. A heterozygote thus has the sickle cell trait but does not suffer from the disease. In fact, as will be seen, the heterozygote has an advantage over individuals with normal haemoglobin in an environment where falciparum malaria is endemic since the heterozygote is resistant to malaria infection. However, sickling can occur in the heterozygote if exposed to a rarified atmosphere such as occurs on high mountains or in unpressurised aircraft at high altitudes or under conditions of anaesthesia.

Other abnormal haemoglobins

Other abnormal haemoglobins can coexist with Haemoglobin-S. An individual who inherits two different abnormal haemoglobins, one from each parent, is referred to as a genetic compound. An example of a genetic compound is that of haemoglobin-F (foetal haemoglobin) and Hb-S. Normally the synthesis of HB-F stops early in life. However in some individuals, high amounts of Hb-F continue to be synthesised in adult life. High persistent foetal haemoglobin (HPFH) is an inherited characteristic. Existence of this abnormality in the Hb-SS homozygote appears to protect the latter from sickle cell disease as foetal haemoglobin can prevent Hb-S cells from sickling. This partly accounts for the variable severity of sickle cell anaemia in Hb-SS homozygotes in different parts of the world.

Gelation of Hb-S

Red cells containing Hb-S become distorted in shape (sickled) when exposed to an environment of low oxygen tension and Hb-S loses its oxygen to form deoxyhaemoglobin-S. When the concentration of deoxyhaemoglobin-S reaches a critical level in the red cell (the socalled minimum gelling concentration (MGC)) the molecules stick together to form long fibrous polymers. The process is known as gelation. Deoxyhaemoglobin-S molecules gel because the presence of

Fig. 14.1. Diagrammatic representation of starch-gel electrophoretic pattern of normal and sickle cell haemoglobins.

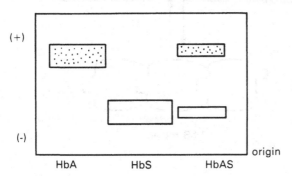

valine in place of glutamate in the β-globin chain gives the Hb-S molecule 'patches' which enable them to 'stick' together (Fig. 14.2). Deoxyhaemoglobin-A molecules do not have *'sticky patches'*. Oxygenated Hb-S molecules have sticky patches, but the complementary site with which the sticky patch has to interact is masked. Hence normal haemoglobin or oxyhaemoglobin-S molecules do not gel. A number of Hb-S molecules become stuck together end to end by a reacting sticky patch with complementary site to form rodlets or needles. Another property which the presence of valine in residue 6 of the β chain confers is that it enables the rodlets to stick together sideways by means of hydrophobic bonds. Up to 14 rodlets can stick together to form tightly packed reversible aggregates. The polymers so formed precipitate out of solution and the red cell becomes distorted into various shapes including the characteristic sickled form.

Sickling is strongly dependent on the concentration of deoxyhaemoglobin-S. The low pO_2 in the capillaries therefore favours the sickling of Hb-S containing red blood cells. Because of the distorted shapes of the sickled cells, the latter become stuck in the capillaries; more oxygen extraction causes a further lowering of intracellular pO_2 which will increase the concentration of deoxyhaemoglobin-S leading to more sickling. Furthermore, sickling increases the viscosity of blood, thereby

Fig. 14.2. Gelation of haemoglobin-S. Deoxyhaemoglobin-S molecules stick together when the 'sticky patch' (S) on the molecule reacts with the complementary site (C) on another molecule.

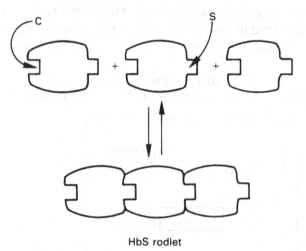

HbS rodlet

increasing the transit time of red blood cells, a factor which can increase the tendency of Hb-S to gel. Also sickled cells passing into an environment of high pO_2 would revert to normal shape and can sickle again in low pO_2. Repeated sickling and unsickling leads to a net loss of water and K^+ from the cell producing a dehydrated cell with increased concentration of Hb-S which enhances the rate of gelation. Thus, sickling once started sets up a vicious cycle.

Sickling is an inherent property of Hb-S, not of the red cell membrane

If a concentrated oxygenated Hb-S solution is transferred into a normal red cell from which the Hb-A has been removed, and the membrane then sealed, and the cell deoxygenated, the haemoglobin-S molecules gel and the cell membrane assumes the characteristic shape of a sickled cell. On the other hand, if a concentrated solution of Hb-A is inserted into the membrane of a 'sickle' cell which is then deoxygenated, the haemoglobin does not gel, and the normal discoid shape of the red cell is retained (Fig. 14.3). This shows that the distortion of shape is brought about by the behaviour of the Hb-S inside the cell.

Irreversibly sickled cells (ISC)

Intracellular polymerisation of the Hb-S leads to functional abnormalities in the red cell membrane which result in increased K^+ loss from, and increased Na^+ movement into, the cell. This is thought to be caused by a defect in the $Na^+ - K^+$ ATP-ase pump. Calmodulin is mobilised, leading to accumulation of Ca^{2+}.

Drug Therapy

There are no specifically effective drugs for the treatment of sickle cell disease. Analgesics are used to relieve the severe pain in joints and limbs which is a characteristic feature of acute sickle cell crisis. Aspirin is commonly used for this purpose and it is possible that apart from its analgesic properties, the patient may also benefit from its anti-inflammatory actions; aspirin blocks cyclo-oxygenase and hence the formation of thromboxane, a powerful stimulant of platelet aggregation. Aspirin thus increases prothrombin time and delays clotting; this would be an advantage in sickle cell disease.

In addition, antibiotics may be used if bacterial infection is a complicating factor and steps are usually taken to prevent parasitic infections such as malaria as these may exacerbate the crisis. Acid–base balance is usually monitored and if acidosis is present, sodium bicarbonate may be given.

Antisickling drugs

The increased knowledge of the processes underlying the sickling phenomenon, has been paralleled by attempts to produce 'antisickling' agents. None of these has found clinical use, partly because of excessive toxicity. Nevertheless, the study of the mechanisms of action of some of these compounds has shown that it is possible to attack the sickling process and prevent it by rationally designed drugs. The Hb-S molecule can be viewed as a potential disease-producing particle with peculiar properties, not possessed by other normal

Fig. 14.3. Membrane distortion in sickling is secondary to change in Hb-S molecule.

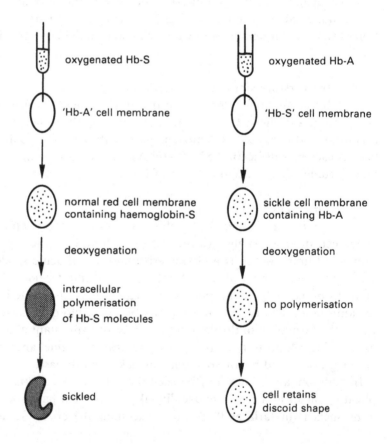

oxygenated Hb-S

'Hb-A' cell membrane

normal red cell membrane
containing haemoglobin-S

deoxygenation

intracellular
polymerisation
of Hb-S molecules

sickled

oxygenated Hb-A

'Hb-S' cell membrane

sickle cell membrane
containing Hb-A

deoxygenation

no polymerisation

cell retains
discoid shape

molecules in the body. Thus, the aim in sickle cell chemotherapy research is to find drugs capable of selectively preventing the Hb-S red blood cell from sickling. Clinically, such agents may act prophylactically to prevent sickling, or be used in the treatment of sickle cell disease if they can reverse the sickling process. This principle is similar to the idea of selective toxicity in the chemotherapy of bacterial and parasitic infections and cancer, discussed elsewhere in this book. The difference is that in sickle cell disease chemotherapy, the aim is to prevent and/or reverse sickling but not to destroy or interfere with vital functions of the Hb-S red blood cells. It is a much more difficult task than killing or preventing the growth of pathogenic micro-organisms.

Targets for drug action in sickle cell disease

From what has been said in relation to the processes of gelation, there are in theory several potential targets for drug action in sickle cell disease. Three which have been explored are listed below.

(1) Direct inhibition of Hb-S polymer formation

Many compounds can apparently inhibit Hb-S polymer formation by complex mechanisms.

(i) Urea

Urea is a well known protein denaturant that can disrupt hydrophobic bonds in many proteins. In 1970, it was discovered that urea could prevent and reverse sickling of Hb-S cells *in vitro*. Because urea is easily permeable through the red cell membrane, metabolically inert, water-soluble, nontoxic in reasonable quantities, and readily excreted, it seemed the ideal substance for clinical trials. Unfortunately, the concentrations at which urea showed any beneficial effects were too high to be tolerated by most patients. High doses of urea turned out to be fatal through acute dehydration.

(ii) Cyanate

Cyanate is known to carbamylate several functional groups of proteins. Potassium cyanate (0.03 M) caused a marked inhibition of sickling, presumably by carbamylation of red cell haemoglobin-S. Unlike the urea effect, carbamylation of Hb-S not only inhibited sickling but also increased the oxygen affinity of Hb-S. Unfortunately, clinical trials revealed that potassium cyanate was ineffective in preventing painful sickle cell episodes. Furthermore, many patients showed symptoms of peripheral neuropathy due to cyanate poisoning.

(2) Increase in the affinity of Hb-S for oxygen

An increase in the affinity of Hb-S for oxygen effectively reduces the concentration of deoxy-Hb-S. Since the concentration of deoxy-Hb-S is critically important for Hb-S polymerisation this should prevent sickling. Many substances have been tested as antisickling agents whose mode of action appears to be, to move the oxygen dissociation curve to the left (see Beddell et al, 1984). In theory, agents of this type can interact with the binding site of 2,3,-diphosphoglycerate (2,3-DPG) by a direct competitive antagonism or by binding at an alternative site on the haemoglobin tetramer in the oxyconformation and producing an allosteric non-competitive antagonism to 2,3-DPG. There is reason to believe that most agents which increase the oxygen affinity of Hb-S, do so by the latter mechanism, that is by allosteric non-competitive alteration of 2,3,-DPG binding sites. 2,3-DPG is present in red cells in the same molecular concentration as haemoglobin and has a large effect on the oxygen affinity of haemoglobin. In the absence of 2,3-DGP, oxygen affinity for haemoglobin is increased by a factor of 26. The physiological function of 2,3-DPG in reducing oxygen binding by haemoglobin is to ensure maximum delivery of oxygen to tissues. By modifying 2,3-DPG binding sites, certain drugs can increase the oxygen affinity of Hb-S.

Fig. 14.4. Acetylation of haemoglobin (Hb).

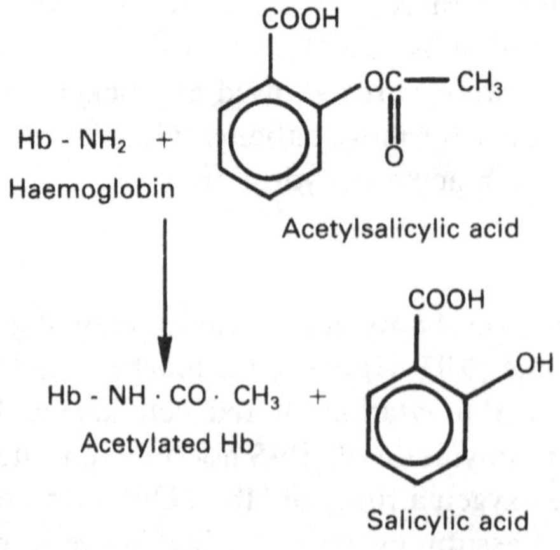

Another target for drug action is the enzyme diphosphoglycerate mutase which regulates the DPG level (Luzzatto & Goodfellow 1989).

(i) *Aspirin and aspirin derivatives*
Aspirin can acetylate amino groups of intracellular Hb-S and increase its affinity for oxygen. However, the extent of acetylation achieved by even a very high concentration of the drug is not sufficient to produce a significant inhibition of erythrocyte sickling. A number of acetylating agents, derived from aspirin, e.g. dibromoaspirin, have been investigated. The compounds acetylate the terminal amino group of the beta chain of both normal and sickle haemoglobins (Fig. 14.4).

Acetylation produces an increase in the oxygen affinity of the molecule as well as directly inhibiting erythrocyte sickling. There is no evidence that aspirin derivatives will be clinically useful as antisickling drugs.

(ii) *Pyridoxine and pyridoxal*
A major limitation of protein-modifying agents such as cyanate and aspirin is their toxicity. In 1974, Benesch had discovered that the aldehyde forms of vitamin B_6 (e.g. pyridoxal) could modify haemoglobin by forming Schiff's bases (Fig. 14.5). Pyridoxal is thought to react specifically with the terminal amino groups of the alpha chains, and to increase the oxygen affinity of haemoglobin-S. As a result, the

Fig. 14.5. Pyridoxylation of haemoglobin.

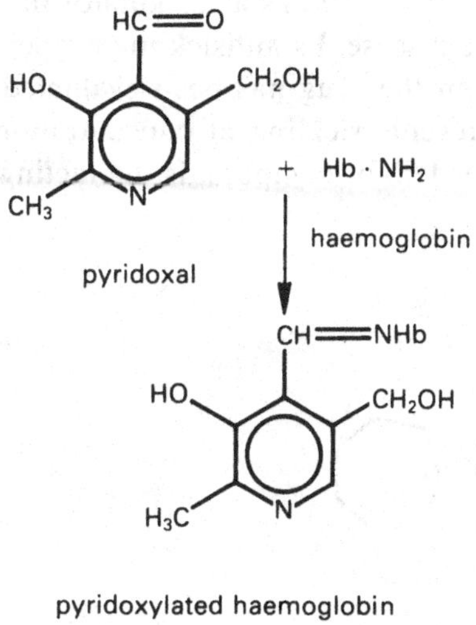

pyridoxal

+ Hb · NH_2

haemoglobin

pyridoxylated haemoglobin

concentration of deoxyHb-S is decreased and this is reflected in a sharply reduced sickled cell count in low pO_2. Other studies have shown that pyridoxine itself is taken up by red cells, where it is converted to pyridoxal. These findings excited some interest because of the low toxicity of this vitamin, but no specific therapy has emerged for this approach.

(3) Red cell membrane

For compounds which interact directly with haemoglobin to be effective, they must be present at intracellular concentrations approximating to that of haemoglobin itself. Such high concentrations are not likely to be achieved without significant toxicity. The search for antisickling compounds has therefore recently focused on the red cell membrane. One rationale for this approach is that substances which can alter membrane permeability and bring about small increases in cell water content are theoretically capable of causing large delays in sickling. Membrane-active agents can also prevent loss of intracellular K^+ by blocking a pH-dependent ouabain–insensitive K^+-channel and entry of Ca^{2+} and so prevent the formation of ISC. Membrane-active drugs offer a potential advantage over drugs which combine with haemoglobin in that the former need not pass through the membrane boundary and could be effective in lower concentrations.

(i) Cetiedil (α-cyclohexyl-3-thiophenacetic acid 2-(hexahydro-1H-azepin-1-yl) ethylester

This compound (Fig. 14.6) was synthesized in France in 1962 and has been used in Europe since 1973 as a vasodilator in the treatment of peripheral ischaemic disease. Its antisickling properties were discovered in 1977. Since then the drug has been evaluated for this purpose. This compound prevents sickling at concentrations much lower than concentrations needed for compounds interacting directly

Fig. 14.6. Cetiedil.

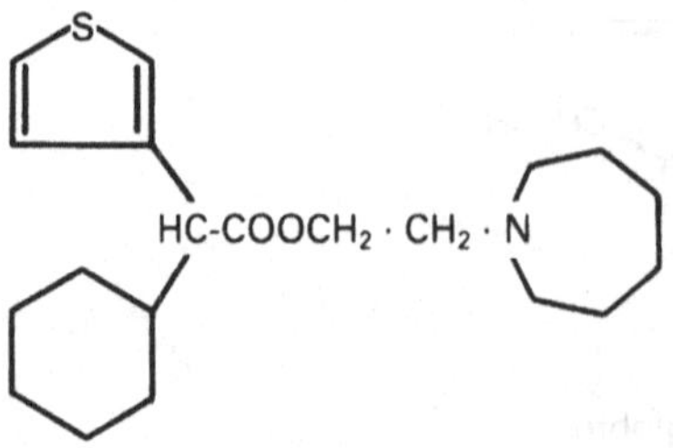

with haemoglobin. *Cetiedil* has no effect on either the oxygen affinity of the sickle cell or the minimum gelling concentration of Hb-S, neither does it alter the solubility of deoxyHb-S. The antisickling effect of cetiedil appears to be secondary to the swelling of the red cell. The drug causes an increase in passive Na^+ movements into the cell (and along with it water) and inhibits increase in K^+ permeability during gelation of Hb-S. The total effect is that the water content of the cell is increased. Cetiedil thus represents an alternative type of antisickling agent, exerting its effect through changes in membrane permeability rather than directly modifying Hb-S.

(ii) *Antipsychotic drugs*

Several antipsychotic drugs have been found to have *in vitro* antisickling effects. The antisickling activities of several compounds such as diazepam, chlorpromazine, pimozide, and penfluridol, have been found to correlate very strongly with their ability to inhibit calmodulin-stimulated phosphodiesterase activity. Some of these compounds are active in extremely low concentrations and can reverse sickling. It is most likely that the action is exerted on the cell membrane, but the mechanism is unknown. Obviously, antipsychotic drugs would not be suitable as therapy in sickle cell disease because of their powerful CNS actions, but non-neuroleptic analogues of these compounds may be usefully investigated as potential antisickling drugs.

(iii) *Fagara extracts and DBA*

In 1971, Nigerian scientists, while testing an aqueous extract of the roots of the Fagara plant (*Zanthoxylum zanthoxyloides*) for antimicrobial activity on blood-agar plates, observed that the extract also prevented red blood cells from haemolysing. Isaacs-Sodeye *et al.* (1975) subsequently showed that the crude extract could also prevent sickling *in vitro*. A limited clinical trial indicated that regular administration of the extract to sickle cell disease patients might reduce the frequency of painful episodes suffered by the patients. It is difficult to establish reliable criteria for subjective assessment of the frequency of sickle cell pain episodes. Nevertheless this report led to a frantic study of both the crude extract and of the chemically defined constituents of the extract for antisickling activity. Zanthoxyllol (Fig. 14.7) was subsequently shown *in vitro* to possess antisickling properties. Laboratory modification of zanthoxyllol yielded the compound 3,4-dihydro-2,2-dimethyl-2H-1-benzopyran-6-butyric acid (DBA), which proved to be a more potent antisickling agent than zanthoxyllol (Ekong *et al.*, 1975).

However, the site of action of DBA and its potential usefulness as an antisickling agent are not known. Natta (1979) has ascribed the following properties to the compound: (i) DBA does not bind covalently to haemoglobin but has a predominant membrane effect. (ii) It inhibits the loss of potassium from deoxygenated Hb-S erythrocytes by an action on the cell membrane. Increased K^+ efflux in deoxygenated Hb-S cells is associated with the attachment of beta and alpha globin chains to the membrane of Hb-S cells. DBA inhibits this aggregation. (iii) DBA increases the incorporation of radioactive aminoacid into globin by an unknown mechanism suggesting that the compound may increase the synthesis of haemoglobin. This interesting compound has also been shown to possess anti-inflammatory, analgesic and antipyretic properties comparable in potency to aspirin (Okpako *et al.*, 1983).

Protective effect of Hb-S in *P. falciparum* malaria

There is evidence that the sickle cell gene protects the heterozygote from *P. falciparum* malaria infection. Part of the evidence for this is that the geographical distribution of the gene is such that high fequency coincides with endemicity of falciparum malaria. Furthermore heterozygotes are observed to suffer falciparum malaria attacks less frequently than normal individuals. There is, however, controversy about the cellular mechanism of the protection. One line of thought is supported by findings by Luzzatto and others that parasitisation of the Hb-S red blood cell caused the cell to sickle more readily than otherwise; since the sickled cell is more liable to haemolysis and removal by the spleen, the cell does not survive long

Fig. 14.7. Zanthoxyllol (upper) and DBA (lower).

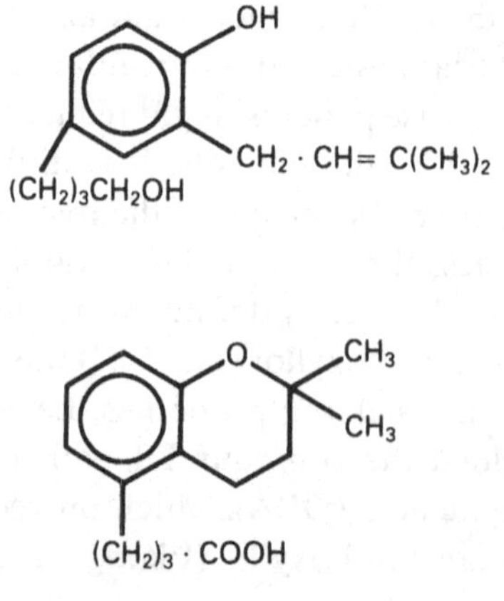

enough for parasite maturation. Hence the heterozygote is protected. It is possible also that the sickle haemoglobin is not a suitable nutrient for the parasite. Another hypothesis comes from the finding of Pasvol that the rate of parasite invasion of Hb-S red cells and of maturation of the parasites in Hb-S containing cells, is less than in normal red cells. However, the reduction in parasite invasion and development occurs only when the pO_2 of the medium is low. However, sickling of the Hb-S cell is not necessary for inhibition of invasion and maturation. All that is needed for inhibition to occur is a tendency towards sickling in an environment of reduced oxygen tension. This mechanism according to Pasvol, can explain why protection is predominantly against *P. falciparum*. Of all human malarias, *P. falciparum* is the only parasite in which the erythrocytic phase includes about 12 h in which the parasite is confined to deep tissues where the pO_2 is low.

14.3   MALARIA
Inhibition of cell invasion

Entry into the interior of specific host cells is obligatory in the development of plasmodia. Inside the cell, the parasite is protected from the host's defences and can exploit the resources available in the host's cell for its growth. Merozoites invade erythrocytes through specific recognition sites present on the red cell membrane. There is also evidence that the entry of sporozoites into liver cells is by way of specific receptors. These developments point to novel ways by which malaria may be controlled. For, if we could prevent invasion, infection would be prevented as the parasites' further development is aborted.

Erythrocyte invasion

Some progress has been made towards identifying the membrane components which serve as receptors for parasite entry into erythrocytes. There are three candidates for the erythrocyte receptor protein, namely, glycophorins, erythrocyte band 3 protein, and Duffy blood group antigen (for *P. vivax* and *P. knowlesi* only). Some of the evidence in support of a role for these proteins is as follows: (i) Invasion of erythrocytes by *P. falciparum* in *in vitro* assays is reduced if the rbc's are genetically deficient in glycophorin; invasion is also reduced if glycophorin is removed from the erythrocyte membrane by digestion with trypsin or neuraminidase, and by addition of isolated glycophorin to the assay medium. (ii) Monoclonal antibody against Rhesus band 3 protein blocks invasion of Rhesus monkey erythrocytes by *P. knowlesi* parasites. (iii) Both human erythrocyte band 3 protein and human glycophorins incorporated into liposomes are potent inhibitors of invasion of human erythrocytes by *P. falciparum*. And (iv) Human erythrocytes lacking Duffy blood group antigen (Duffy-negative erythrocytes) are resistant to invasion by merozoites of the primate parasite, *P. knowlesi*, whereas Duffy-positive human erythrocytes and Rhesus monkey erythrocytes are invaded by *P. knowlesi* merozoites.

Hepatocyte invasion

Sporozoites invade liver cells by a complicated mechanism. The parasites do not become attached to liver cells directly by way of recognition sites present in these cells, as is the case with merozoites. Sporozoites gain entrance into liver cells by becoming firmly bound to serum glycoproteins for which receptors and transport mechanisms exist on liver cell membranes. These glycoproteins (those with mannose and glacatose as terminal residues) thus serve as the carriers for sporozoites into liver cells.

The evidence for this theory is as follows: Sporozoites incubated in serum can take up, and become firmly bound to, glycoproteins having mannose and galactose terminal residues. The binding is species specific; the rodent parasite, *P. berghei berghei* can bind glycoproteins from rodent serum but not from primate serum, and *vice versa* with the primate parasite *P. knowlesi*. It is also known that there are mannose receptors in Kupffer cells and galactose receptors on hepatocyte plasma membranes. Circulating glycoproteins with galactose terminal residues are taken up and bound by hepatocytes.

The importance of these proteins lies not only in their potential as targets for inhibition of cell invasion, but also the specificity of these receptors helps to explain plasmodium life cycles and why different malarias infect different species.

Drug targeting with liposomes

So far in this book we have talked about selective toxicity in terms of using chemicals to harm the parasite but not the host by exploiting vulnerable pathways or enzymes in the parasite. It is not always possible to find a chemical substance which is toxic to the pathogenic organism but completely harmless to the host. To maximise the benefit of potentially toxic drugs, one approach is to deliver the drug directly to where the parasite is located so that there is minimum exposure to the drug, of cells in other parts of the body. This is known as drug targeting. Targeting can substantially increase the therapeutic index of the drug.

Liposomes

Targeting of a drug can be achieved by transporting it with a carrier. When water-insoluble lipids (phospholipids e.g. cholesterol phosphatidylcholine, phosphatidic acid) are mixed with water, highly ordered multilamellar structures are formed called liposomes which persist in excess water. These can be reduced to smaller unilamellar residues by suitable treatment such as sonication. Liposomes of different sizes can now be prepared to incorporate water-soluble drugs. Alternatively, lipid-soluble drugs can be embedded in the lipid phase of liposomes. Depending on their route of administration, and structural characteristics (e.g. stability, size, surface charge, lipid composition) liposomes can be made to transport drugs into various cell types in the liver, spleen, lungs, lymph nodes, etc. Liposomes (without drug) containing glycolipids with terminal galactose residue can interfere with sporozoite invasion of hepatocytes. The possibility that liver cells take up these liposomes specifically has been exploited by incorporating into the liposomes a drug (primaquine) which is known to act against the exoerythrocytic stages of the plasmodia. Although primaquine so encapsulated was no more effective than the free drug in infected mice, it was 4 times less toxic. Targeting can thus have the advantage of increasing the therapeutic index of a drug and making it more useful. The advantages of successful targeting of primaquine to the liver cells are great, especially in African patients where drug induced haemolysis precludes primaquine use in G6PD deficiency.

14.4   LEISHMANIASIS
Inhibition of purine salvage enzymes

Protozoan parasites are unable to synthesise purine nucleotides. These parasites use various purine salvage enzymes which can transfer phosphate groups from a variety of monophosphate esters to purine nucleosides to convert them to nucleotides. Among the Leishmania, the salvage enzyme purine nucleoside phosphotransferase (PNP) has been identified. This enzyme can be inhibited by purine nucleoside analogues such as allopurinol riboside and thiopurinal riboside (Fig. 14.8). These compounds are potent leishmanicides *in vitro* and *in vivo*. This is a useful approach to the development of new chemotherapeutic agents since the purine nucleoside analogues are nontoxic to the mammalian host due to lack of PNP enzyme in the latter.

Drugs targeting

A major new approach in the chemotherapy of leishmaniasis is the use of liposomes to target drugs at the parasite. The *L. donovani* parasite which causes visceral leishmaniasis is restricted to cells of the reticuloendothelial system (liver, spleen, and bone marrow). Because of their location in deep organs these parasites are quite often difficult to treat. On the other hand, after i.v. injection, liposomes are rapidly cleared from the circulation by phagocytic cells of liver and spleen. Advantage is being taken of this in the development of a drug-targeted treatment of visceral leishmaniasis. Antimonial compounds are incorporated into liposomes and administered intravenously. In the treatment of *L. donovani* in mice, liposome-encapsulated sodium stibogluconate is up to 700 times as effective as the free drug. This approach should provide an effective and safe way of using these highly toxic drugs.

14.5   TRYPANOSOMIASIS

Inhibition of glycolysis in trypanosomes

Bloodstream forms of trypanosoma are entirely dependent on glycolysis for their energy needs. A detailed study of glycolysis in these parasites has presented two possible ways of drug attack on them:

The glycosome

Under aerobic glycolysis in trypanosomes, one glucose molecule generates only two ATP molecules. This low energy yield makes it

Fig. 14.8. Allopurinol riboside (left) and thiopurinal riboside (right).

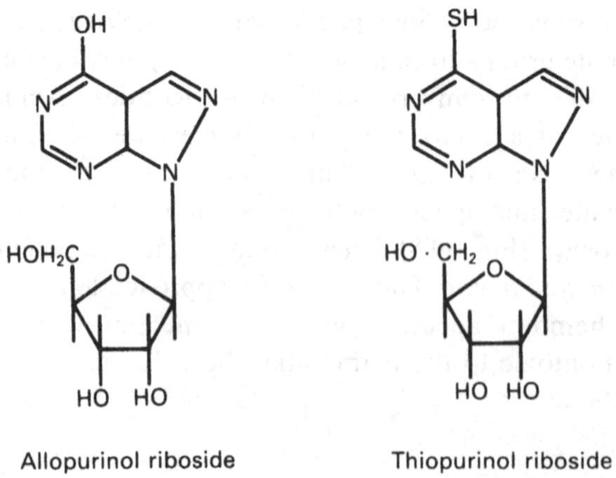

Allopurinol riboside   Thiopurinol riboside

necessary for the parasite to have an extremely high rate of glycolysis in order to meet the contingencies of an equally high rate of cell division. The rate of glycolysis in *T. brucei* is 50 times that in mammalian cells and the cell divides every seven hours. This high rate of glycolysis is made possible not only by the abundant supply of glucose in the host blood but also by the clustering of most of the glycolytic enzymes of the parasite in a membrane-bound organelle called a *glycosome*. The glycosome evolved to optimise conditions for glycolysis by creating a compartment where high concentrations of substrate and enzymes are maintained. The organelle has its own transport system which enables it to concentrate necessary metabolic intermediates. Since there is no organelle equivalent to the glycosome in mammalian cells, and since most of the glycolytic enzymes are concentrated there, this organelle is a potential chemotherapeutic target.

Inhibition of specific enzymes in trypanosome glycolytic pathway

Glycolysis in trypanosomes involves two enzymes, an NAD^1-dependent glycerol-3-phosphate dehydrogenase and a glycerol-3-phosphate oxidase. The oxidase can be blocked by the oxidase inhibitor, salicylhydroxamic acid (SHAM). This compound prevents O_2 uptake by bloodstream African trypanosomes and is a potent inhibitor of parasite glycolysis *in vitro*. It is, however, inactive *in vivo* because when the aerobic glycolytic pathway is blocked by SHAM, the parasites switch on an alternative pathway. Glycerol inhibits this alternative pathway by mass action and a combination of SHAM and glycerol has been found to be lethal *in vitro* and *in vivo* to African trypanosomes. Unfortunately, the concentration of SHAM/glycerol required to produce a radical cure is very high and very toxic. Attempts are now being made to produce practical therapeutic regimens using polyols other than glycerol and hydroxamates other than SHAM.

Other possible sites of drug action
Ornithine decarboxylase

Polyamines are found in virtually all living cells. They are required for cellular proliferation and differentiation. The major polyamines in trypanosomes are putrecine and spermidine. These are made from ornithine by ornithine decarboxylase. This enzyme can also act on the compound α-(difluoromethyl) ornithine (see below), which it converts to a product which inhibits DNA synthesis and is therefore toxic to the parasite.

$$\text{CHF}_2$$
$$|$$
$$\text{NH}_2\text{–CH}_2\text{–CH}_2\text{–CH}_2\text{–C–COOH}$$
$$|$$
$$\text{NH}_2$$

α–(difluoromethyl) ornithine

ornithine
decarboxylase

$$\text{CHF}_2$$
$$|$$
$$\text{NH}_2\text{–CH}_2\text{–CH}_2\text{–CH}_2\text{–CH}$$
$$|$$
$$\text{NH}_2$$

toxic product

α-(difluoromethyl) ornithine has been found to have good activity against African trypanosomes in infected animals and *in vitro* against *P. falciparum* schizogony.

Intracellular hydrogen peroxide

Trypanosomes lack the enzyme catalase. Therefore the production and concentration of H_2O_2 in these organisms is of interest since hydrogen peroxide is a normal product of aerobic metabolism and is known to be cytotoxic. Most cells are protected from H_2O_2 cytotoxicity by the enzyme catalase or by glutathione (GSH) peroxidase. The concentration of H_2O_2 in trypanosomes is several times higher than in mammalian cells due to lack of catalase to break it down. The parasite should also be more susceptible to any increase in intracellular H_2O_2 than mammalian cells. Indeed, naphthoquinones have been found to increase intracellular H_2O_2 of trypanosomes and are lethal to *T. cruzi* and *T. brucei in vitro*. Unfortunately, naphthoquionnes show little activity *in vivo* because of poor pharmacokinetics, but increasing intracellular H_2O_2 remains a possible target for drug action.

Variant specific antigen (VSA)

African trypanosomes have evolved an ingenious device by which they combat the host's immune response. The disease is characterised by periods of high parasitaemia in blood followed by periods of little or no parasitaemia. Each episode of high parasitaemia represents the appearance of a new antigenic type possessing a distinct glycoprotein 'coat' covering the cell surface membrane. The glycoprotein coat of one variant is immunologically distinct from that of the previous or future variant and is referred to a variant specific antigen

(VSA). VSA's have been studied extensively so that the molecular basis of antigenic variation in trypanosomes is becoming clear. It is now known for example that the VSA consists of a single glycoprotein with a molecular weight of about 65000; glycoproteins of different trypanosomal variants differ in amino acid composition, conformational features and N-terminal aminoacid sequences. A single trypanosome is capable of making hundreds of immunologically different glycoproteins. Since the process is unique to trypanosomes, its inhibition can form the basis for the development of selectively toxic chemotherapeutic agents. For example, if a drug could be found which prevented the synthesis and assembly of variant specific glycoproteins, the drug would cure infection not by destroying the parasite but by enabling the body's immune defences to deal with the infection.

FURTHER READING
Beddell, C.R., Goodford, P.J., Kneen, G., White, R.D., Wilkinson, S. & Wootton, R. (1984). Substituted benzaldehydes designed to increase oxygen affinity of human haemoglobin and inhibit the sickling of sickle erythrocytes. *Br. J. Pharmac.* 82, 397–407.

Benesch, R., Benesch, R.E., & Young, S. (1974). Chemical modifications that inhibit gelation of sickle haemoglobin. *Proc. Natl. Acad. Sci. USA* 71, 1504–5.

Berkowitz, L.R. & Orringer, E.P. (1982). Effects of cetiedil on monovalent cation permeability in the erythrocyte: an explanation for the efficacy of cetiedil in the treatment of sickle cell anaemia. *Blood Cells* 8, 283–8.

Ekong, D.E.U., Okogun, J.L., Enyinihi, V.U., Balogh-Nair, V., Nakanichi, K. & Natta, C. (1975). New antisickling agent 3,4-dihydro-2,2-dimethyl-2H-1-benzopran-6-butyric acid. *Nature* 258, 743–6.

Fleming, A.F. (1982) (ed.). *Sickle-cell Disease. A handbook for the General Clinician.* Churchill Livingstone, London.

Herrick, J.B. (1910). Peculiar elongated and sickle-shaped red blood corpuscles in a case of severe anaemia. *Archives of Internal Medicine* 6, 517–52.

Ingram, V.M. (1965). A specific chemical difference between the globins of normal human and sickle cell anaemia haemoglobin, *Nature.* 178, 792–4.

Isaacs-Sodeye, W.A., Sofowora, E.A., Williams, A.O., Marquis, V.O., Adekwale, A.A. & Anderson, C.O. (1975). Extract of *Fagara xanthoxyloides* root in sickle cell anaemia. Toxicology and preliminary clinical trials. *Acta Haemotologica* 53, 158–84.

Luzzatto, L. & Goodfellow, P. (1989). Sickle cell anaemia – a simple disease with no cure. *Nature* 337, 17–18.

Luzzatto, L., Nwachuku-Jarret, E.S. & Reddy, S. (1970). Increased sickling of parasitised erythrocytes as mechanism of resistance against malaria in the sickle cell trait. *Lancet* i, 311–22.

Manning, N.J., Ceramic, A., Gillette, P.N., de Furia, F.G. & Miller, R.D. (1973). Cyanate inhibition of red blood cell sickling. In *Sickle Cell Disease*

– Diagnosis, Management, Education and Research (eds. H. Abramson, J.F. Bertles & D.L. Wethers). The C.V. Mosby Company.

Natta, C.L. (1979). DBA: effects on sickle cells and sickle haemoglobin biosynthesis. In Development of Therapeutic Agents for Sickle Cell Disease, eds. J. Rosa, Y. Benzard & J. Hercules, P.169. Elsevier/North Holland Press, Amsterdam, New York.

Newton, B.A. (1983). New strategies in the search for antiprotozoal drugs. In Chemotherapeutic Strategies, ed. D.I. Edwards & H.R. Hiscock, p.87. The Macmillan Press Ltd., London & Basingstoke.

Okpako, D.T., Oriowo, M.A., Okogun, J.I., Ekong, D.E.U. & Enyenihi, V.U. (1983). 3,4-Dihydro-2, 2-dimethyl-2-M-1-benzopyran-6-butyric acid. Its preparation from zanthoxyllol and its anti-inflammatory and related pharmacological properties. Planta Medica 47, 112–16.

Pasvol, G. (1980). The interaction between sickle haemoglobin and the malaria parasite Plasmodium falciparum. Trans. Roy. Soc. Med. Hyg. 74, 701–5.

Pauling, L., Itano, H.A., Singer, S.J. & Wells, I.C. (1949). Sickle cell anaemia, a molecular disease. Science, 110, 543–8.

Perutz, M.F. & Mitchinson, I.M. (1950). State of haemoglobin in sickle cell anaemia. Nature 166, 677–9.

Schmidt, W.F., Asakura, T. & Schwarts, E. (1982). The effect of cetiedil on red cell membrane permeability. Blood Cells 8, 289–98.

Walder, J.A., Zaugg, R.H., Iwaoka, R.S., Watkin, W.G. & Klotz, I.M. (1977). Alternative aspirins as antisickling agents. Acetyl-3,5-dibromosalicylic acid. Proc. Natl. Acad. Sci. USA 74, 5499–503.

PART VI
Systematic Pharmacology

15

Drug targets in the nervous system

15.1 INTRODUCTION

The nervous system consists of the central and peripheral divisions. Although impulses arising in the central nervous system (CNS) do influence the functions of the peripheral nervous system (PNS), a major part of the PNS is autonomous. In the absence of CNS control, organs such as the heart, gastrointestinal tract and glands can function under the influence of the autonomic nervous system (ANS). The other reason why we can think of the PNS separately from the CNS is that the outflow of impulses from the CNS can be interrupted at the periphery by drugs that do not enter the CNS.

The CNS consists of the brain and spinal cord; the PNS consists of the efferent nerves of the ANS and the efferents in the motor nerves supplying skeletal muscles. The ANS is in turn made up of the sympathetic and parasympathetic branches. Afferent sensory fibres conducting impulses to the brain are also targets for the drug action. These are mainly concerned with the senses and reflex systems.

Another component of the ANS is the adrenal medulla which is innervated by the splanchnic nerve.

15.2 THE AUTONOMIC NERVOUS SYSTEM

The ANS is the efferent motor supply to smooth muscles (e.g. gut, blood vessels, bladder, etc.), heart and glands. The nerve fibres (preganglionic) leave the CNS and relay with a second group of nerve cells (ganglia) whose nerve fibres (postganglionic) are mainly unmyelinated. These continue to the effector (the cell or organ that responds to the stimulation of its efferent nerve). In contrast, the motor nerve supply to striated muscle runs all the way from the CNS to the effector. In mammals, preganglionic fibres of the sympathetic system leave the thoracic and lumbar segments of the spinal·cord through ventral roots to relay with chains of sympathetic ganglia (Fig. 15.1). These chains lie on each side of the spinal cord ventral to the vertebral column. At the relay station, the preganglionic fibre meets the sympathetic cell body (sympathetic ganglion) from which postganglionic fibres run to effectors. Preganglionic fibres of the parasympathetic on the other hand leave the CNS through cranial nerves (e.g. vagus) and the sacral segments of the spinal cord. The parasympathetic cell bodies (ganglia) with which the preganglionic fibres synapse are embedded in, or close to, the effector organs which they innervate.

Fig. 15.1. Diagrammatic representation of the functional organisation of the peripheral nervous system. Cranial, thoracolumbar and sacral outflows of the autonomic nervous system are represented: P = parasympathetic and S= sympathetic. Solid lines are used to represent preganglionic, splanchnic efferents (SP) to the adrenal medulla (AM) and motor efferents to skeletal muscle (SM). Dashed lines represent postganglionic fibres. The paravertebral ganglionic chain is represented by PVG.

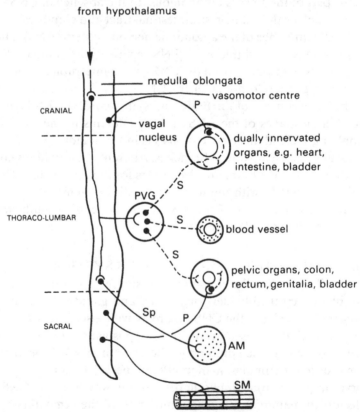

Parasympathetic and preganglionic sympathetic fibres are cholinergic (that is, they release acetylcholine when stimulated). Postganglionic sympathetic fibres are almost all noradrenergic, that is, their neurotransmitter is noradrenaline. An exception is the sympathetic nerve to sweat glands where the postganglionic nerve transmitter is acetylcholine. The splanchnic nerve to the adrenal medulla releases acetylcholine which in turn releases adrenaline and noradrenaline.

Sensory afferent fibres which are linked to internal receptors concerned with the reflex activities of the ANS are also components of the ANS. Examples are the afferent fibres to the vasomotor centre in the medulla that are linked to barareceptors in the carotid. These receptors can sense arterial pressure changes and send impulses to the vasomotor centre which then activates the sympathetic outflow. The CNS coordination of the ANS occurs in the hypothalamus, medulla and spinal cord.

Functions of the ANS

The physiological function of the parasympathetic system can be roughly said to be the conservation and restoration of energy whereas the sympathetic is concerned with the expenditure of energy when the animal is under stress. For example, activation of the parasympathetic system slows the heart, lowers blood pressure, increases secretion and motility in the gastrointestinal tract, aids absorption of nutrients, and empties the bladder and rectum. In general the sympathetic system has effects opposite to those of the parasympathetic. The sympathetic system is responsible for unconscious adjustments to changes in body temperature, blood sugar, vascular responses to haemorrhage, exercise, change in posture and oxygen need. In 'fright, fight or flight', the sympathetic system and adrenal medulla are activated; the heart rate increases rapidly, blood pressure rises, blood vessels in the skin and splanchnic areas are constricted and blood is shunted to skeletal muscle, the heart and brain; blood sugar rises and bronchi and pupils dilate.

The muscles of the small intestine receive a motor supply from the vagus (parasympathetic) and an inhibitory supply from the sympathetic. There is in addition a local nerve network (Auerbach's plexus), which, even when the muscle is separated from the CNS, can execute the reflexes concerned with peristalsis and propulsion of gut contents. In hollow organs such as the bladder, stimulation of the sacral nerves (parasympathetic) causes contraction of the body of the bladder (detrusor) and a relaxation of its sphincter, so that micturition takes place. Stimulation of the sympathetic produces the opposite effect. Some organs are innervated by only one division of the ANS, e.g. uterus, adrenal medulla; most arterioles (except those supplying the genital organs) are innervated only by the sympathetic, while glands of the stomach and pancreas are innervated only by the parasympathetic.

Neuroeffector junction

In the nervous system, the nerve does not fuse with the effector cell. The narrow gap between the nerve ending and the effector cell is called the neuroeffector or synaptic junction. Some texts use the term 'neuromuscular junction' for autonomic nerve junctions; it is better to use 'neuroeffector junction' for autonomic nerve junctions with, e.g. smooth muscle, and to reserve the term 'neuromuscular junction' for motor-nerve–skeletal muscle junctions in the somatic nervous system.

Transmission of impulse from nerve to effector organ

When autonomic nerves are stimulated, the effector organs which they innervate respond in a characteristic way (Table 15.1). It is now firmly established that this response is caused by a chemical substance released from the end of the nerve. Substances which mediate the effect of nerve stimulation are called neurotransmitters. Acetylcholine (ACH) and noradrenaline (NA) are neurotransmitters at different points in the ANS (see above).

The idea that nerve function is mediated by chemical substances is important in medicine; drugs can be used to modify the action of a neurotransmitter by inhibiting its release, by interfering with its synthesis or catabolism, or by preventing the action of the transmitter on the neuroeffector organ. Until the late 19th century, it was thought that transmission of excitation from nerve terminals to effector cells was produced electrically by action currents. Then, following the work of Langley who drew attention to the similarity between the effects of extracts of the adrenal medulla and of sympathetic nerve stimulation, Elliot in 1904 proposed that sympathetic nerves might release an adrenaline-like substance in close contact with effector cells. Elliot considered this to be the chemical step in the process of transmission. This was one of the earliest statements of the neurotransmitter hypothesis. More than fifty years later Von Euler showed categorically that noradrenaline is the principal neurotransmitter in postganglionic sympathetic nerves.

Again, following Dale's observation that acetylcholine *mimicked* the

Table 15.1 *Responses of effector organs to autonomic nerve stimulation*

Organ	Sympathetic	Parasympathetic
BLOOD VESSELS		
Skins, splanchnic areas	constriction	
Coronary	dilatation	Nil (except in a few special cases, e.g. blood vessels of the genital organs which are dilated)
Skeletal muscle	dilatation	Nil
EYE		
Iris	contraction of radial muscle (mydriasis)	contraction of circular muscle (miosis)
Ciliary muscle	Nil	contraction
SKIN		
Sweat secretion	increase (cholinergic)	Nil
Salivary glands	slight viscid secretion	profuse watery secretion
STOMACH		
Motility	inhibition	stimulation
Secretion	inhibition	stimulation
Sphincter	inhibition or contraction	inhibition or contraction
INTESTINAL MOVEMENTS	inhibition	stimulation
LUNGS		
Bronchial muscle	relaxation	contraction
Bronchial secretion	–	stimulation
BLADDER		
Fundus	relaxation	contraction
Sphincter	contraction	relaxation
HEART		
Rate	increase	decrease
Force	increase	–

responses produced by parasympathetic nerve stimulation (he coined the term 'parasympathomimetic' to describe this action of acetylcholine), Dale and Otto Loewi proved that acetylcholine is the neurotransmitter in cholinergic nerves. For this Dale and Loewi shared the Nobel Prize in 1936.

Criteria to be met for a substance to be accepted as a neurotransmitter

The criteria include:

(1) The substance must be recovered from the perfusate of an innervated organ during periods of nerve stimulation.

(2) The substance must produce responses identical with those produced by stimulation of the appropriate nerve; the response to nerve stimulation and to applied substance should be modified (blocked or potentiated) in the same manner by drugs. Thus, eserine potentiates the response of mammalian hearts to vagal stimulation as it does the action of ACH. Atropine, a muscarinic receptor antagonist, prevents the response of the heart to vagal stimulation and injection of ACH. Similarly, cocaine (uptake inhibitor), and phentolamine, respectively potentiate and block the responses of sympathetically innervated organs to nerve stimulation and injected noradrenaline.

(3) Enzymes responsible for the synthesis of the neurotransmitter (e.g. dopamine-β-hydroxylase or cholineacetylase) and for the breakdown or removal of the substance after its release (e.g. acetylcholinesterase or uptake mechanisms), must be present at the nerve ending or close to the nerve ending.

Noradrenaline and acetylcholine are now generally accepted as neurotransmitters in many efferent fibres of the peripheral nervous system. Certain nerves which are components of the ANS are, however, nonadrenergic noncholinergic (NANC), i.e. the neurotransmitter of these nerves is not known, but it can be shown that it is neither noradrenaline nor acetylcholine. There is evidence that some NANC nerves release adenosine triphosphate (ATP) and Burnstock has described such nerves as purinergic, but the idea that such a widely occurring purine can be a neurotransmitter is not yet universally accepted.

Transmission of impulse from preganglionic terminals to postganglionic neurones

A word needs to be said about transmission of impulses from the preganglionic nerve terminal to the postganglionic cell body. The most important neurotransmitter at this synapse for sympathetic and parasympathetic efferents is ACH. The receptors which ACH stimulates to set off impulses in the postganglionic nerve fibre are called nicotinic (a term historically associated with the fact that low concentrations of nicotine applied to autonomic ganglia produced a response in the effector similar to that produced by stimulation of the preganglionic nerve). Note that the ACH receptors at the motor-end-plate (see section 17.3) of skeletal muscle fibres are also called nicotinic receptors. The two sets of nicotinic receptors can be distinguished in terms of drugs which block them. Also tetramethylammonium and dimethylphenylpiperazinium (DMPP) can activate ganglionic nicotinic receptors, but not the motor-end-plate receptors.

Events at the ganglionic synapse may be complex. There is evidence that there exists a small intensely fluorescent (SIF) interneurone in which the ACH receptor is muscarinic (that is, it can be blocked by low dose of atropine) and the postganglionic fibre of the SIF interneurone (see Fig. 15.2) is thought to release dopamine or noradrenaline which then acts on adrenoceptors on the postganglionic neurone to cause an increase in cyclic AMP and hyperpolarisation. There also exist muscarinic receptors on the postganglionic cell body which ACH, released from the pre-ganglionic nerve terminal, can stimulate. Most of these studies have been conducted on sympathetic nerves, but events in parasympathetic nerves may be similar.

The adrenal medulla

The adrenal medulla contains large amounts of adrenaline and noradrenaline contained in *chromaffin* granules, so called because

Fig. 15.2. Transmission of impulses from preganglionic nerve terminals to postganglionic neurones: SIF, small intensely fluorescent interneurone; N, nicotinic receptor; M, muscarinic receptor; A, adrenoceptor; DA, dopamine; NA, noradrenaline; ACH, acetylcholine.

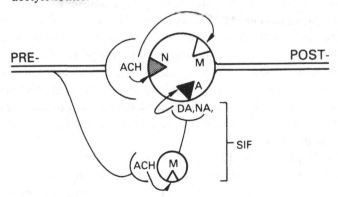

oxidation of the granules by dichromate produces a characteristic brown colour. The chromaffin cells of the adrenal gland are innervated by the splanchnic nerve, stimulation of which causes the release of acetylcholine which in turn causes the release of adrenaline and noradrenaline into the adrenal vein and into the circulation. The ACH receptor on the chromaffin cells is similar to nicotinic receptors on postganglionic cell bodies and can be blocked by hexamethonium. The enzyme, phenylethanolamine N-methyl transferase, which converts noradrenaline to adrenaline (see page 352) is abundant in the adrenal medulla. Chromaffin cells may be considered as modified postganglionic sympathetic ganglion cells which liberate adrenaline into the circulation to act as a hormone rather than as a transmitter.

15.3   TRANSMISSION AT THE NEUROMUSCULAR JUNCTION
Anatomy

The efferent motor nerve to skeletal muscle does not synapse at ganglia, but runs directly from the central nervous system to skeletal muscle fibres. As the nerve approaches the muscle fibre, it loses its myelin sheath. Within the skeletal muscle the motor axon breaks up into several branches and each terminal branch innervates a single muscle fibre. An axon together with its branches and the muscle fibres which they innervate constitute a motor unit which functions as a single unit (Fig. 15.3).

The position of the muscle fibre apposite to the motor nerve ending is the motor-end-plate. This is where the highest concentration of receptors can be found. Stimulation of motor-end-plate receptors by ACH causes an increase in permeability of the membrane to cations especially Na^+ and Ka^+ ions. The influx of Na^+ causes a depolarisation of the membrane. The ACH receptor is thus linked to ion channels which become open when the receptor is activated. Most mammalian skeletal muscle fibres have one motor-end-plate whereas some amphibian and avian skeletal muscle fibres have multiple motor-end-plates. Examples are the rectus abdominis of frog and toad and the biventer cervicis in the chick. These muscles respond by a contracture to drugs which activate the nicotinic receptors in these end-plates to produce depolarisation.

When the nerve supply to mammalian skeletal muscle is cut (denervation), e.g. the phrenic nerve to rat diaphragm, the muscle responds by contracture to acetylcholine due to growth of new receptors in response to denervation. The three preparations just mentioned above are used in class experiments to demonstrate the action of drugs on neuromuscular transmission.

Release of ACH

The transmitter at the neuromuscular junction is ACH packaged·in vesicles in the efferent nerve terminals. Normally, the vesicles release their contents continuously and randomly. The ACH thus released produces quantal changes in potential of the postsynaptic membrane called miniature end-plate poetentials (m.e.p.p.). Each

Fig. 15.3. Innervation of skeletal muscle fibres by motor efferents. In focal innervation (a), as in most mammals each muscle fibre is innervated by a branch of the motor efferent. In multiple innervation (b), each muscle fibre is supplied by several branches of the motor efferent.

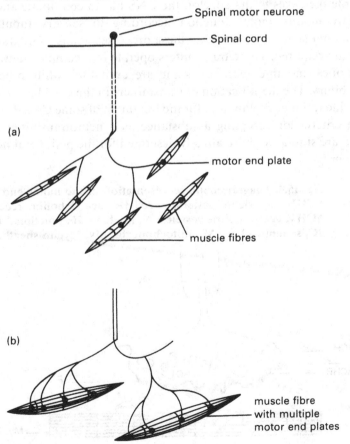

quantum represents the contents of a single vesicle containing about 10000 molecules of ACH. When the nerve is stimulated, the impulse arriving at the nerve terminal causes a transient increase in permeability of the terminal nerve membrane to Ca^{2+}. This causes an explosive release of ACH from about 100 vesicles. ACH diffuses across the synaptic cleft to combine with receptors in the postsynaptic membrane. This causes a large end-plate potential (e.p.p.) which can be recorded by intracellular electrodes. The e.p.p. gives rise to a propagated muscle action potential, activation of the contractile mechanism and a twitch response or tetanic contractions, if the impulses arrive at high frequencies.

15.4   CENTRAL NERVOUS SYSTEM

The central nervous system (CNS) consists of the spinal cord and the brain. Unlike the peripheral nervous system which conveys simple messages to the effector, the CNS has to coordinate and constantly modify motor function according to sensory inputs and hormonal signals. To integrate these processes, many more transmitters are required. These transmitters operate in a complex network of neurones and interneurones: some are excitatory, while others are inhibitory. The identification of transmitters in the CNS has helped to provide rational explanation for the treatment of some CNS disorders. The criteria for accepting a substance as a neurotransmitter in the CNS are similar to those already described for the peripheral nervous system.

Fig. 15.4. Diagrammatic representation of the motor end plate. ACHE, acetylcholinesterase; ACHR, acetylcholine receptors; ACHV, acetylcholine vesicles; N, nucleus; JF, junctional folds; SC, synaptic cleft; M, mitochondria; My, Myelin sheath.

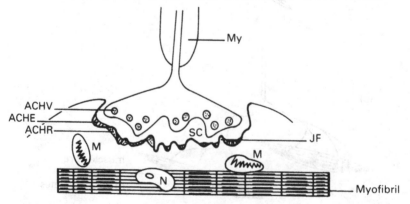

Table 15.2   *Occurrence of ACH, dopamine (DA), noradrenaline (NA) and 5-hydroxytryptamine (5-HT) in different areas of the brain*

Brain region	ACH	DA	NA	5-HT
Cerebral cortex	+	+	+	+
Basal ganglia				
(caudate nucleus)	+++	+++	−	−
Hypothalamus	+	+	+++	++
Brain stem	+	+	++	++
Spinal cord	+	−	+	+

Concentrations: +++, high; ++, moderate; +, significant; −, insignificant compared to concentrations in other tissues.

The main techniques used in the identification of neurotransmitters in the CNS are the following.

(a) *In situ* demonstration of the substance in tissue slices by histochemical flourescence and autoradiography;

(b) immunoflourescence of associated enzymes;

(c) uptake of radiolabelled transmitter in brain slices or synaptosomes; and

(d) receptor binding.

The effects of the substances when applied directly to discrete areas of the brain can be studied. This technique involves the use of a syringe fixed to a stereotaxic manipulator which by the use of a set of predetermined coordinates allows introduction of the chemical into a preselected area of the brain. This technique is known as *micropipette iontophoresis*. The animal response to such an injection can be measured, and by the use of selective antagonists, the role of such substances in CNS function can be inferred.

Acetylcholine

Acetylcholine occurs in many parts of the brain (Table 15.2). High concentrations are found in the caudate nucleus. In these regions too, are high concentrations of choline acetyltransferase and muscarinic and nicotinic receptors. Acetylcholine usually excites central neurones, but inhibitory effects have also been shown in the hypothalamus. Specific areas of the brain where ACH occurs are discussed below.

(a) *Reticular activating system*. The cholinergic neurones liberate acetylcholine in proportion to the state of wakefulness, i.e., high release in wakefulness and less in sleep and least when the animal is heavily anaesthetised, e.g. with barbiturates.

(b) *Corpus striatum.* The caudate nucleus contains a high concentration of ACH mainly derived from neurones originating in the thalamus. The activity of ACH in this part of the brain is essential for the control of motor cortical activity and coordination. Any imbalance between this cholinergic (muscarinic) system and the opposing dopaminergic one results in motor disorder such as Parkinsonism or Huntington's chorea. Tremor occurs when ACH action predominates.

(c) *Hypothalamus.* Cholinergic neurones in the hypothalamus liberate ACH which stimulates nicotinic receptors in the neurohypophysis to release vasopressin and oxytocin.

Aminoacids

Three aminoacids are commonly considered to be neutrotransmitters in the CNS. These are glycine, γ-aminobutyric acid (GABA) and L-glutamic acid (see Table 15.3). Glycine and GABA are inhibitory; L-glutamic acid is excitatory. A fourth amino acid, L-aspartic acid, has also been found in moderately high concentrations in the posterior horn of the spinal cord and is considered a putative neurotransmitter. GABA has been extensively studied. The enzymes L-glutamic acid decarboxylase which converts L-glutamic acid to GABA, and GABA transaminase which inactivates GABA, are found at the locations of high GABA concentration. Specific uptake mechanisms have also been identified for various aminoacids in the CNS. GABA and gylcine inhibit neurones by increasing membrane permeability to chloride and potassium ions. Their actions are similar but they are concentrated in different parts of the CNS, glycine being more highly concentrated in the spinal cord while GABA is concentrated in the supraspinal regions of the CNS. Strychnine is a specific antagonist of glycine receptors and picrotoxin and bicuculline are specific antagonists of GABA receptors.

Catecholamines, 5-HT and histamine

Noradrenergic, dopaminergic, and tryptaminergic neurones have been demonstrated by the technique of fluorescence. Tissue slices are treated with formaldehyde vapour under carefully controlled conditions to form isoquinolines which are fluorescent. Table 15.2 shows

Table 15.3   *Occurrence of amino acids in different areas of the brain*

Brain region	Glycine	GABA	L-Glutamic acid
Cerebral cortex	–	+	+
Basal ganglia			
caudate nucleus	–	+	+
globus pallidus	–	+++	–
Hypothalamus	–	++	+
Brain stem	+	+++	+
Spinal cord	+++	+	+

Concentrations: +++, high; ++, moderate; +, significant; –, insignificant compared to concentrations in other tissues.

the occurrence of NA, DA and 5-HT in different regions of the brain. The associated biosynthetic and metabolising enzymes have also been found to be closely associated with the sites at which the putative transmitters are highly concentrated.

The three transmitters can affect the limbic system which is important in the action of psychotropic agents (see Chapter 18). There is evidence that noradrenergic neurones in the brainstem are involved in cardiovascular and respiratory control. DA receptors are present in the chemoreceptor trigger zone which activates the vomiting centre. Chlorpromazine and metoclopramide block these receptors and are used as antiemetics. Histamine has been identified in many regions of the brain but its role as a CNS transmitter has not been as well established as that of the other putative transmitters. It is probably an excitatory transmitter acting on H_1-histamine receptors. Most H_1-receptor antagonists which enter the CNS cause sedation in man (see Chapter 24.3).

Polypeptides

Several polypeptides have been identified in the CNS. Vasopressin and oxytocin occur in the hypothalamo-pituitary axis. Their transmitter role in the CNS has yet to be defined. Another peptide found in the CNS is substance P originally isolated from the gastrointestinal tract. High amounts occur in the substantia nigra and parts of the spinal cord. Substance P has been implicated as a transmitter in sensory terminals. Capsacin, the irritant principle in pepper (*Capsicum*), can deplete the spinal neurones of substance P. Somatostatin and neurotensin are other peptides found in the spinal cord.

Extracts of the hypothalamus contain β-endorphins which produce marked analgesia similar to that produced by morphine when injected into the third ventricle of cats. The term endorphin is used to imply that these peptides are endogenous peptides activating classical opiate morphine receptors. Methionine-enkephalin and leucine-enkephalin ((met)enkephalin and (leu)enkephalin) are two pentapeptides differing only in one aminoacid and are found in regions of the brain with high concentrations of opiate receptors. These endogenous peptides have similar aminoacid sequence to the β-endorphins but are not derived from them. The endorphins occur mainly in relation to endocrine function. The enkephalin peptides occur widely in the CNS and myenteric plexus of the gut and are implicated in pain mechanisms and pain relief.

The essential features of impulse transmission from nerve to muscle have been described for different arms of the nervous system. Based on the fundamental principles enunciated here, the pharmacology of drugs acting on the nervous system is described in the chapters that follow.

FURTHER READING
Goodman, L.S.,& Gilman, A., Rall, T.W. & Murad, F., eds. (1985). *The Pharmacological Basis of Therapeutics*, 7th edn. Macmillan, London.
Katz, B. & Miledi, R. (1972). The statistical nature of the acetylcholine potential and its molecular components. *J. Physiol.*, **224**, 665–99.
Ryall, R.W. (1979). *Mechanisms of Drug Action on the Nervous System*. Cambridge University Press, Cambridge, London.

16

Noradrenergic mechanisms

16.1   INTRODUCTION

Noradrenaline (NA) is synthesised and stored at the terminals of postganglionic sympathetic nerves. When released the transmitter can act, depending on the effector, on four different types of adrenoceptors, to produce a variety of effects. What the student should know after reading this chapter are: the principal steps and the major enzymes involved in the biosynthesis of NA; how NA is stored in, and released from, sympathetic nerve terminals; the uptake processes responsible for its removal from the site of action; and the enzymes which catalyse its breakdown. These are the principal targets of drug action. The reader should know the type of drug that affects each mechanism and the clinical conditions in which such drugs are indicated (see also Chapter 4).

Although NA is the neurotransmitter at peripheral sympathetic nerve terminals, the mechanisms enumerated above are also affected by dopamine, adrenaline and synthetic drugs such as isoprenaline. The basic structure common to these amines is the catechol nucleus. They are therefore commonly referred to as catecholamines. The term sympathomimetic amine is used to describe all amines which have properties similar to those of noradrenaline, whether they are catecholamines or not.

16.2   BIOSYNTHESIS OF CATECHOLAMINES

A schematic representation of the major stages in catecholamine (CA) biosynthesis is shown in Fig. 16.1. Something must be known about each of the enzymes involved in CA biosynthesis.

Tyrosine hydroxylase (TH)

The main dietary precursor of catecholamines is tyrosine. Dietary phenylalanine can be converted to tryosine in the liver by the enzyme phenylalanine hydroxylase. Tyrosine hydroxylase is present exclusively in sympathetic nerve terminals and other catecholamine-

Fig. 16.1. Biosynthesis of catecholamines. The enzymes which catalyse the different stages are: (1) tyrosine hydroxylase; (2) aromatic L-aminoacid decarboxylase (dopa decarboxylase); (3) dopamine β-hydroxylase; (4) phenylethanolamine-N-methyltransferase (PNMT).

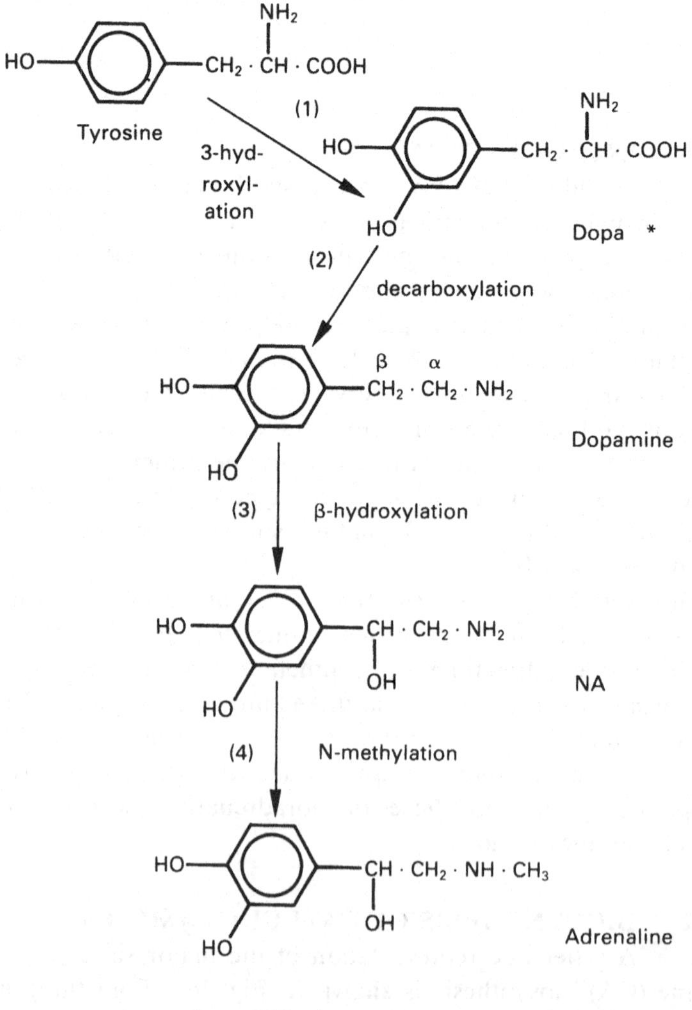

* = Dihydroxyphenylalanine

containing structures. This enzyme can also hydroxylate phenyl-alanine to make tyrosine in sympathetic nerves. Normally, this reaction is of no importance, but in phenylketonuria (a disease condition associated with a genetic deficiency in phenylalanine hydroxylase), the formation of tyrosine from phenylalanine in sympathetic nerves becomes an important pathway for catecholamine biosynthesis.

The conversion of tyrosine to dopa is the rate-limiting step (the slowest rate) in the whole process. It is normally controlled by end-product feedback, i.e. NA inhibits it when the cytoplasmic concentration of the transmitter reaches a critical value. Prolonged sympathetic nerve stimulation and treatment with resperine (which cause loss of NA from nerve ending stores, see below) increase the activity of TH. Alphamethyl-p-tyrosine blocks TH activity and has been found useful in the treament of phaeochromocytoma, a tumour of adrenal medulla associated with a high rate of synthesis and secretion of catecholamines.

L-aminoacid decarboxylase (LAAD)

LAAD, also known as dopa decarboxylase is found in sympathetic nerves as well as in serotonergic nerves, that is, nerves in which 5-hydrotryptamine (serotonin) is thought to be a neurotransmitter. The enzyme converts dopa to dopamine and 5-hydroxytryptophan to 5-hydroxytryptamine in their respective neurones. Conversion of dopa to dopamine is rapid so that dopa is hardly detectable in sympathetic nerves. Postmortem examination of patients who have died of Parkinson's disease has shown that the level of dopamine within the basal ganglia complex (the caudate nucleus and corpus striatum) of the brain is reduced. Parkinson's disease is characterised – clinically – by three extrapyramidal symptoms: akinesia (difficulty in initiating skeletal muscle movement), rigidity of skeletal muscles, and tremor. L-DOPA is used in its treatment. The drug is converted to dopamine and therefore increases to normal, the concentration of dopamine in the basal ganglia. L-DOPA is used in combination with carbidopa, a dopa decarboxylase inhibitor which does not cross the blood–brain barrier. By inhibiting peripheral dopa decarboxylase, carbidopa ensures that most of the L-DOPA administered reaches the basal ganglia for conversion to dopamine. The extrapyramidal side effects of several psychotropic drugs are attributed to their depletion of dopamine (reserpine) or blockade of dopamine receptors (chlorpromazine, haloperidol). There is also evidence that some atropine-like drugs used in the treatment of Parkinson's disease, e.g., etrophine, block dopamine uptake. This amine is therefore probably of critical importance in the control of motor behaviour of extrapyramidal origin.

Dopamine-β-hydroxylase
Dopamine-β-hydroxylase is found in NA-containing granules in sympathetic nerves where it converts dopamine to NA (see Fig. 16.1). It is released with NA during sympathetic nerve stimulation. Since the enzyme is not taken back into the nerve, high levels in circulation is evidence of high sympathetic nerve activity.

Phenylethanolamine-N-methyltransferase (PNMT)
PNMT catalyses the N-methylation of NA to form adrenaline. It is found in the central nervous system. Adrenaline therefore occurs in the brain. In the periphery, it is found in chromaffin tissue – mainly the adrenal medulla. It is not found in peripheral sympathetic nerves. The small percentage of adrenaline released from sympathetic nerve terminals is due to uptake from the blood via uptake₁ (see below).

16.3   STORAGE AND RELEASE OF CATECHOLAMINES
Noradrenaline is stored in granules (chromaffin granules) contained within membrane-bound vesicles. The granules also contain ATP, a high molecular weight protein called chromogranin, and lipids. NA is complexed to ATP. This complex together with chromogranin form a non-diffusible stable storage unit within the granule. The membrane of the granule has a special pumping mechanism that concentrates NA in the granule where the amine is protected from monoamine oxidase. This pump is blocked by reserpine which thus exposes NA to MAO and eventually depletes the nerve ending of NA.

When an impulse arrives at the end of the sympathetic nerve, NA is released unto receptors at the postsynaptic membrane (Fig. 16.3). The mechanism of release is thought to be by a process of *exocytosis*: the membrane of the NA-containing vesicle fuses with the nerve cell membrane (Fig. 16.2). At the point of fusion an opening occurs and the soluble contents of the vesicle are emptied into the synaptic cleft. The opening is sealed and presumably the vesicle is reloaded with newly synthesised NA or NA taken up after release (see Fig. 16.3). Calcium is required for the release process.

The physiological control of NA release is achieved by at least three mechanisms.

Negative feedback control by NA stimulating presynaptic alpha adrenoceptors

There is abundant evidence that when the concentration of NA at the synaptic cleft reaches a critical value, NA stimulates alpha-adrenoceptors present on the nerve to inhibit further release of NA. These receptors are classified as α_2-adrenoceptors. Clonidine, an antihypertensive drug is thought to lower arterial blood pressure by stimulating α_2-adrenoceptors in the CNS. Another example is guanfacine which is thought to stimulate peripheral alpha$_2$-adreno-

Fig. 16.2. Release of NA by exocytosis: (1) Nerve at rest. When the nerve is stimulated (2) membrane of NA-containing vesicle fuses with nerve cell membrane; at the point of fusion an opening occurs (3) through which the soluble contents of the vesicle are emptied into the synaptic cleft (4). The opening is resealed and the empty vesicle may be refilled (5) with NA.

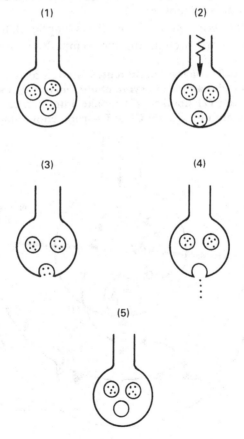

ceptors to reduce NA release. Blockade of these receptors on the other hand, increases the output of NA during sympathetic nerve stimulation.

Negative feedback control by prostaglandins acting on the sympathetic nerve terminal

Prostaglandins E_1 and E_2 in low concentrations inhibit NA release from sympathetic nerves, but do not, at these concentrations, affect the response of the effector to NA. It is suggested that prostaglandins may be physiological modulators of NA release. There is no evidence that sympathetic nerves release prostaglandins, but NA can release prostaglandins from effector cells, which may diffuse back to affect NA release from the neurone. The physiological significance of this mechanism is not known.

Positive feedback control by NA acting on presynaptic beta-adrenoceptors

At low concentrations in the synaptic cleft, NA stimulates beta-adrenoceptors present on the sympathetic nerve terminal to

Fig. 16.3. Diagrammatic representation of release and reuptake of catecholamines in sympathetic nerves: ▲, catecholamine; (1) uptake₁; (2) uptake₂; (3) uptake into storage vesicles. MAO = monoamine oxidase; COMT = cathechol-O-methyltransferase.

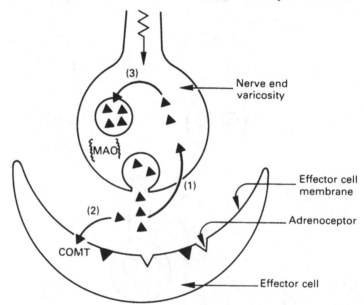

increase NA output per impulse. The physiological significance of this mechanism is not known, but it is thought that beta-adrenoceptor antagonists (beta-blockers) used in the treatment of hypertension may act by blocking presynaptic-beta-adrenoceptors to *reduce* NA release from sympathetic nerves. This has been offered as an explanation for their antihypertensive effects.

16.4   ADRENOCEPTORS

Noradrenaline can activate alpha-adrenoceptors (alpha$_1$ and alpha$_2$) and beta-adrenoceptors (beta$_1$ and beta$_2$). The receptors are classified on the basis of the selectivity of agonist and antagonist drugs (see page 10, Chapter 4 where classification of receptors is discussed in detail). Adrenoceptor subclassification extends further than differences in drug affinity; activation of each receptor subtype also leads to different intracellular events. Activation of alpha$_1$-adrenoceptors leads to increased phosphoinositide (PI) hydrolysis. Phosphoinositol-4, 5-biphosphate (PIP$_2$) is hydrolysed to diacylglycerol (DAG) and inositol-1,4,5-triphosphate (IP$_3$). DAG and IP$_3$ are second messengers acting to stimulate protein kinase C and to mobilise intracellular Ca^{2+}. PI hydrolysis is regarded as the signal transducer for receptors which mediate cellular responses via mobilisation of intracellular Ca^{2+}. On the other hand, alpha$_2$-adrenoceptors are coupled to adenylate cyclase by a guanine nucleotide binding protein (Ni) whose activation leads to a decreased activity of the enzyme (contrast beta-adrenoceptors) and a reduction in cyclic GMP production.

16.5   UPTAKE OF CATECHOLAMINES

The idea that the sympathetic neurotransmitter might be taken up into storage after release was first suggested by Burn. Iversen studied *uptake* in detail. Three major processes can be identified.

Neuronal uptake or uptake$_1$

This is the uptake of NA from the extracellular space into adrenergic neurones. Up to 75–80% of released NA is taken back into the sympathetic neurone for storage. The physiological function of uptake$_1$ is to remove NA from its site of action and so terminate its action. This function is analogous to that of acetylcholinesterase in cholinergic nerves (see later). Uptake$_1$ is an active energy-requiring process with a higher affinity for NA than adrenaline. Isoprenaline is not a substrate for uptake$_1$. Thus there are structural requirements for binding to uptake sites. Uptake₁ operates at both peripheral and central adrenergic neurones. The clinical significance of uptake₁ is that many drugs interact with the process to produce powerful pharmacological effects, for example the following:

(*a*) *Cocaine* is a powerful inhibitor of uptake₁ and so produces sympathomimetic effects such as blanching (due to vasoconstriction) when it is used as a local anaesthetic in the eye. This effect is due to accumulation of NA released from sympathetic nerves. This mechanism also accounts for cocaine's stimulant action in the CNS. Noradrenaline and adrenaline are associated with arousal states in the CNS.

(*b*) *Indirectly acting sympathomimetic amines* such as tyramine and ephedrine enter adrenergic neurones by the uptake₁ process to release NA from storage sites.

(*c*) *Adrenergic neurone blockers* (see later) are taken up and concentrated in sympathetic nerve endings by the uptake₁ process. Therefore, substances which block or compete for uptake₁ sites, such as amphetamine and imipramine, reduce or abolish the hypotensive effects of neurone blockers.

Extraneuronal uptake or uptake₂
Uptake₂ is the uptake of catecholamines into sites other than sympathetic nerve terminals, e.g. smooth muscles of blood vessels and heart muscle. Its characteristics are different from those of uptake₁ in the following ways.

(*a*) Uptake₂ operates at much higher catecholamine concentrations (you need a lot more NA to activate it) and has a higher capacity (can take up more) than uptake₁.

(*b*) Isoprenaline and adrenaline have higher affinities for uptake₂ than NA. Note the reverse structural requirements for uptake₂ compared with uptake₁.

(*c*) Catecholamines taken up into smooth muscles and the myocardium are rapidly metabolised by catechol-oxygen-methyltransferase (COMT).

The physiological function of uptake₂ is mainly to remove and destroy circulating catecholamines (adrenaline and NA) administered exogenously or released from the adrenal medulla. Uptake₂ is blocked by steroids (oestradiol, corticosterone), phenoxybenzamine, metanephrine and inhibitors of COMT. Thus the actions of NA on the cardiovascular system are potentiated by steroids and COMT inhibitors, e.g. catechol and thajuplicin.

Uptake of NA into storage vesicles (Intraneuronal uptake)

NA entering the sympathetic nerve is rapidly taken up into intracellular storage vesicles which are present in the cytoplasm. This is also an energy-requiring process which enables NA to enter storage vesicles against a concentration gradient. Inside the vesicle, NA is complexed to ATP and stored in granules and protected from monoamine oxidase (MAO). Uptake into storage vesicles is powerfully inhibited by *reserpine, tetrabenazine,* and *segontin.* These drugs therefore allow NA to be deaminated by MAO, thereby leading to a depletion of NA stores. These drugs do not inhibit uptake₁.

Dopamine uptake

Dopamine is actively taken up by dopaminergic neurones in the CNS. This uptake is inhibited by amphetamine but not by imipramine or desipramine, showing that the structural requirements are different from uptake₁ requirements. Dopamine uptake is also inhibited by a variety of anticholinergic drugs, e.g. benztropine, used in the treatment of Parkinson's disease. These drugs thus have dual mode of action, namely they reduce cholinergic activity and enhance dopamine activity. (See Table 16.1).

16.6   ENZYME DEGRADATION OF CATECHOLAMINES

A schematic representation of the main stages is shown on Fig. 16.4. Monoamine oxidase (MAO) removes the amino group with subsequent oxidation of the side chain to aldehyde which is further oxidised to carboxylic acid or reduced to a primary alcohol (glycol). Catechol-oxygen-methyltransferase (COMT) acts on catecholamines to convert the phenolic OH group on the *meta*-position to a methoxyl group producing normetanephrine. Compounds having OH groups in the *ortho* or *para* position are not substrates for COMT. The combined effects of both enzymes give rise to 3-methoxy, 4-hydroxymandelic acid (vanillylmandelic acid), VMA; more should be said about these enzymes.

Table 16.1 *Properties of catecholamine uptake processes*

Uptake	Concentration of amine required to activate	Physiological function of process	Substrate affinity rank order	Specific inhibitor	Site of uptake	Fate of uptaken amine	Capacity
Uptake 1	low	Recycling of neuronal NA	NA > adrenaline > isoprenaline	cocaine, imipramine	From synaptic cleft into nerve cell	stored	low
Uptake 2	high	Removal of circulating CA	isoprenaline > adrenaline > NA	metanephrine, oestradiol, phenoxybenzamine	From circulating into non-nervous tissue	inactivated by COMT	high
Storage vesicle uptake	low	Protection of CA from MAO	NA > adrenaline	reserpine, tetrabenazine	From cytosol to storage vesicle	stored	low
Dopamine uptake	low	Protection of DA from MAO	DA > NA > adrenaline	amphetamine, benztropine	Dopaminergic neurones in CNS	stored	low

DA = dopamine; CA = catecholamine; MAO = monoamine oxidase; COMT = catechol-O-methyltransferase.

Monoamine oxidase (MAO)

The term MAO represents a number of isoenzymes found in mitochondria of sympathetic nerve cells, liver, and gastrointestinal tract and other nerve cells in the limbic system. The physiological role of MAO in sympathetic nerves is to mop up NA spilling over from storage vesicles. MAO is not located at the postsynaptic membrane. Therefore this enzyme does not serve the purpose of inactivating NA released from the sympathetic nerve.

Points of clinical significance to note about MAO are:

(a) MAO can be inhibited by a wide variety of drugs such as tranylcypromine, pargyline and phenelzine. These substances

Fig. 16.4. Breakdown of noradrenaline. Dopamine and adrenaline undergo corresponding catabolic reactions. The enzymes are: (1) monoamine oxidase (MAO); (2) catechol-oxygen-methyltransferase (COMT). VMA is 3-methoxy, 4-hydroxymandelic acid (Vanillylmandelic acid).

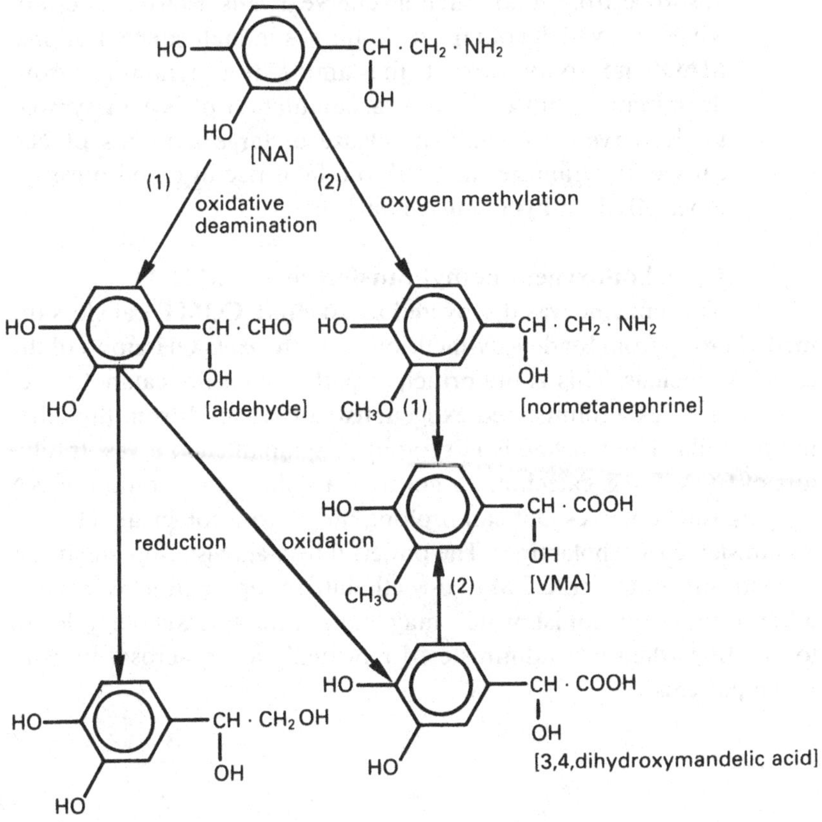

increase the concentration of monoamines in the brain and are used in the treatment of psychotic disorders such as depression. Paradoxically, some of them, e.g. pargyline, also lower blood pressure. The mechanism of action is not known. They may increase the concentration of NA and dopamine at sympathetic ganglia (see page 343) and thereby act as ganglion-blocking drugs or they may increase the concentration of other monoamines in sympathetic nerves and when these are stimulated, compounds such as dopamine which are less potent than NA as vasoconstrictors are released along with NA thereby *diluting* the action of NA (a false transmitter effect).

(b) Normally, sympathomimetic amines such as tyramine present in foods, do not enter the circulation, because they are deaminated by MAO present in the gastrointestinal tract and in the liver. However in patients taking MAO inhibitors (MAOI), large amounts of vasoactive monoamines can be absorbed from foods such as cheese, beans, Marmite, certain wines, etc. which contain such amines in high concentrations. MAOI not only protect the amine (e.g. tyramine) from deamination, but can cause accumulation of NA in sympathetic nerves. The sudden release of large amounts of NA caused by tyramine can lead to a fatal rise in blood pressure especially in a hypertensive patient.

Catechol-oxygen-methyltransferase (COMT)

This enzyme was discovered by Axelrod. COMT transfers the methyl group from S-adenosylmethionine to the *meta* OH group of the catechol nucleus. This is the principal pathway for the catabolism of catecholamines administered exogenously or released from the adrenal medulla. The enzyme is not found in sympathetic nerves. Inhibitors of COMT, e.g. catechol, do not increase the concentration of NA in sympathetic nerves, but can prolong the pharmacological action of administered catecholamines. The powerful beta-agonist, isoprenaline, is a good substrate for COMT. o-Methylated isoprenaline is a beta-adrenoceptor antagonist, which may explain the tolerance developed to the drug when it is administered repeatedly as an aerosol in asthmatic patients.

16.7 EFFECT OF DRUGS ON ADRENERGIC TRANSMISSION

Several useful drugs affect the different mechanisms we have described. The drugs are used in the treatment of cardiovascular diseases such as hypertension and cardiac arrhythmias. It is advisable to read Chapter 15 and the preceding sections of this Chapter before reading this section, for clearer understanding of the mechanism of action of the drugs mentioned here. Note also that some of the drugs mentioned here are discussed again under other systems, e.g. the cardiovascular system. Their use in the treatment of cardiovascular diseases is based on the mechanisms described here.

Drugs affecting storage of NA

The storage process can be inhibited by reserpine. This is an alkaloid obtained from the roots of *Rauvolfia serpentina*, a climbing plant indigenous to India. Reserpine can also be obtained from the Nigerian species of rauvolfia *R. vomitoria*, roots and bark of which have been used for the treatment of psychoses by traditional Yoruba healers long before the advent of modern medicine. Several alkaloids can be extracted from the plant, but reserpine is the most active and clinically useful (see also Chapter 1). The primary action of reserpine is to deplete tissue stores of their catecholamines and 5-hydroxytryptamine and dopamine content. All organs are affected: the brain, the heart, blood vessels, and the adrenal medulla. The mechanism of depletion has been described, i.e. blocking of the uptake of NA into storage vesicles and exposure of the amine to MAO deamination. Consequently, after reserpine treatment, indirectly acting sympathomimetic amines, e.g. tyramine, are ineffective. The transient rise in blood pressure which accompanies the injection of NA-releasing drugs such as amphetamine, is not observed with reserpine. This is because reserpine produces NA depletion intraneuronally rather than by release of NA unto receptors. What appear outside the neurone after reserpine treatment are deaminated products.

Another effect of reserpine is that the sensitivity of effector organs, e.g. heart and blood vessels, to NA is increased. This *supersensitivity* is not due to block of uptake, because after reserpinisation, sympathetic nerves can concentrate NA in the cytosol if MAO is inhibited. Neither is it due to depletion of NA since supersensitivity can be demonstrated before significant NA depletion has occurred. Reserpine seems to facilitate the mobilisation of intracellular calcium by NA.

Resperine has been used in the treatment of psychoses, e.g. schizophrenia, and in the control of blood pressure, usually in combination with a thiazide diuretic, and in hyperthyroidism associated with overactivity of the sympathetic nerve.

Toxic effects with large doses of reserpine are consistent with its pharmacoloical actions, e.g. depression with tendency to suicide, Parkinsonian syndrome due to depletion of dopamine in the basal ganglia, diarrhoea, increased gastric secretion, and peptic ulceration due to increased activity of the parasympathetic nervous system, and impairment of ejaculation.

Drugs affecting NA release

NA release can be triggered by a nerve impulse or by a drug, e.g. tyramine. Such drugs produce effects which are similar to those produced by nerve stimulation or NA. They are called indirectly acting sympathomimetic amines and are discussed under a separate heading. NA release triggered by nerve impulse can be inhibited by a number of drugs used in the treatment of hypertension; they are known as nor-adrenergic neurone blockers. Examples are bretylium guanethidine, bethanidine, and debrisoquine (Fig. 16.5).

Some noradrenergic neurone blocking drugs are selectively concentrated in sympathetic nerve endings by the uptakeı process. Once inside the neurone, the drugs prevent, by an unknown mechanism, the release of NA. The drugs may stabilise the nerve terminal and prevent the entry of calcium. Bretylium, the first of these drugs to be used clinically, has no effect on NA stores but blocks NA release; it is now obsolete. The mechanism of action of guanethidine is by slow deple-

Fig. 16.5. Noradrenergic neurone blockers.

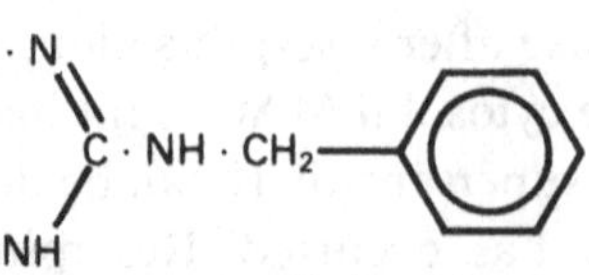

Debrisoquine

Bethanidine

tion of NA stores in sympathetic nerves, but lowering of arterial blood pressure occurs before a significant NA depletion has occurred. NA depletion cannot therefore account for the hypotensive action of guanethidine. For all neurone blockers, the fundamental action is inhibition of NA release. Possibly, noradrenergic neurone blockers displace NA within the neurone and are released by sympathetic nerves thereby acting as false transmitters.

These drugs do not act on NA receptors. Since they occupy uptake sites and thereby compete with NA for uptake into storage, they cause supersensitivity to circulating catecholamines. Note also that these drugs do not block the release of catecholamines from the adrenal medulla. Increasing sensitivity of adrenoceptors to medullary catecholamines may account for the tolerance which develops to some of these drugs, e.g. bretylium.

Another point of clinical importance to note is that neurone blockers enter the nerve cell cytoplasm by uptake₁. Consequently, if they are given simultaneously with uptake₁ inhibitors such as imipramine, the hypotensive action of the drug is prevented.

Drugs acting at adrenoceptors

Drugs acting at adrenoceptors either stimulate the receptors and cause effects similar to those of the neurotransmitter or block the receptors to prevent the response of the effector organ to the neurotransmitter when it is released from the nerve or when the transmitter or a drug acting like it is administered exogenously. Drugs which stimulate the adrenoceptor may act directly, indirectly, or have mixed direct and indirect actions.

Directly and indirectly acting sympathomimetic drugs

Directly acting sympathomimetic amines stimulate alpha and/or beta adrenoceptors; indirectly acting sympathomimetic drugs produce effects which are due to NA released from sympathetic nerves. Table 16.2 shows the structures of some phenylethylamine derivatives. There is some relationship between structure and direct/indirect activity. In general compounds with the catechol nucleus (catecholamines) have direct sympathomimetic effects; for example NA, adrenaline, isoprenaline and dopamine. In this series, the substitution on the nitrogen atom (R_5) determines the receptor preferentially stimulated, i.e. the larger the substituent group, the greater the activity at beta-adrenoceptors. Hence at these receptors the rank order of activity is isoprenaline > adrenaline > noradrenaline. This should not be taken

Table 16.2 *Directly and indirectly acting sympathomimetic amines*

$$\text{(benzene ring)} - \overset{\beta}{C}H \cdot \overset{\alpha}{C}H \cdot NH$$

	R_1	R_2	R_3	R_4	R_5	
Noradrenaline	OH	OH	OH	H	H	
Adrenaline	OH	OH	OH	H	CH_3	
Isoprenaline	OH	OH	OH	H	$CH(CH_3)_2$	
Dopamine	OH	OH	H	H	H	
Phenylephrine	H	OH	OH		CH_3	
Metaraminol	H	H	OH	CH_3	CH_3	
Tyramine	OH	H	H	H	H	} Indirectly
Amphetamine	H	H	H	CH_3	H	} acting

to suggest that NA is a weak beta agonist; NA is the natural beta₁
agonist.

Compounds in which one or both phenyl hydroxy groups are miss-
ing are either predominantly indirectly acting or have mixed direct
and indirect actions. Phenylephrine acts mainly on alpha₁ adrenoceptors, ephedrine has mixed actions but tyramine and amphetamine
act indirectly.

Two further points to note are the relationships of structure to
enzyme inactivation. Catechol-oxygen-methyltransferase (COMT) will
only attack compounds with the catechol nucleus, i.e. *both* R_1 and R_2
are OH substituted. Hence, of the compounds listed in Table 16.2, only
NA, adrenaline, isoprenaline and dopamine are COMT substrates.
This point is important later when considering beta-agonists used in
the treatment of asthma. Monoamine oxidase attacks the nitrogen end
of the molecule, but the compound is not a good substrate if the substitution on the Nitrogen atom (R_5) is too bulky, e.g. isoprenaline, or if the
alpha carbon atom (R_4) has a methyl substitution on it, e.g. ephedrine
and amphetamine. These compounds are therefore active after oral
administration.

The following characteristics of indirectly acting sympathomimetic
drugs should be noted.

(a) The drugs are taken up into noradrenergic neurones by the
   uptake₁ process and they release NA on to adrenoceptors.
(b) When they are repeatedly administered, the response obtained
   diminishes with successive applications, i.e. they exhibit
   tachyphylaxis.

(c) They are inactive after chronic sympathetic denervation, depletion of NA stores with reserpine or in the presence of noradrenergic neurone blockers; under all these conditions, the sensitivity of effector organs to directly acting sympathomimetic amines is increased, i.e. denervation supersensitivity occurs.

Sympathomimetic amines are used as bronchodilators in the treatment of asthma (see later) and as vasoconstrictors, e.g. *phenylephrine* (neophryn) is used as a nasal decongestant in nasal drops and as a mydriatic for diagnostic examination of the retina. *Orciprenaline* (alupent) has marked beta-adrenoceptor stimulant action and is used as a bronchodilator in the treatment of asthma. *Ephedrine* is an alkaloid occurring naturally in the plant *Ephedra sinica*; it stimulates the heart and dilates bronchioles, and is used as a mydriatic, nasal decongestant and in the treatment of bronchial asthma. *Amphetamine* or its dextrorotatory form, *dexamphetamine*, and the methyl derivative, *methylamphetamine*, lack a phenyl OH substitution and are therefore highly lipid-soluble, and centrally active. The amphetamines are widely abused as CNS stimulants. Therefore their clinical use is highly restricted in many countries.

The drugs mentioned so far cause vasoconstriction by stimulating alpha-adrenoceptors located on the postsynaptic membrane (alpha$_1$-adrenoceptors). Some drugs used in the treatment of hypertension (see later) owe their action to stimulation of alpha$_2$-adrenoceptors located either on pre- or post-synaptic membrane. An example is alpha-methylnoradrenaline in which a methyl group is substituted on the alpha carbon atom (R$_4$ see Table 16.2). The prodrug is alpha-methyldopa (methyldopa); this is taken up into sympathetic nerves and converted to alpha-methylnoradrenaline by dopa decarboxylase and dopamine-β-hydroxylase. Alpha-methylnoradrenaline is stored in sympathetic nerves and released on nerve stimulation. Its hypotensive effect is exerted in the CNS where it stimulates alpha$_2$-adrenoceptors to cause a fall in peripheral resistance. Another example is *clonidine* which stimulates alpha$_2$-adrenoceptors in the vasomotor centre to inhibit efferent sympathetic tone and so reduce peripheral resistance.

Effects of adrenoceptor activation
Important sites of catecholamine action are discussed below.

(a) Heart and blood vessels
NA causes a sharp rise in blood pressure after i.v. injection.

This is followed by a baroreceptor-mediated reflex bradycardia, so that cardiac output falls, but peripheral resistance is increased despite the fall in cardiac output. This is because NA produces a powerful constriction of the vessels in the skin and splanchnic areas by stimulating alpha-adrenoceptors which are abundant in these vessels. Adrenaline also raises the blood pressure, but the cardiac output is increased due to a powerful increase in force of contraction *and* rate of beating. Despite this, the overall perhipheral resistance may fall because adrenaline dilates skeletal muscle, coronary, and probably CNS blood vessels by stimulating beta-adrenoceptors present in these vessels. Isoprenaline produces a potent stimulant effect on myocardial beta-adrenoceptors causing an increase in cardiac output and pulse pressure. Despite this the overall effect of isoprenaline is a fall in blood pressure because the drug dilates skeletal muscle blood vessels by its action on beta-adrenoceptors.

Catecholamines increase the rate of impulse formation in the sinoatrial node, and so increase the heart rate (chronotropic effect). The drugs also increase the rate of impulse conduction in the Purkinje fibres. High concentrations of catecholamines in the heart give rise to cardiac arrhythmias. For this reason adrenaline and isoprenaline should never be given by i.v. injection.

Catecholamines increase the force of contraction (ionotropic effect) of the myocardium; of the three catecholamines, isoprenaline, adrenaline and NA, isoprenaline is the most potent. NA is also a potent activator of cardiac beta-adrenoceptors. Its apparent relatively lower activity is due to its high affinity for uptake$_1$ sites in cardiac tissues which are densely supplied by sympathetic nerves. After blockade of uptake$_1$, NA is equally as potent as adrenaline in stimulating cardiac beta-adrenoceptors.

(b) *Smooth muscles*

The smooth muscles of the bronchi contain beta-adrenoceptors which are stimulated by adrenaline and isoprenaline to produce bronchodilation. These and similar drugs are used in the treatment of bronchial asthma. Smooth muscles of the gastrointestinal tract are relaxed by catecholamines. Adrenaline and NA contract gastrointestinal tract sphincters. The human uterine smooth muscle contains beta-adrenoceptors which mediate relaxation on stimulation by isoprenaline and such-like drugs. The beta$_2$-agonist salbutamol (see Chapters 4 and 24) is used to treat threatened abortion. On the eye, NA and adrenaline contract the dilator pupillae by an action on alpha-adrenoceptors.

(c) *Hyperglycaemic action*

Adrenaline causes hyperglycaemia (increase in blood sugar) by stimulating glycogenolysis. The first step in this complicated reaction is the activation of the membrane enzyme adenylcyclase following receptor occupation by agonist. Adenylcyclase converts ATP to cyclic-3, 5-adenosine monophosphate (cyclic AMP or cAMP) which in turn converts inactive to active phosphorylase; the latter catalyses the breakdown of glycogen to yield glucose. The action is mediated by beta-adrenoceptors (adrenaline and isoprenaline being more potent than NA) and is blocked by propranolol. The activation of adrenylate cyclase by beta-adrenoceptor agonists is widespread. It has been observed in smooth and cardiac muscle where the effector organ response is thought to be due to the action of the phosphodiester, cAMP, which has thus been referred to as the *second messenger*. Initially, it was thought that adrenylate cyclase might be the beta-adrenoceptor. But is was soon discovered that other drugs, e.g. endocrine hormones such as hydrocortisone, histamine, prostaglandins, and other transmitters can also activate adenylate cyclase to increase intracellular cAMP. Glycogenolysis itself can be induced via activation of adenylate cyclase by glucagon and somatotrophin. These other effects are resistant to propranolol. It is now thought that the different hormone receptors are regulatory subunits on the enzyme (see Fig. 16.6).

Fig. 16.6. The formation of cyclic AMP: a = PGE$_2$; b = transmitter; c = hydrocortisone; d = histamine.

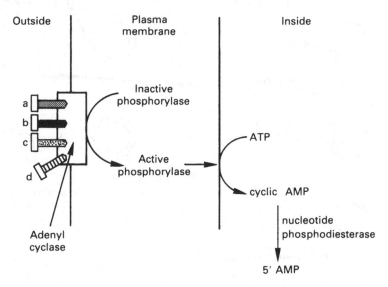

Alpha-adrenoceptor antagonists

Several drugs block alpha-adrenoceptors (Fig. 16.6) and so prevent the vasoconstrictor and other alpha-receptor mediated effects of sympathetic nerve stimulation and of circulating catecholamines. Alpha-adrenoceptor antagonists do not effectively lower blood pressure (b.p) in hypertension, but they can produce a sudden fall in b.p when administered intravenously to patients with phaeochromocytoma in whom the level of circulating catecholamines is high. This is because alpha-adrenoceptor blocking drugs are more effective in antagonising the effects of circulating catecholamines than the effects of NA released from noradrenergic nerves. It may also be because ATP is released from sympathetic nerves to contract vessels. The rapid fall in b.p. provides a diagnostic test for phaeochromocytoma. Phentolamine is usually used for this test.

Presynaptic alpha₂-adrenoceptors

The reason that most alpha adrenoceptor blockers are not effective in essential hypertension is because they also block

Fig. 16.7. Structures of some alpha-adrenoceptor antagonists.

IRREVERSIBLE

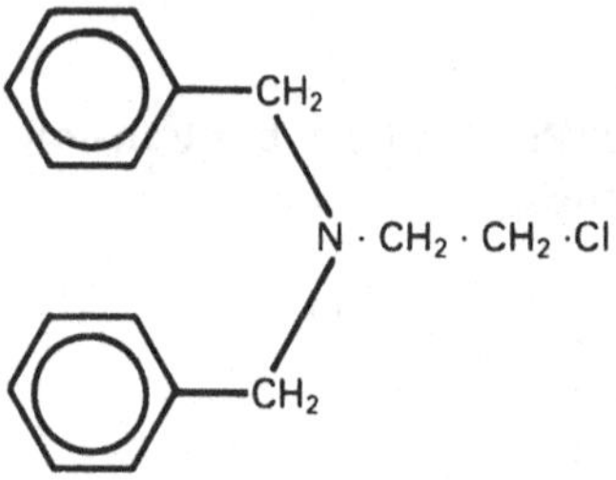

REVERSIBLE

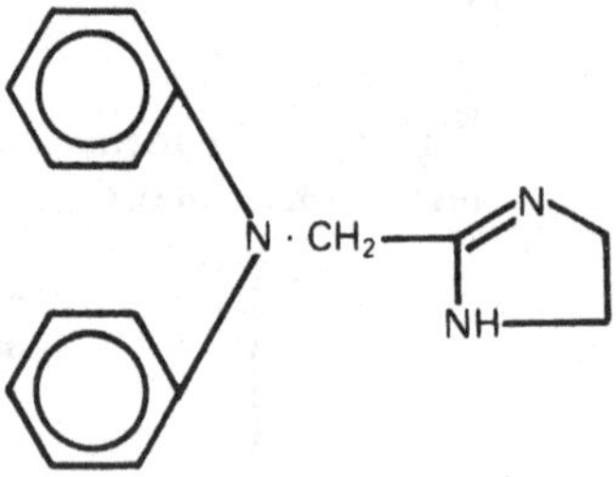

Dibenamine

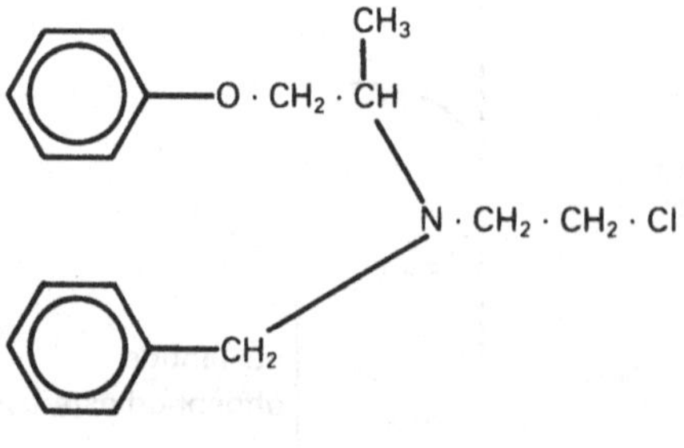

Phentolamine

Phenoxybenzamine

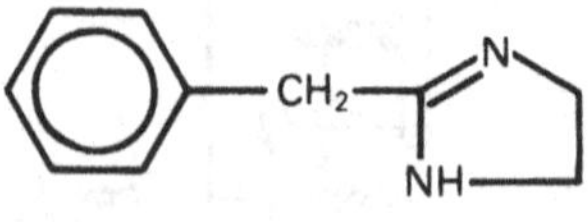

Tolazoline

presynaptic alpha₂-adrenoceptors (see page 103) which would increase the amount of NA released by sympathetic nerves. This is counter-productive in two ways. The increased NA may effectively overcome the alpha-receptor blockade at the postsynaptic membrane. Secondly the initial fall in peripheral resistance caused by these drugs leads to a reflex tachycardia, and since the cardiac receptors are not blocked by this class of antagonists, there are increased cardiac output and alarming palpitations. The blood pressure may soon rise to its previous high level. The antihypertensive drug *prazosin* has a preference for postsynaptic alpha₁-adrenoceptors and therefore does not increase the sympathetic output of NA in the heart; the drug is reputed to cause minimal tachycardia and palpitations. Tachycardia is a beta-adrenoceptor mediated effect; therefore a useful drug would be one which combines beta- and alpha-adrenoceptor blocking properties. Such a drug is *labetolol*. In animal experiments labetolol is more potent at blocking beta- than alpha-adrenoceptors. A decrease in peripheral resistance caused by this drug is not accompanied by tachycardia; rather there is a fall in cardiac output due to blockade of cardiac beta-adrenceptors. Interestingly, West Indian and West African black hypertensives are reported to be resistant to the antihypertensive action of labetolol compared to Caucasion hypertensives. The reason for this difference is not known. Remembering that blacks are resistant to the antihypertensive action of beta-adrenoceptor blockers (see chapter 8), it may be inferred that the major component of the antihypertensive effect of labetolol is due to beta-adrenoceptor blockade, bearing in mind that the drug is more potent at blocking beta- than alpha-adrenoceptors.

The alpha-adrenoceptor blocking drugs are used in the diagnosis of phaeochromocytoma (phentolamine), in the treatment of peripheral vascular disease (Regnauld's disease) (phenoxybenzamine, tolazoline), and in the treatment of hypertension (prazosin, labetolol and ergot alkaloids). Common side effects due to blockade of alpha-adrenoceptors are, for instance postural hypotension and failure of ejaculation. (See Fig. 16.7).

Beta-adrenoceptor antagonists

These are structurally related to isoprenaline. The pharmacological basis for their subdivision into beta₁ and beta₂ is discussed in Chapter 4. The drugs have various other actions such as intrinsic sympathomimetic activity (partial agonism), membrane-stabilising activity (local anaesthetic action), and lipid solubility (this determines

Table 16.3   *Properties of some beta-adrenoceptor antagonists*

Non-selective (β₁, β₂) antagonists	Membrane stabilising (local anaesthetic) activity	Intrinsic sympathomimetic (partial agonist) activity	Lipid solubility (CNS penetration)
Propranolol			
R (−)	+	0	high
S (+) (lacks receptor-blocking action)	+	0	high
Timolol	0	0	moderate
Alprenolol	+	+	high
Pindolol	+	+	moderate
Sotalol	0	0	low
Cardioselective (predominantly β₁) antagonists			
Atenolol	0	0	low
Metoprolol	+	0	high
Acebutalol	+	+	high
Practolol	0	+	low

Note: (i) Cardioselectivity is not absolute. In large doses cardioselective antagonists can also block beta₂-adrenoceptors and can cause bronchospasm in asthmatics.
(ii) Beta-adrenoceptor antagonists with partial agonist activity cause less bradycardia and less cardiac output reduction than those without this activity.

whether they act on the CNS) see Table 16.3. There is no correlation between membrane-stabilising activity and beta-adrenoceptor blockade or lowering of blood pressure. For example, sotalol has beta-blocking and blood pressure lowering action but no local anaesthetic action. Further points to note are as follows:

(a) Beta-adrenoceptor antagonism is particularly demonstrable when the sympathetic tone is high.

(b) Membrane-stabilising activity may be of additional advantage when the drugs are used in the treatment of cardiac arrhythmias.

(c) The non-selective beta-adrenoceptor antagonists can precipitate dangerous bronchospasm in asthmatics due to blockade of beta₂ adrenoceptors on bronchiolar smooth muscle; latterly some socalled beta₁ selective antagonists have also shown this effect. In large doses these drugs also block beta₂ receptors.

Additionally, the bronchioles contain a small proportion of beta₁ adrenoceptors which mediate dilatation. All beta-blockers should be used with great care, especially in patients with heart disease in which these drugs may slow down the rate of impulse conduction so much as to cause heart block and heart failure.

(d) These compounds are used in a wider range of disease conditions than the alpha blockers, e.g. in hypertension, angina pectoris, cardiac arrhythmias, glaucoma, and hyperthyroidism.

Another important consequence of beta-adrenoceptor blockade is potentiation of insulin response in diabetes. Normally the hypoglycaemic effect of insulin is opposed by liver and muscle glycogenolysis. These are beta-receptor mediated. Blockade of beta-receptors in the diabetic being treated with insulin may precipitate a hypoglycaemic coma; his doctor may not know this in time because the usual tachycardia and tremor which accompany hypoglycaemia are also blocked by the beta-receptor antagonist.

17

Cholinergic mechanisms

17.1   INTRODUCTION
From the point of view of drug action, three sites of ACH release in the peripheral nervous system are important. These are the following.

  (i) Ganglia (both sympathetic and parasympathetic).
 (ii) Neuromuscular junction. And
(iii) All postganglionic parasympathetic nerve endings and exceptionally the sympathetic nerve ending to sweat glands. ACH is also released by the splanchnic nerve to the adrenal medulla. Although the catecholamine-releasing action of ACH in this gland can be blocked by ganglion blockers (e.g., hexamethonium), this site of drug action is not therapeutically important. When released ACH produces a variety of effects (depending on the effector organ) by activating different types of receptors. The action of ACH is terminated through its rapid hydrolysis by acetylcholinesterase (ACHE) which is present in high concentrations at the postsynaptic membrane wherever ACH is a transmitter. An exception seems to be the ganglia where the presence of ACHE is hard to demonstrate and where diffusion from the synaptic cleft followed by hydrolysis by plasma cholinesterase, may be the major mechanism for the termination of ACH. After reading this chapter, the student should know how ACH is synthesised and released, the different types of receptors which it can activate, the characteristics of ACHE, and the classes of drugs that affect these mechanisms.

17.2   ACH BIOSYNTHESIS AND RELEASE
ACH is synthesised in cholinergic neurones from choline and acetic acid under the influence of choline acetyltransferase and stored

in vesicles for subsequent nerve impulse-mediated release (see section 15.3). ACH release is triggered by impulses (Na^+ ions in, K^+ ions out) transmitted along the cholinergic nerve. ACH release by the process of exocytosis involves Ca^{2+} entry into the axonal cytoplasm. After release ACH is hydrolysed to choline and acetic acid; choline is pumped back into the nerve for reuse in ACH synthesis. These events at the cholinergic neurone can be blocked by a number of substances of scientific and possibly warfare, but not therapeutic, interest.

Impulse transmission along the axon can be inhibited by several naturally occurring substances which block Na^+ and K^+ channels. Examples are given below.

   (i) *Tetrodotoxin* (TTX), obtained from puffer fish, acts like a local anaesthetic, but more powerful, being 10^4 times more potent than procaine. Because TTX can block Na^+ and K^+ channels in nerves at much lower concentrations than those required for the same purpose in muscle cells, the compound is a useful experimental tool for distinguishing between neurogenic and myogenic contractions.

  (ii) *Saxitoxin*, a shell fish poison,

 (iii) *Chiriquitoxin*, a tropical frog skin poison; both of these block Na^+ and K^+ channels in nerves,

  (iv) *Batrachotoxin*, is a South American frog skin poison, forces Na^+ channels to stay permanently open and prevents impulse conduction.

   (v) *Botulinum toxin*, from *B. botulinus* prevents ACH release at the nerve terminal.

  (vi) *Black widow spider venom* (α-latrotoxin) prevents the storage of ACH in vesicles (cf. reserpine in sympathetic neurones). Since ACH is released only in its packaged form, α-latrotoxin prevents release even if ACH is present in the nerve cytosol.

 (vii) Chelating agents may prevent ACH release by removing Ca^{2+}, e.g. the neuromuscular blocking action of streptomycin and its potentiation of neuromuscular blocking drugs may be due to chelation of Ca^{2+} ions.

(viii) Hemicholinium-3 (HC-3) causes transmission failure by inhibiting the uptake of choline. Choline acetyltransferase is not inhibited; consequently, neuromuscular transmission block by HC-3 is reversed by choline.

17.3   CHOLINERGIC RECEPTORS

The most important drugs are those which produce therapeutic benefits by interacting with the different receptors activated by ACH at its different sites of release. These are nicotinic and muscarinic receptors (see section 15.2). Most of the drugs acting at nicotinic receptors are antagonists, whereas muscarinic agonists as well as antagonists have therapeutic uses.

Structural requirements for successful interaction with cholinergic receptors

The pharmacological properties of ACH are due primarily to its strongly basic cationic quaternary nitrogen. This positive charge is essential for the interaction of ACH with a negatively charged site on the receptor, i.e. the anionic site. The oxygen atoms of the ketone and ether tend to negativity; they interact with corresponding positive sites on the receptor, i.e. the esteratic site (see Fig. 17.1).

Some further points can be made about the structural requirements for successful interaction with cholinergic receptors.

(a) Formylcholine (in which the CH_3 group in the acetyl moiety is replaced by H) is an agonist at muscarinic receptors, but weaker than ACH. As the substituent group gets bulkier, the compound loses activity so valerylcholine is an antagonist

(b) (Table 4.1b).

In ACH, the distance between CH_3 and $-N^{(+)}-$ is 5 atoms long (Table 17.2) and this is optimal for muscarinic agonist activity. Thus tetramethylammonium is inactive.

(c) There must be at least two methyl groups attached to the $-N^{(+)}-$. Ethyl cannot replace methyl.

(d) NH_2- can replace CH^3- on the acetyl moiety as in carbachol and bethanecol.

Clinically useful compounds which stimulate cholinergic receptors are shown in Fig. 17.2. Methacholine, bethanecol and pilocarpine stimulate muscarinic receptors only. Carbachol stimulates both

Fig. 17.1 Interaction of ACH with cholinergic receptor (hypothetical).

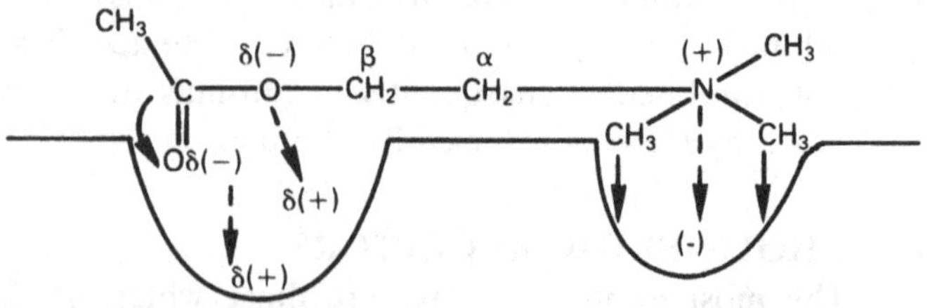

nicotinic and muscarinic receptors. These compounds are resistant to cholinesterase and are active when given orally or by injection. Some cholinergic receptor stimulants are alkaloids, e.g. pilocarpine (from *Pilocarpus jaborandi*), arecoline (from *Areca catechu*), muscarine (from *Amanita muscaria*, the most poisonous mushroom known), and nicotine. The synthetic compounds are used for the termination of paroxysmal tachycardia (methacholine), emergency treatment of glaucoma (carbachol and bethanecol), and post-operative urinary retention (bethanechol). Effects with large doses include bronchoconstriction and cardiovascular collapse.

The alkaloids are not choline esters and are therefore not substrates

Fig. 17.2. Choline esters. Note the horizontal bar indicating the 5-atom distance.

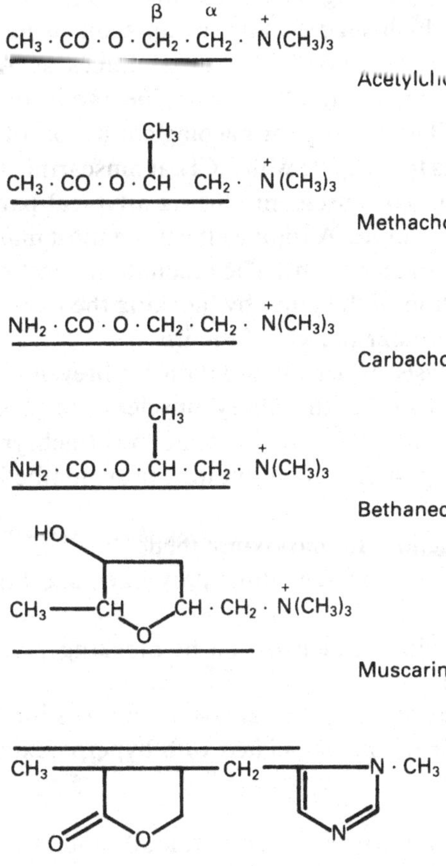

Acetylcholine

Methacholine

Carbachol

Bethanechol

Muscarine

Pilocarpine

for cholinesterases. The most useful is pilocarpine, e.g. to produce miosis and hence counteract atropine-induced mydriasis or reduce intraoccular pressure in glaucoma. Arecholine can be used to expel ascaris or tapeworms in domestic animals. Nicotine produces complex effects due to stimulation and inhibition of autonomic ganglia and CNS effects; its inhalation in tobacco is partly responsible for the habituation produced by cigarettes, but the carcinogenicity is not attributed to the alkaloid but to the products of slow combustion, e.g. tar.

Muscarinic receptor antagonists

The classic muscarinic receptor antagonist is atropine. The group of drugs which antagonise muscarinic receptors are therefore also referred to as *atropine-like drugs* or *parasympatholytic* because they abolish the effects of parasympathetic nerve stimulation. Some structures are shown in Fig. 17.3. Note the five-atom chain also in these compounds which suggests that the antagonists too may interact with the muscarinic receptor with similar forces as ACH. *Atropine* is a racemic mixture of d-and l-hyoscyamine and is an ester of tropic acid and tropine. The main pharmacological action of atropine in therapeutic doses is to compete with ACH at muscarinic receptors in glands, heart and smooth muscle, producing a typical parallel shift of ACH dose–response curves. Atropine effects are most marked in organs with high parasympathetic tone. They include the following.

(a) Dilation of the pupil by blocking the parasympathetic tone to the circular muscle of the iris.

(b) Paralysis of accommodation by preventing parasympathetic contraction of the ciliary muscles of the eye (see section 17.5).

(c) Reduction of glandular secretions (lachrymal, salivary, bronchial, gastric) and of sweating (a sympathetic cholinergic function).

(d) Reduction in parasympathetic tone of smooth muscles of bronchi, stomach, alimentary tract, and bladder (urinary and gall).

(e) Induction of tachycardia by blocking vagal inhibition of the heart.

In toxic doses, atropine reveals a central stimulant effect, causing excitement or mania associated with hyperpyrexia.

Uses

Atropine can be given by mouth and is also easily absorbed from the mucous membrane of the conjunctiva. It is used for the following purposes.

(1) Premedication
    (a) to reduce bronchial and salivary secretions especially when ether is used as a general anaesthetic,
    (b) to prevent bronchospasm in light anaesthesia, and
    (c) to prevent bradycardia normally caused by most inhalation anaesthetics, e.g. halothane.
(2) Atropine is given before neostigmine when the latter is used to terminate the action of tubocurarine. The nicotinic action of tubocurarine is needed in this instance, and atropine is used to block the unwanted muscarinic effects. Atropine is used for the same purpose when neostigmine is employed in the treatment of myaesthenia gravis (see page 393).
(3) It is used to control overactive bowels and in the treatment of peptic ulceration. Atropine must not be given to patients with raised intraoccular pressure as then it may precipitate glaucoma.

Fig. 17.3. Structures of some muscarinic receptor antagonists.

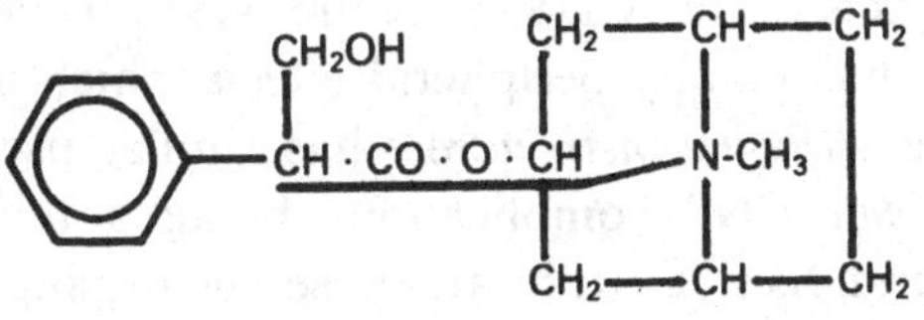

Atropine

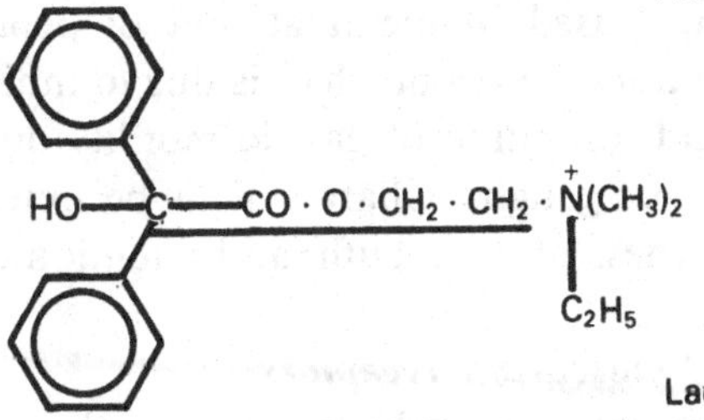

Lachesine

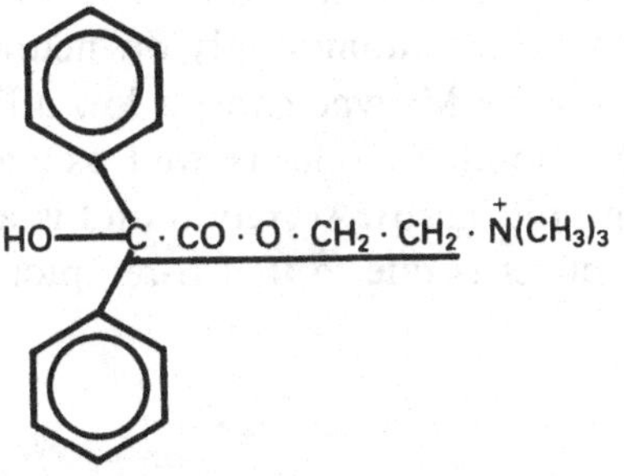

Benzilylcholine

(4) When dropped into the conjunctiva (1% solution), atropine produces a long-lasting mydriasis, paralysis of pupillary reaction to light, and paralysis of accommodation. With the eye in this state it is easy to examine the ocular fundus. Homatropine is preferred because it is shorter acting. Atropine is used to rest an inflamed eye.

(5) Atropine is used in the treatment of organophosphorus anticholinesterase poisoning.

Hyoscine (scopolamine)

The principal difference between hyoscine and atropine is that hyoscine is not a central stimulant, but can quieten mania and produce amnesia; used to relieve motion sickness and in the treatment of Parkinsonism. In this condition it reduces tremor, and salivation.

Synthetic atropine-like drugs

The 5-atom rule applies in most of these compounds (see Fig. 17.3). In addition they possess a quaternary nitrogen and therefore have minimal effects on the CNS. They are used for their peripheral effects. *Lachesine* has mainly peripheral effects which are similar to those of atropine. *Atropine methonitrate* has similar uses to those of atropine with fewer CNS complications being a quaternary ammonium compound. Its side effects are those due to ganglion and neuromuscular blockade. *Propantheline* (probanthine) is a quaternary ammonium compound used in the treatment of peptic ulcer and pylorospasm. Its usefulness in peptic ulcer is due to inhibition of gastric acid secretion and inhibition of gastric motility due to block of muscarinic receptors and ganglia. Characteristic peripheral effects are blurring of vision, dryness of the mouth, and retention of urine.

Subclasses of muscarinic receptors

Muscarinic receptors have been subdivided into M_1 and M_2 subtypes on the basis of their relative affinities for the competitive antagonist pirenzepine. M_1-receptors exhibit a high binding affinity for pirenzepine and are found predominantly on neural tissue, e.g. autonomic ganglia, whereas the M_2 type show a low affinity for this agent and are found in smooth muscle as well as neural tissues. Pirenzepine selectively inhibits gastric secretion and is a useful antiulcer drug. Possibly this effect is due to its M_1-receptor blockade at autonomic ganglia.

Nicotinic receptor antagonists

Nicotinic receptors are present at sympathetic and para-sympathetic ganglia, and at the motor end plates of nerve–skeletal muscle junctions, and on chromaffin cells in the adrenal medulla.

Ganglionic-blocking drugs

Transmission across the ganglionic synapse is complex involving nicotinic and muscarinic receptors and dopamine receptors (Fig. 15.2). Although the involvement of these mechanisms in ganglionic transmission can be demonstrated experimentally, activation by ACH of nicotinic receptors on the membrane of the postsynaptic ganglion is the most important mechanism by which the impulse in the preganglionic fibre is transmitted to the postganglionic fibre. Ganglionic nicotinic receptor blockers can thus interrupt transmission at this site, whereas classical muscarinic receptor antagonists, in general, do not. Ganglionic blocking drugs are sometimes useful as therapeutic agents. The classic example is hexamethonium (C6) whose action may be used to describe the characteristics of ganglion blockade:

(a) C6 does not cross the blood–brain barrier, it has no action on the CNS; therefore its effect on the ANS is entirely peripheral.

(b) It does not prevent conduction along nerve trunks.

(c) C6 does not reduce the amount of ACH released from preganglionic nerve terminals and it does not prevent the effect of postganglionic stimulation; the effector organ responds normally to the appropriate neurotransmitter. These points show the site of action of C6 to be the nicotinic receptors on the ganglion cell membrane. C6 combines with these receptors and competitively blocks ACH release from the preganglionic nerve.

Pharmacological actions of ganglion blocking drugs

Bear in mind that the drugs interrupt transmission at both sympathetic and parasympathetic nerves; therefore their effects reflect blockade of the functions of both systems. The drugs lower blood pressure; they can therefore be used in the treatment of hypertension when this is due to excessive activity of the sympathetic nervous system. Ganglion blockade causes a fall in blood pressure because the resistance vessels in skin and splanchnic areas are innervated by sympathetic nerves only.

The effect of ganglionic blockade is most pronounced in conditions of increased vasomotor tone such as occurs in change of posture. Consequently postural hypotension is a common side effect of all ganglion blockers. A patient whose blood pressure is stabilised on a ganglion blocking drug may faint on getting up from bed. The sympathetic reflex (initiated by baroreceptors in the carotid) which prevents gravitational pull of blood downwards from the brain is no longer effective. Other undesirable side effects of ganglion blockers are due to their action on parasympathetic ganglia. These constitute the most serious objections to the clinical use of ganglion blocking drugs. They include: blurred vision, reduced glandular secretion (dry mouth, dry skin), constipation, paralytic ileum, difficulty in micturition and impotence. Hexamethonium is too short acting to be useful. Other examples are discussed below.

Pentolinium (ansolysen)

Like hexamethonium, is a competitive antagonist of ACH, more potent and longer acting and useful in emergency treatment of hypertension; it is given by subcutaneous injection.

Chlorisondamine (ecolid)

Is a bisquaternary ammonium compound with a long duration of action (12–24 h) and is more active than pentolinium.

Mecamylamine (inversine)

Is a secondary amine, rapidly and completely absorbed from the gastrointestinal tract, has a gradual onset and longer duration of action than the quaternary ammonium compounds named above; also it blocks neuromuscular transmission and can therefore potentiate the muscle relaxant effects of tubocurarine. Mecamylamine is not a competitive antagonist; it appears to desensitise nicotinic receptors. It can be used to control blood pressure, but because it penetrates the blood–brain barrier, it produces CNS side effects, e.g. tremor and mental confusion.

Pempidine

Is a tertiary amine and is also completely absorbed from the gastrointestinal tract after oral ingestion; it has similar properties to mecamylamine.

Neuromuscular blocking drugs

The events leading to skeletal muscle contraction can be affected by drugs acting at presynaptic and postsynaptic sites. Substances acting at presynaptic sites are described under section 17.2.

The clinically useful drugs are those acting at the postsynaptic motor end plate. These drugs interact with nicotinic receptors to competitively occlude ACH or to depolarise the membrane and/or desensitise the receptors.

Competitive block of ACH receptors

The combination of ACH with receptors at the motor end plate causes *depolarisation* (i.e. an increase in the resting potential) which leads to muscle contraction. Competitive neuromuscular blockers, e.g. gallamine, d-tubocurarine, combine with end plate receptors without producing a depolarisation and hence no build up of end plate potential occurs. These drugs thus compete with ACH on the 'lock and key' principle. Another type of neuromuscular blocker combines with the end plate receptor and causes depolarisation, but subsequent repolarisation is incomplete so that after a period of exposure to the drug (about 60 s) the resting potential is raised and ACH released from the motor nerve ending can no longer cause a depolarisation, and the muscle is paralysed.

Suxamethonium as an example of this type of activity is described later, but the essential difference between it and tubocurarine is depicted in Fig. 17.4.

Some characteristics of tubocurarine block are listed below.

(a) Neuromuscular block is not preceded by initial stimulation.

(b) After intravenous injection, skeletal muscles are blocked at different rates: eyelid muscles, neck, limbs, trunk and finally the respiratory muscles, i.e. intercostal and the diaphragm muscles, are blocked in that order.

(c) The threshold amount of ACH for the initiation of muscle contraction is raised; the corollary is that drugs such as neostigmine which increase the concentration of ACH at the motor end plate can overcome the block.

(d) During development of the block, the response of the muscle to tetanic nerve stimulation (about 100 pulses per second) is not sustained (Fig. 17.4). Since some of the receptors are occupied by d-tubocurarine molecules, then the threshold for ACH contraction is high. In tetanic nerve stimulation, the amount of ACH released falls off with time as release exceeds synthesis; even with continued stimulation, the amount of ACH released rapidly falls below the threshold for muscle stimulation.

(e) As in (d) above, the twitch response following a tetanic stimulus is potentiated because the large amount of ACH released

Fig. 17.4. Neuromuscular block by (a) d-tubocurarine (d-tc), and (b) suxamethonium (sux). Note: the response to tetanic nerve stimulation (TET) is poorly maintained *during development* of the d-tc block, but there is post-tetanic potentiation (PTP); the block is reversed by neostigmine (NEOS). In (b), there is initial stimulation, a well maintained response to TET, and no PTP. The block is deepened by NEOS. (Redrawn from Grundy (1985), see p. 463 in Ch.20 for reference).

(a)

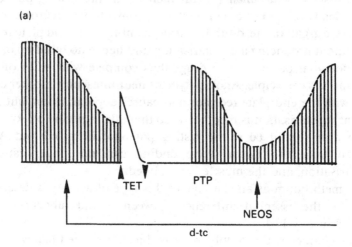

(b)

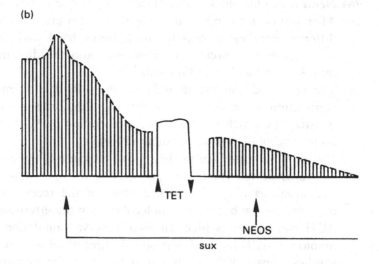

during tetanus causes d-tubocurarine molecules to be displaced from the receptors.

The following important points of clinical interest should be noted.

(a) Tubocurarine is potentiated by inhalation anaesthetics such as ether and by streptomycin which have curare-like action of their own. Children are more sensitive to this effect than adults.

(b) Tubocurarine may not be effective in patients with obstructive jaundice because the drug forms an insoluble complex with high molecular weight bile acids of which serum concentrations are high in this condition.

(c) Tubocurarine is a fairly potent ganglion blocker. This may partly account for its lowering of arterial blood pressure. Another action related to its hypotensive action is that it can release histamine from mast cells and other storage sites. Anaesthetists should watch out for this hypotensive effect which may be particularly marked with halothane as this substance possesses ganglion blocking action of its own.

(d) Histamine liberation by tubocurarine may lead to dangerous bronchospasm in asthmatics undergoing surgery. Gallamine is less potent as a histamine liberator and is therefore preferred under these circumstances.

Gallamine (Fig. 17.5)

This is a synthetic neuromuscular blocker similar in action to tubocurarine. It is different from tubocurarine in the following respects.

(a) Gallamine is much less potent than tubocurarine, requiring a dose of 80–120 mg in the adult.

(b) Gallamine has atropine-like action on the heart, producing tachycardia; this action is possibly due to block of cardiac (M_2) muscarinic receptors for which gallamine is regarded as a selective antagonist.

(c) Gallamine does not release histamine. It may therefore be used instead of tubocurarine in asthmatics.

Pancuronium

This is a bisquaternary ammonium steroid synthesised in 1964. It is about 5 times more potent than tubocurarine in competitive blockade of neuromuscular transmission. It has minimal cardiovascular actions (i.e., no action on cardiac muscarinic receptors or ganglionic transmission); and it does not release histamine. It is therefore indicated for patients with cardiovascular complications.

Atracurium

This is a short-acting competitive type neuromuscular blocker similar in its range of effects to pancuronium. It is preferred to tubocurarine when hypotensive and histamine releasing effects are undesirable.

Fig. 17.5. Structures of some major competitive neuromuscular-blocking drugs.

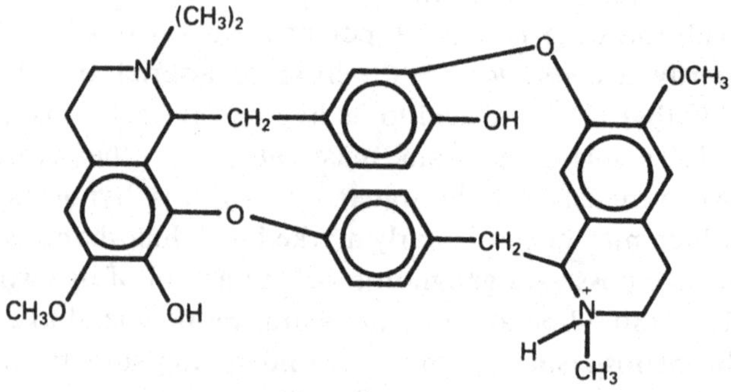

d- Tubocurarine

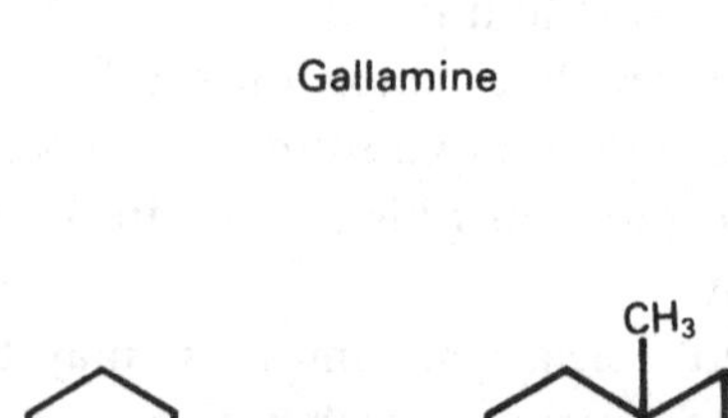

Gallamine

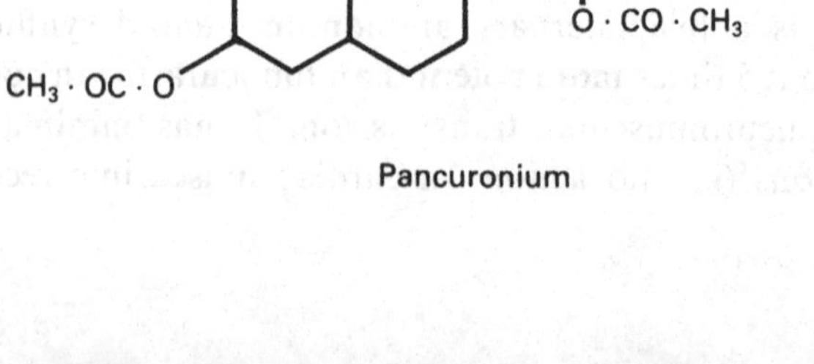

Pancuronium

Depolarisation or desensitisation block

Some drugs combine with ACH receptors at the motor end plate and produce first a depolarisation of the cell membrane, and then subsequently a block of neuromuscular transmission. Examples are decamethonium and suxamethonium. A study of the structural requirements for interaction with nicotinic receptors by Paton and Zaimis established that in the methonium series, bistrimethyl ammonium compounds of the type $(CH_3)_3 \overset{+}{N} - (CH_2)_n - \overset{+}{N} (CH_3)_3$, the n value for optimum blocking action at nicotinic receptors in ganglia was 6 (i.e., hexamethonium) and that at skeletal muscle motor end plate receptors it was 10 (i.e., decamethonium) (Fig. 17.6). In decamethonium, the distance between the two $\overset{+}{N}$, is estimated to be about 1.2 nm, (about 10 atoms) and is approximately the same in suxamethonium (remember the 5-atom distance in ACH; suxamethonium is virtually two ACH molecules joined together). Note that many competitive antagonists (Fig. 17.5) also have two $\overset{+}{N}$ which are approximately 10 atoms apart.

The mechanism of action of depolarising agents is not fully understood but it definitely involves interaction with the end plate

Fig. 17.6. The effect of methylene chain length on the blocking activity of *bis*trimethyl ammonium compounds $[(CH_3)_3.N.(CH_2)_n.\overset{+}{N}(CH_3)_3]$ at (a) autonomic ganglia, and (b) skeletal muscle motor end plate. Nicotinic receptor blocking activity is plotted against number (n) of methylene (CH_2), groups in the chain (see text). This graph is diagrammatic to show that optimum blocking activity is achieved at (a) and (b) with different chain lengths.

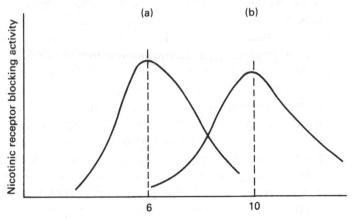

receptors and depolarisation of the end plate membrane as indicated by the following characteristics.

(a) Block is preceded by initial stimulation (muscle fasciculation). This is of short duration as neuromuscular block follows immediately.

(b) The block can be reversed by tubocurarine which reduces the end plate potential. This fact is of no practical importance in reversing the effect of excess depolarising agent. There is no practical antidote to these agents. Fortunately the most widely used, suxamethonium, is short-acting due to hydrolysis by plasma cholinesterase.

(c) In multiply innervated skeletal muscles, e.g. chick biventer cervices, toad rectus abdominis or denervated mammalian skeletal muscle, where there are numerous motor end plates per muscle fibre, suxamethonium causes a contracture similar to ACH; this is blocked by tubocurarine. The responses of the chick biventer and toad rectus are used experimentally to differentiate between depolarising and competitive blockers. Following an intravenous injection, day-old-chicks die in *spastic* paralysis with suxamethonium and *flaccid* paralysis with tubocurarine. (a), (b) and (c) above point to interaction of depolarising blockers with end plate receptors.

(d) During the development of the block by suxamethonium, the response to tetanic nerve stimulation is sustained. This is because the drug raises the resting end plate potential and inhibits repolarisation. At this stage even few ACH molecules can trigger a sustained contraction.

(e) Increasing the concentration of ACH during a depolarisation block can only increase the block as ACH causes further depolarisation (Fig. 17.4). Thus one explanation of muscle paralysis caused by suxamethonium is that the drug causes a persistent depolarisation of the motor end plate which leads to inactivation of the sodium pump required for the propagation of action potential in muscle fibres. Alternatively, ACH receptors become *desensitised* after interaction with a depolarising blocker, so that even when the muscle has repolarised, ACH cannot activate the receptors. Thesleff has shown that in some cases muscular paralysis can persist after membrane repolarisation. *Suxamethonium* (Fig. 17.7) is the depolarising agent mostly in use as a muscle relaxant. Its short duration of action makes it suitable for procedures such as the introduction of a bronchoscope which requires brief relaxation of the muscles of the larynx. It can also be used in conjunction with thiopentone to reduce muscle movement in electroconvulsive therapy.

The initial fasciculation caused by suxamethonium can give rise to considerable postoperative pain in the head, neck and trunk. The drug stimulates ganglia and may thus raise the arterial blood pressure. It may also stimulate muscarinic receptors to cause salivation, increased bronchial secretion and bradycardia. These effects are blocked by atropine. In a small number of patients genetically deficient in plasma cholinesterase, apnoea may be prolonged (see page 184).

There is evidence that during prolonged exposure to a depolarising blocker, the characteristics of the block can change, later showing properties displayed by competitive blockers. This is described as the dual mode of action. The clinical significance of this is not known. *Benzoquinonium* is a synthetic muscle relaxant with depolarising and competitive block properties. Table 17 1 is a summary of competitive and depolarising characteristics in neuromuscular block.

17.4 ACHE INHIBITORS (ANTICHOLINESTERASES)

Two classes of drugs inhibit acetylcholinesterase (ACHE). These are: (a) *carbamates* – reversible anticholinesterases, e.g. physostigmine (contains a tertiary nitrogen group) neostigmine, and pyridostigmine (both contain quaternary N^+ ions) (see Fig. 1.3); and (b) *organophosphorus compounds* – irreversible anticholinesterases, e.g. diisopropylphosphorofluoridate (DEP), malathion, tetraethylpyrophosphate (TEPP), and octamethylpyrophosphoramide (OMPA). All these are used in agriculture as insecticides.

Mechanism of action of ACHE inhibitors

Acetylcholine binds to ACHE at two sites on the enzyme: the *anionic* site and the *esteratic* site (see Fig. 17.8a). The anionic is the weaker of the two bonds so that after hydrolysis of ACH, the 'Choline – enzyme' complex rapidly dissociates to free the anionic site. The esteratic site remains acetylated for a little longer; deacetylation of this site is the final step in the action of the enzyme.

The quaternated carbamates edrophonium, neostigmine, and pyridostigmine (Fig. 17.8b) bind to the enzyme also at the anionic and esteratic sites. In the case of physostigmine which contains a tertiary nitrogen group (pK_a 8.0), the molecule is protonated at the body fluid

Fig. 17.7. Structures of some depolarising blockers.

$(CH_3)_3 \overset{+}{N} \cdot CH_2 \cdot CH_2 \cdot CH_2 \cdot CH_2 \cdot CH_2 \cdot CH_2 \cdot CH_2 \cdot CH_2 \cdot CH_2 \cdot CH_2 \cdot \overset{+}{N}(CH_3)_3$

Decamethonium

$(CH_3)_3 \overset{+}{N} \cdot CH_2 \cdot CH_2 \cdot O \cdot CO \cdot CH_2 \cdot CH_2 \cdot CO \cdot O \cdot CH_2 \cdot CH_2 \cdot \overset{+}{N}(CH_3)_3$

Suxamethonium

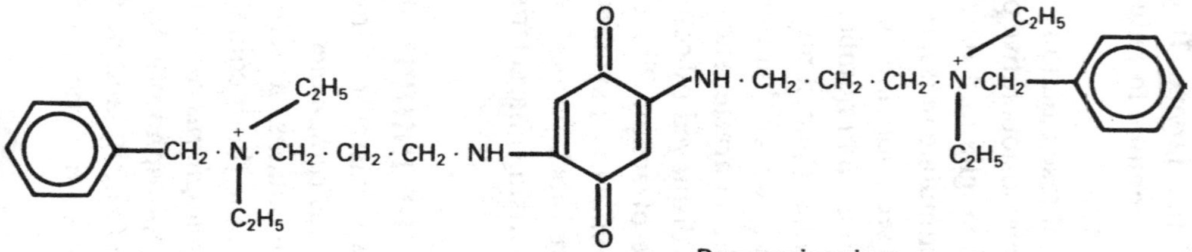

Benzoquinonium

Table 17.1 *Differential effects of tubocurarine and suxamethonium in skeletal muscle*

Characteristics	d-Tubocuravine	Suxamethonium
Initial fasciculation	absent	present, brief
Muscle paralysis due to:	competitive antagonism	depolarisation followed by desensitisation
End plate potential	decreased to zero	raised, falls to zero
Effect of anticholinesterase, e.g. neostigmine on block	relieves block	increases block
Effects:		
(a) on day-old chicks	flaccid paralysis	spastic paralysis-
(b) on toad rectus muscle (see text)	none, but blocks ACH- or Sux-induced contracture	contracture
During partial block:		
(a) tetanic nerve stimulation	rapidly fading response	well-maintained response
(b) post-tetanic potentiation	present	absent

pH (7.4), so that interaction with the negatively charged anionic site also occurs. The esteratic site is carbamylated. Dissociation from the anionic site is rapid but decarbamylation is about a million times slower than deacetylation. Access of the substrate to the enzyme site is thus prevented and ACH accumulates.

The organophosphorus compounds interact with the enzyme only at the esteratic site to form initially a reversible complex, but after about 1 h an irreversible covalent bond is formed. The duration of action of this class of ACHE inhibitors can be days, weeks or even months and depends on the time taken for a new enzyme to be formed and for the drug to be eliminated from the body. The organophosphorus compounds are noted more for their toxicology than for their therapeutic applications; they are used widely as insecticides in agriculture and accidental poisoning occurs frequently. The symptoms of poisoning are due to accumulated ACH: copious salivation, sweating, bronchoconstriction, increased gastrointestinal motility (diarrhoea), bradycardia, and muscle fasciculation.

Treatment must include administration of atropine to block muscarinic effects. The phosphorylated enzyme can be reactivated by a nucleophilic reagent (these react at centres of low electron density).

An example is *pralidoxime* (PAM) (Fig. 17.9). This reacts with the anionic site of ACHE and by orientation of the oxime group, the latter displaces the phosphoryl group from the esteratic site, thereby reactivating the enzyme. An 'aged' phosphorylated enzyme is more difficult to reactivate with a nucleophilic reagent than a recently phosphorylated enzyme. Nucleophilic agents should not be used in the treatment of overdosage with physostigmine or neostigmine.

Some uses of ACHE inhibitors

Other fundamental points about ACHE inhibitors can be brought out by considering their major uses, under (a) and (b) below.

Fig. 17.8. (a) Schematic representation of interaction of ACH with ACHE at anionic and esteratic sites. (b) Molecular structures of carbamate inhibitors of ACHE. Vertical broken line in (a) indicates point of hydrolysis of ACH and ACHE inhibitors.

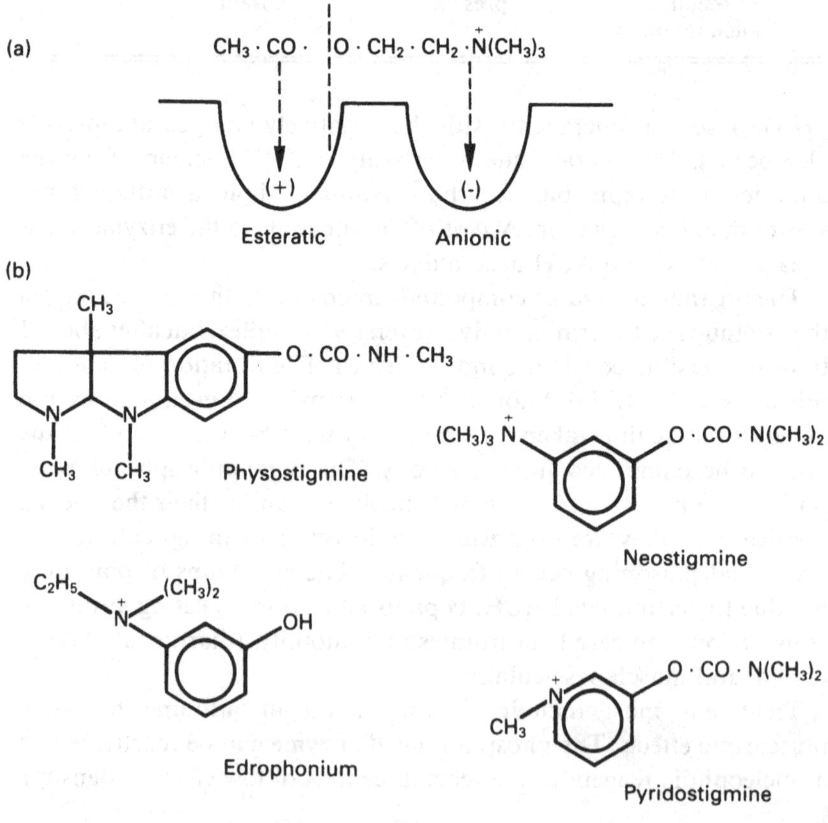

(a) Systemic applications

The carbamates with quaternary nitrogen groups, e.g. neo-stigmine, and pyridostigmine are preferred to physostigmine because the latter with a tertiary nitrogen crosses the blood–brain barrier and causes CNS side effects. The clinical situations in which systemic anticholinesterases are required include the following.

Postoperative reversal of tubocurarine block
This is often necessary to restore spontaneous respiration.

Myaesthenia gravis
This is a disease characterised by weakness of skeletal muscle, a common feature being drooping eyelids and difficulty in swallowing or talking. Some patients benefit from treatment with ACHE inhibitors because these drugs increase the concentration of ACH at the motor end plate, and in the case of the carbamates with quaternary nitrogen (neostigmine and pyridostigmine), the drugs also directly stimulate the nicotinic receptors at the skeletal muscle motor end plate (but not at ganglia). Note the clinically important point that when anticholinesterases are used in the above situations, the effect is required at nicotinic receptors of skeletal muscle end plates. Therefore the patient should be protected from accompanying muscarinic effects by prior administration of atropine. Neostigmine can also be used to produce muscarinic effects as in the treatment of *paralytic* ileus and

Fig. 17.9. Cholinesterase reactivators.

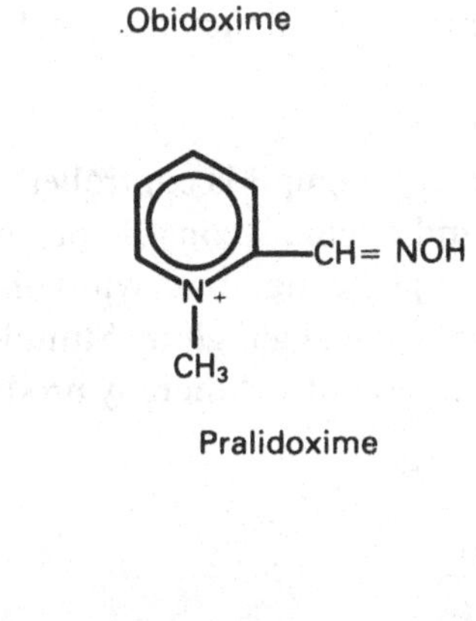

Obidoxime

Pralidoxime

post operative urinary retention. Because physostigmine can enter the CNS more easily than other carbamates, it may be used to counteract the CNS effects of atropine overdose.

(b) Topical applications

An important topical use of ACHE inhibitors is in the eye in the following circumstances.

To counter the effects of atropine

This may often be necessary to correct long-lasting blurred vision after atropine administration. Physostigmine is preferred because it penetrates the mucous membrane of the conjuctiva better than neostigmine or pyridostigmine.

In the treatment of glaucoma

This is a disease characterised by an increase in intraocular tension. By contracting the circular muscles of the iris, ACHE inhibitors widen the angle of filtration, open the canal of Schlemm and permit the drainage of aqueous humour away from the posterior chamber to the anterior chamber of the eye. This reduces intraocular pressure. For the reason stated above, physostigmine is preferred. DFP can also be used; its intraocular pressure-lowering effect lasts 2-3 weeks.

17.5   ACTION OF AUTONOMIC DRUGS ON THE EYE

Much of the pharmacology of the autonomic nervous system can be learnt by studying the action of drugs on the eye. The muscles of the iris are innervated by sympathetic and parasympathetic nerves and drugs can be applied topically and their effects observed directly.

Two sets of muscles in the eye respond to autonomic nerve stimulation or to drugs acting on the ANS. These are the *iris* which controls the size of the pupil and the *ciliary* muscles which control the curvature of the lens and hence the focal point.

The iris

The size of the pupil is controlled by the iris which consists of radial (dilator) and circular (constrictor) muscles. The dilator muscles are innervated by postganglionic sympathetic nerves which originate from the superior cervical ganglion. Stimulation of these nerves causes the radial muscles to contract thereby producing a dilation of the pupil (Fig. 17.10).

The constrictor muscles of the iris are innervated by postganglionic parasympathetic nerves which originate in the ciliary ganglion. Preganglionic fibres to the ciliary ganglion run in the 3rd nerve. Stimulation of this nerve causes a contraction of the circular (constrictor) muscles resulting in constriction of the pupil. These muscles also act in response to the amount of light prevailing.

Oculomotor centre

An oculomotor centre in the brain stem also has controlling influence on the size of the pupil. The main function of the oculomotor centre is to constrict the pupil, acting through the parasympathetic nervous system. The oculomotor centre is in turn controlled by impulses from higher (cortical) centres. If cortical impulses are blocked, there is constriction of the pupil. This happens in sleep and deep anaesthesia. Morphine stimulates the oculomotor centre directly causing constriction of the pupil (pin-point pupil seen in morphine addicts).

Accommodation

Accommodation is focussing for near vision. There is an increase in the curvature of the lens and therefore the focal length is reduced. The mechanism of accommodation is as follows: The lens is attached to the ciliary body by suspensory ligaments. When the eye is set for distant vision, the ciliary muscle is relaxed and the suspensory

Fig. 17.10. Muscles of the iris. Circular (constrictor pupillae) muscles (CM) are innervated by parasympathetic postganglionic nerves from the ciliary ganglion. The radial (dilator pupillae) muscle (RM) are innervated by sympathetic postganglionic nerves from the superior cervical ganglion. These muscles control the size of the pupil (P).

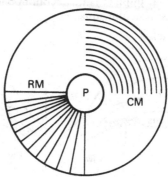

ligaments exert tension on the lens which becomes flattened. There is reduced curvature and increased focal length. The tension in the suspensory ligaments is reduced when the ciliary muscles contract. The curvature of the lens is increased, so there is reduced focal length. The eye is thus accommodated for near vision (see Fig. 17.11 for diagrammatic representation).

The ciliary muscles receive parasympathetic innervation only. When these muscles contract, the ciliary body moves inwards and by decreasing the tension on the suspensory ligaments, the curvature of the lens is increased.

Effects of drugs on accommodation

Stimulation of the 3rd nerve, or application of acetylcholine-like drugs to the conjunctiva, e.g. pilocarpine, carbachol, or anti-cholinesterases such as eserine, contract the ciliary muscles and produce accommodation for near vision. In contrast, drugs which block muscarinic receptors such as atropine, or hyoscine or those which block ganglia such as hexamethonium, mecamylamine or pempidine prevent contraction of the ciliary muscles and paralyse accommodation. Sympathomimetic drugs which dilate the pupil do not paralyse accommodation because they have no effect on ciliary muscle, although they may limit the extent of accommodation.

Fig. 17.11. Mechanism of accommodation. In (a), the ciliary muscles (CM) are relaxed; there is tension in the suspensory ligaments (SL). The lens is flattened (i.e., reduced curvature and increased focal point; the eye is set for distant vision). In (b), the ciliary muscles are contracted; the suspensory ligaments are not tensed. The lens is rounded (i.e., increased curvature and reduced focal point; the eye is accommodated for near vision). Note that the pupil (P) and accommodation are controlled by different sets of ocular muscles.

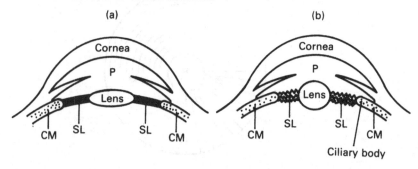

Intraocular pressure

The aqueous humour is a fluid secreted by the epithelial cells covering the ciliary body. It is contained in the posterior and anterior chambers of the eye. The two chambers are separated by the iris. The fluid passes over the lens through the pupil into the anterior chamber. It is drained away through the filtration angle into the canal of Schlemm. Dilatation of the pupil (mydriasis) entails a folding of the iris and withdrawal into the filtration angle. The filtration angle is narrowed and access to the canal of Schlemm and hence drainage is made more difficult. Thus, drugs which dilate the pupil are likely to cause an increase in intraocular pressure and may precipitate glaucoma in susceptible patients. In contrast, drugs which constrict the pupil (miosis) open the access to the canal and so ease the pressure (Fig. 17.12).

Action of other drugs on the eye

Physostigmine (eserine)

A 1% solution applied topically into the conjunctiva constricts the pupil, and contracts the ciliary muscle thereby producing a spasm of accommodation. In this state when far and near points are identical, objects appear enlarged (macropia). For reasons already stated, neostigmine is not suitable for topical application.

Diisopropylfluorophosphonate (dyflos)

An irreversible anticholinesterase, has similar effects to eserine but is more potent and longer acting. Sometimes used topically as a 0.1% solution in oil in the treatment of glaucoma. Dyflos is too toxic for routine use.

Fig. 17.12. Movement of aqueous humour (AH) in posterior and anterior chambers of the eye. Note that a contraction of the dilator pupillae (mydriasis) will pull back the muscles of the iris, decrease the angle of filtration and block the canal of Schlemm. CB = ciliary body.

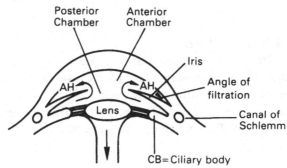

Pilocarpine

Is a parasympathomimetic alkaloid. It stimulates muscarinic receptors on the iris and ciliary muscles. It can be used in the treatment of glaucoma.

Acetazolamide

Is an inhibitor of carbonic anhydrase and is used in the treatment of glaucoma because it is thought that the enzyme, carbonic anhydrase, is concerned with the production of aqueous humour.

Atropine

A 1% solution applied topically to the conjunctiva produces effects which are opposite to those of parasympathomimetic drugs. The pupil dilates, and the near point recedes until accommodation is completely paralysed. Objects appear smaller in size (micropia). Accommodation paralysis produced by atropine may last for days. The dilated pupil allows light to enter the eye freely, resulting in photophobia. Atropine is used in ophthamology for the following:

   (a) By dilating the pupil and paralysing accommodation, it allows an accurate determination of refraction.
   (b) Dilatation of the pupil permits examination of the fundus of the eye.
   (c) By preventing contractions of the ciliary muscle, atropine ensures rest in an inflamed eye.

The main disadvantage of atropine is its effect on intraocular pressure especially in the elderly, in whom atropine may precipitate glaucoma.

Homatropine

Has similar effects to atropine, but is shorter acting and therefore preferred in cases where raised intraocular pressure is suspected. Other drugs with similar effects to atropine are lachesine and hyoscine. (Other atropine-like drugs used in ophthamology are discussed on page 379).

Adrenergic drugs

Adrenaline produces only a transient mydriasis. It is said to relieve intraoccular pressure either by its vasoconstrictor effect or by reduction of aqueous humor formation.

Ephedrine, amphetamine, and phenylephrine are more active on local application. They produce dilatation of the pupil without paralysis of accommodation.

18

Anaesthesia

18.1   LOCAL ANAESTHETICS

Local anaesthetics are substances which produce short/moderate lasting, reversible blockade of pain impulses peripherally at concentrations of the drug which do not damage either the nerve or surrounding tissues. Examples are shown in Fig. 18.1.

There are three parts to the structures:

The *hydrophobic* end contains in all the examples given a benzene ring. This part is poorly ionised at body pH and is helpful in the penetration of the nerve membrane.

The *intermediate chain* is a major determinant of the duration of action. The esters are relatively rapidly hydrolysed by plasma cholinesterase and ACHE; the amides are more slowly inactivated by hepatic microsomal enzymes. Metabolism is significant only in infiltration and conduction anaesthesia and is minimised in these cases by the addition of a low concentration of a vasoconstrictor agent, e.g. procaine may be combined with adrenaline.

The hydrophilic end is usually a secondary or tertiary amine with a pK_a in the range 7.5 - 9.0. Changing the pH therefore significantly affects the degree of ionisation of this part of the molecule.

Studies of anaesthetic action of ionised and unionised forms of the drugs suggest that *inside* the nerve the ionised molecule is the *active* form, whereas the molecule has to be mostly unionised to penetrate the nerve cell membrane.

Mechanism of action

The nerve impulse is initiated by membrane depolarisation which produces a rapid inward movement of Na^+ ions (this generates the action potential). This is followed by a slower outward K^+ ion current which repolarises the axon membrane so that it is ready to respond to the next stimulus. Local anaesthetics prevent conduction in excitable tissues by blocking the entry of Na^+ ions   during the generation of the action potential. This effect is dose dependent. As the concentration of drug is increased there is a progressive decrease in the rate of rise of the spike potential (Fig. 18.2). This also leads to a reduction in the conduction velocity because the less intense the

Fig. 18.1. Structures of some local anaesthetics.

DRUG	STRUCTURE	ESTER/AMIDE

Procaine	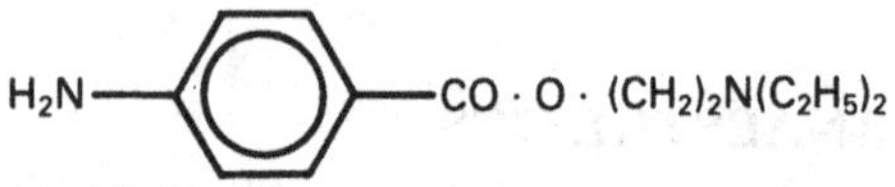 H_2N— ⬡ —$CO \cdot O \cdot (CH_2)_2N(C_2H_5)_2$	Ester
Benzocaine	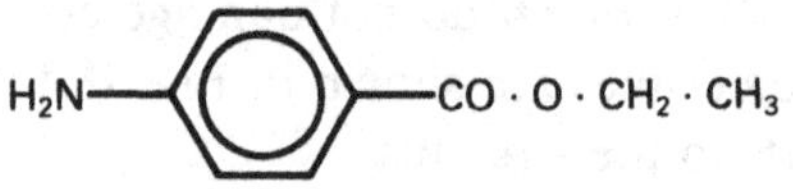 H_2N— ⬡ —$CO \cdot O \cdot CH_2 \cdot CH_3$	Ester
Lignocaine	CH_3 / ⬡ —$NH \cdot CO \cdot CH_2 \cdot N(C_2H_5)_2$ / CH_3	Amide
*Bupivacaine	CH_3 / ⬡ —$NH \cdot CO$— ⬡N— / CH_3 C_4H_9	Amide
Tetracaine	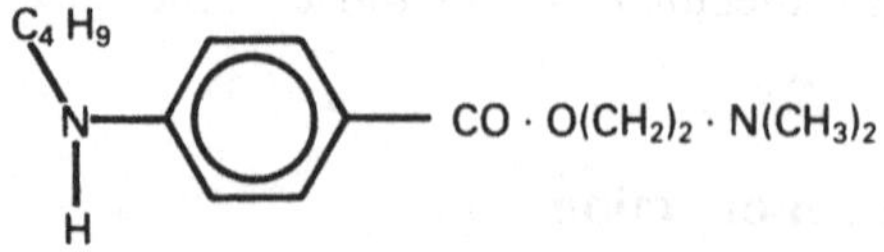 C_4H_9 N— ⬡ —$CO \cdot O(CH_2)_2 \cdot N(CH_3)_2$ H	Ester

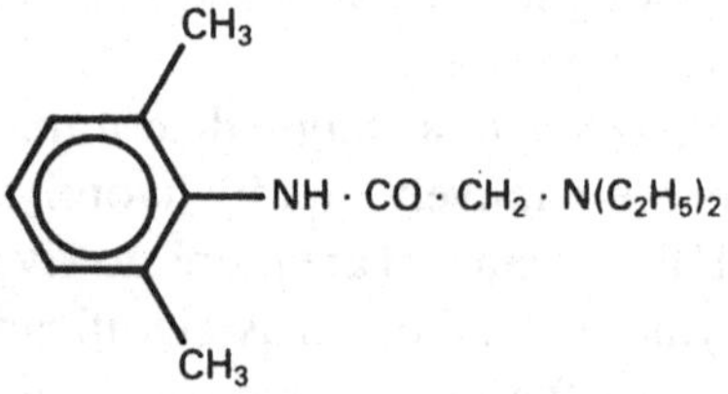

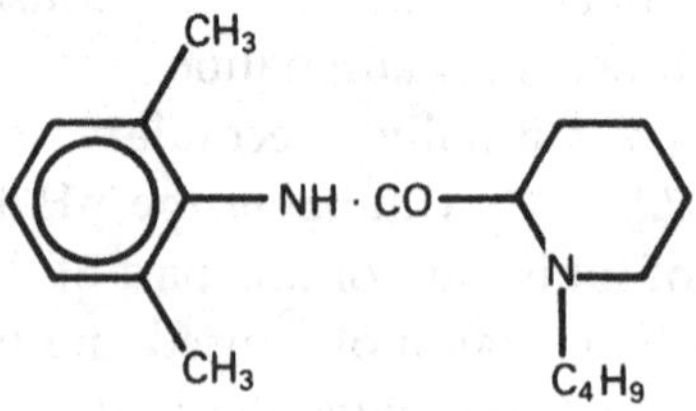

*Mepivacaine has an N-methyl substituent in place of the butyl (C_4H_9) group in bupivacaine

depolarisation at any point, the shorter the range of local circuits induced. At sufficiently high concentrations of drug, local depolarisation fails to trigger a spike potential resulting in conduction block. The effect on K^+ ion conductance is insignificant.

At sufficiently high doses local anaesthetics can block conduction in all excitable membranes; in therapeutic doses, however, the small sensory nerves are preferentially blocked because the thicker the nerve fibre the higher is the concentration of drug required to block it. Local anaesthetics act most effectively on unmyelinated nerves where Schwann cells do not provide a barrier to diffusion. In myelinated nerves, local anaesthetics act only at the nodes of Ranvier. In the rest of the nerve, Schwann cells have encircled the axon with layers of dense lipid that constitute a diffusion barrier to drugs. At the nodes, the myelin is interrupted.

Individual local anaesthetics

It is useful to consider the properties of some local anaesthetics to bring out the point that not all drugs which block nerve conduction as described above may be clinically useful in all cases where local anaesthesia is required. Also, different local anaesthetics are used to produce different types of local anaesthesia (see Table 18.1) and this depends on the individual properties of the drugs. In reading this section, the reader should bear in mind that local anaesthesia can be

Fig. 18.2. The effect of increasing concentrations of a local anaesthetic (C_1–C_3) on action potentials in an excitable membrane. C_0 is the action potential before the addition of local anaesthetic. Note the decline in both the size, and the rate of rise, of the spike as the concentration of drug increases (diagrammatic).

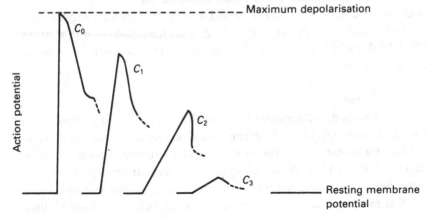

Table 18.1   *Some common ways by which local anaesthesia may be induced*

Method of application	Type of local anaesthesia produced	Drug type
Topical application to mucous membranes, e.g. eye, nose, throat	Surface anaesthesia	Cocaine, tetracaine, lignocaine
Subcutaneous injection around nerve terminals	Infiltration anaesthesia	procaine, lignocaine (combined with adrenaline 5 µg ml^{-1})
Deeper subcutaneous injection around nerve trunk	Conduction anaesthesia (Field)	Procaine, lignocaine (may be combined with adrenaline 5 µg ml^{-1})
Lumbar puncture into the cerebrospinal fluid (intrathecal)	Spinal (subarachnoid) anaesthesia	Procaine, lignocaine tetracaine
Via a sacral foramen into the epidural space	Caudal (epidural) anaesthesia	Lignocaine, bupivacaine, chloroprocaine, (may be combined with adrenaline)

achieved by means of cold, application of pressure on nerve trunks, or ischaemia. Drugs are by far the most used agents. Generally, any protoplasmic poison can anaesthetise tissues locally, but the ideal local anaesthetic should (a) reversibly paralyse sensory nerve endings without injuring surrounding tissues; (b) be non-irritant; (c) have a short onset and a reasonably long duration of action; (d) not produce vasodilation with consequent rapid diffusion from the site of action and systemic toxicity; and (e) be active after topical and hypodermic application. Not all the available drugs are ideal. Note also that drugs like tetrodotoxin which block Na^+ channels are fundamentally similar to local anaesthetics.

Cocaine

This is an alkaloid which occurs in the leaves of *Erythroxylum coca* and other species of *Erythroxylum*. Cocaine is an ester of benzoic acid and a nitrogen-containing base with a structure which is fundamentally similar to those of synthetic local anaesthetics already described. Cocaine is a potent local anaesthetic, but because of its CNS stimulant action, tendency to cause addiction, and high abuse potential, the drug is restricted to topical application in surface anaesthesia; even then, the use is severely restricted. Apart from its anaesthetic properties, cocaine has a number of important other actions. On the CNS, cocaine is a stimulant, manifesting initially in a sense of well-being and euphoria, accompanied by excitement, talkativeness and restlessness. With high doses, stimulation is followed by depression of all vital centres in the CNS. Low doses of cocaine can also cause depression in the novice. The euphoria and stimulant effects are due to potentiation of the actions of catecholamines in the CNS (NA and dopamine) through inhibition of uptake; this is probably not the whole story as tricyclic antidepressants (imipramine) which are potent inhibitors of uptake, do not produce euphoria and are not abused. Cocaine is abused extensively in Europe and North America. The high demand for this drug in these societies and consequently its high cost, have made trafficking in cocaine an international problem (see later under Drug abuse). On the sympathetic nervous system, cocaine potentiates responses to sympathetic stimulation by blocking uptake (see Chapter 16). In the eye the drug thus produces mydriasis, vasoconstriction and sensitisation to NA. It is the only local anaesthetic with these effects.

Procaine
Procaine (see Fig. 18.1) was synthesised in 1905 and is still a useful local anaesthetic. The important features are:
 (a) Procaine is hydrolysed, yielding para-aminobenzoic acid (PABA) which may inhibit the action of sulphonamides. This may be of clinical importance.
 (b) Procaine may interfere with the chemical determination of sulphonamides in solution.
 (c) Procaine causes vasodilation, hence it is usually given with adrenaline (1 : 200 000).
The main shortcomings of procaine are:
 (a) Being a vasodilator means that in the absence of a vasoconstrictor agent, procaine is rapidly absorbed into the circulation and hydrolysed by plasma cholinesterase.
 (b) Hypersensitivity to procaine is commonly encountered.

Lignocaine
This is one of the most widely used local anaesthetics. It is superior to procaine in many respects:
 (a) It has a shorter onset of action and a more intense and a

longer duration of effect than procaine and is more diffusible, hence better for topical use.

(b) Lignocaine does not dilate blood vessels, although its duration of action is usually increased by the addition of a vasoconstrictor.

(c) Being an amide, it can be used in place of procaine – like local anaesthetics where hypersensitivity is a problem (see also Table 18.1 and Fig. 18.1). In addition to its use as a local anaesthetic, lignocaine is used as an antiarrhythmic agent.

18.2   GENERAL ANAESTHETICS

These are employed to produce general unconsciousness immediately prior to and during a surgical operation. General anaesthesia is preceded by premedication. Two types of general anaesthetics are used, namely those given by inhalation and those given by intravenous injection.

Premedication

Premedication is the treatment given to the patient before being taken to the theatre. It may include:

(a) A sedative

This is used to calm the patient without producing sleep. Usually nowadays a benzodiazepine, e.g. diazepam is used, instead of morphine or other opioid. The aims in pre-anaesthetic sedation are: to relieve anxiety before anaesthesia; to reduce the amount of general anaesthetic required to induce and to maintain unconsciousness; and, possibly, to produce post-operative sedation.

(b) An antimuscarinic agent, e.g. atropine or hyoscine

This is necessary to reduce salivary and bronchial secretions especially when ether is used as inhalation anaesthetic. Ether is irritant to the mucosae and stimulates the vagus; it is virtually obsolete. The inhalation anaesthetics, e.g. halothane, currently in use do not have ether's irritant properties; but antimuscarinic agents are still used to: prevent bradycardia due to vagal stimulation of cardiac muscle (e.g., halothane); to reduce post-operative vomiting; and to produce amnesia (hyoscine).

Intravenous anaesthetics

These are given intravenously to induce rapid anaesthesia

which is then maintained by another anaesthetic or are used for operations of brief duration.

(a) Barbiturates

Barbituric acid was synthesized in 1864 by condensing urea and malonic acid. It is not itself an anaesthetic but is the parent of a long line of derivatives which are (Fig. 18.3). Many barbiturates are too long acting (e.g., phenobarbitone) to be useful as anaesthetics; subanaesthetic doses are used as sedative/hypnotic or antiepileptic (see pages 441–2).

The first really useful, short-acting barbiturate was thiopentone. Even shorter acting and used widely as anaesthetics are methohexitone and thiohexitone. It has previously been pointed out that the short duration of action of thiopentone is due to its redistribution between brain tissues and peripheral sites. With methohexitone and thiohexitone metabolism is the limiting factor. Although barbiturates are active after oral administration; they must be given intravenously for the induction of anaesthesia. The rate of absorption from the oral route after a non-toxic dose is too low for anaesthetic purposes.

The main advantage is that barbiturates produce a rapid and smooth induction, speedy recovery and lack any stimulant effect on bronchial and salivary glands. The main problems are laryngospasm, bronchospasm, severe fall in arterial blood pressure, and respiratory depression. They should be used only with great care in patients with cardiovascular or respiratory disorders. Barbiturates have no analgesic properties (on the contrary, they may increase pain sensation).

(b) Eugenols, e.g. propanidid

These are esters and are rapidly hydrolysed by plasma and liver esterases. They are therefore extremely short acting. Unlike the barbiturates, propanidid rarely causes bronchospasm or laryngospasm.

(c) Soluble steroids, e.g. alphaxalone

These are short-acting anaesthetics which also produce good muscle relaxation.

(d) Dissociative anaesthetics, e.g. cyclohexylamine (ketamine)

These are arylcycloalkylamines which induce a state of sedation and marked analgesia. They are called dissociative anaesthetics because they produce a strong feeling of dissociation from the

Fig. 18.3. Barbituric acid and the structures of some barbiturates derived from it. Useful barbiturates are commonly made by substitutions at the oxygen numbered 1 and the hydrogens numbered 2-5. The barbiturates in this figure have been arranged in order of decreasing duration of action when administered to man.

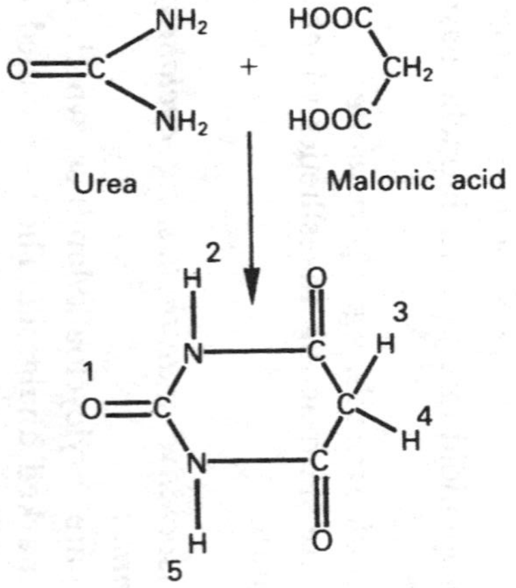

Barbiturate	Substitutions				
	1	2	3	4	5
Phenobarbitone	O	H	$-C_2H_5$	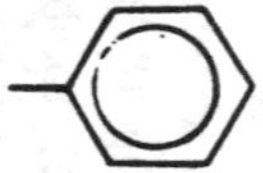 (methyl-substituted benzene ring)	H
Hexobarbitone	O	$-CH_3$	$-CH_3$	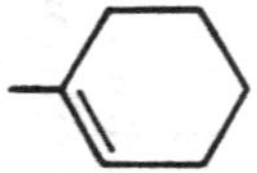 (methyl-substituted cyclohexene ring)	H
Thiopentone	S	H	$-C_2H_5$	$-CH \cdot (CH_2)_2CH_3$ with $-CH_3$	H
Methohexitone	O	$-CH_3$	$-CH_2 \cdot CH= CH_2$	$-CH \cdot C \equiv C \cdot CH_2 \cdot CH_3$ with $-CH_3$	H
Thiohexitone	S	H	$-CH_2 \cdot CH= CH_2$	$-CH \cdot C \equiv C \cdot CH_2 \cdot CH_3$	H

surrounding environment in the patient. The first drug of this kind was phencyclidine, which is now obsolete as it caused severe and prolonged psychological effects including mania and hallucinations. These effects are less marked with ketamine. With this drug there is no muscle relaxation but it produces analgesia. One of its main advantages is that it causes minimal effects on the cardiovascular system and may therefore be preferred to other anaesthetics in those patients with cardiac disease or in the elderly.

Inhalation anaesthetics
(a) Nitrous oxide (N_2O)
This gas is compressed into a liquid form and stored in cylinders. It may be used: as the sole anaesthetic agent, mainly for dental and outpatient operations; to induce anaesthesia before continuing with another anaesthetic agent, e.g. ether, halothane; to maintain anaesthesia in major surgery in combination with other drugs; or to produce analgesia in labour in a mixture with an equal part of air or oxygen. In all cases nitrous oxide is given as a mixture with oxygen to prevent hypoxia, the proportion varying from 50 – 80% depending on the surgical procedure and other clinical considerations.

(b) Halothane ($F_3C. CHBr.Cl$)
This is a volatile liquid that is vapourised by a special device and applied in open or closed circuits including soda lime for the absorption of carbon dioxide. Important characteristics are: its slower onset of action than N_2O; similarity to nitrous oxide in being non-irritant; it lowers arterial blood pressure due to block of autonomic ganglia, cardiac depression and inhibition of vasomotor centre; it sensitises cardiac ventricles to the dysrrhythmic effects of circulating catecholamines; it depresses respiration, (therefore one must assist respiration); and it depresses hepatic function. An alternative anaesthetic in patients with liver disease is enflurane (which also depresses respiration).

(c) Other inhalation anaesthetics
Diethylether (ether) a volatile anaesthetic, is practically obsolete because: it is explosive and highly inflammable when mixed with oxygen; its use entails prolonged induction and recovery; it is irritant – post-operative nausea and vomiting are common; it stimulates salivary and bronchial secretions (this can be prevented by premedication with

atropine); and it stimulates the vagus to cause bradycardia (this can also be prevented by atropine premedication).

Its main advantage is that it is cheaper than halothane or the other newer inhalation anaesthetics and it can be administered without special equipment. It possesses reasonable analgesic and muscle relaxant properties. These are no longer special advantages since analgesics and muscle relaxants can be used to supplement anaesthetics lacking these properties.

Other more or less obsolete inhalation anaesthetics are ethylchloride, vinyl ether, cycloproprane, and chloroform. These agents cause serious severe cardiovascular side effects such as cardiac dysrhythmias by sensitising the cardiac muscle to circulating catecholamines which the agents themselves may release from the adrenal medulla. Chloroform is toxic to the liver.

Mechanisms of anaesthesia

The action of general anaesthetic agents cannot be explained on the basis of their interaction with a single receptor molecule or its subtypes as can now be done for a good many other drugs. This is apparent from an inspection of the chemical structures of these agents which range from inert gases (e.g. xenon) to such complex molecules as steroids. Several attempts have been made in the past to explain the phenomenon of anaesthesia on the basis of the physical and chemical characteristics of the agents. This gave rise to a number of physicochemical theories; all these assume a non-specific action of the agents on cell membranes. Some are mentioned below but no attempt is made at exhaustive discussion.

Lipid solubility theory

Overton and Meyer were among the earliest to draw attention to lipid solubility as the determining factor in anaesthesia. It has since been pointed out that lipid solubility of the anaesthetic agent is an important factor in gaining access to brain structures or even cell membranes where the agents work, but does not represent a fundamental mode of action.

Critical volume theory

This was proposed by Mullins who suggested that when anaesthetics dissolve in cell membranes, they cause these membranes to expand. When the expansion reaches a critical volume, normal membrane properties are disrupted and anaesthesia ensues. Some anaesthetics do cause expansion and disorganisation of the membrane.

Clathrate hypothesis

This was proposed by Pauling. It suggests that general anaesthetics form hydrates (clathrates or structured water) in cell membranes and thereby alter membrane function. These clathrates are supposed to be stabilised by linkages with protein side chains. There are several observations which make physicochemical theories generally unacceptable. Examples of these are as following. (a) In a homologous series, anaesthetic potency may increase in parallel with a physicochemical characteristic such as lipid solubility, up to a point beyond which anaesthetic potency may decrease, but the lipid solubility may continue to increase in the series.

(b) The theories fail to explain why some substances should be anaesthetics whereas compounds closely related to them may be without potency or even be antagonists, e.g. $CF_3.CH.CLBr$ (halothane) is an anaesthetic whereas $CF_3.CH_2.Br$ is a convulsant, and alphaxalone is a steroid anaesthetic whereas Δ-16-alphaxalone is an antagonist of alphaxalone. This is despite the fact that these pairs of compounds possess almost identical physicochemical properties.

(c) General anaesthetics are known to have differential effects in different parts of the CNS, which should not be the case if their action were due to a non-specific interference with membrane function. For example, halothane is a potent anaesthetic as well as having good analgesic properties whereas barbiturates are potent anaesthetics but may be anti-analgesic.

There is some evidence that anaesthetics may act specifically on certain neurones within the CNS rather than non-specifically on all membranes; multisynaptic pathways of the reticular-activating system are more susceptible to the action of anaesthetics than non-synapsing pathways. General anaesthetics depress central neurones by affecting both pre- and postsynaptic mechanisms but the presynaptic site is more susceptible to anaesthetic block. The effect is not like that of local anaesthetics on sensory fibres where conduction is blocked. There is evidence that some anaesthetics (barbiturates) decrease ACH release. The drugs may also act rather specifically at postsynaptic sites, e.g. general anaesthetics are known to depress the excitation of cerebral cortical neurones caused by iontophoretically administered ACH without any effect on similar excitation caused by glutamate. A depression of ACH action is important since ACH function in the cerebral cortex is thought to be important in maintaining consciousness. Another factor is that general anaesthetics may not only block excitatory transmission as above, but may also increase transmission at inhibitory neurones where GABA is thought to be a transmitter.

The drugs used as anaesthetics differ from most other drugs discussed in this book in one important respect. Their action is not associated with a specific enzyme, receptor, neurotransmitter, or specific cellular mechanism, so may thus appear to be non-specific; but this is as far as our knowledge of their action goes. There is clearly some degree of selectivity. Some neuronal membranes at different sites are susceptible to the action of anaesthetics more than others. This may be because certain membrane processes are more important for the function of some cells in maintaining consciousness than for others. Such a selectivity is only marginal with existing anaesthetics which can depress all neuronal functions in concentrations only slightly higher than those required to induce unconsciousness.

19

Pain and inflammation

19.1 INTRODUCTION

Pain and inflammation are treated together in this chapter in the section on nervous system because many pain-producing substances are generated during inflammation reactions. Also many drugs used in the treatment of inflammation (e.g. nonsteroidal anti-inflammatory agents) are also analgesic. Pain will be discussed first.

19.2 THE PHYSIOLOGICAL BASIS OF PAIN

The sensation of pain is initiated in peripheral receptors (nociceptors) by stimuli which are sufficiently intense to cause tissue damage. The function of pain, then, is to draw attention to injury and through the reflexes elicited to protect the injured part or do something about it. Some of the nociceptors respond only to painful stimuli; the impulses generated as a result are conveyed to the CNS in special afferent pain fibres. When pain fibres enter the spinal cord, they make extensive synaptic connections in the dorsal horn, ascend the spinal cord and synapse extensively in the reticular formation and thalamus. Projections then advance to the cerebral cortex. Thus, many parts of the brain may be involved in the perception of pain. Nociceptors and the afferent pain fibres are present everywhere – skin, muscle, blood vessels, meninges, etc.

Pain may be crudely regarded as consisting of two components, namely, the primary sensation and the individual's reaction to the sensation. Beecher observed that soldiers wounded in battle may construe the wound as a welcome occurrence, for it means release from an intolerable situation; under such conditions, the pain may be completely ignored. Sportsmen may also ignore a great deal of pain while actually in competition. The pain is experienced only afterwards. Strong emotional experience can dominate the CNS and block pain. Hence small doses of morphine can relieve pain of pathological origin in most humans but experimentally-induced pain may not be affected by similar doses.

19.3   MEASUREMENT OF ANALGESIC POTENCY

Substances which prevent or modify the sensation of pain are analgesics and substances which intensify the pain sensation are hyperalgesics. There is no recording technique or other objective device to measure pain specifically. The measurement of pain is thus subjective. Experimental pain can be evoked by one of the following:

(a) *Mechanical pain*: can be evoked by applying pressure on a rat's tail until the animal squeaks or withdraws the tail.

(b) *Electrical pain*: can be induced by application of electrical stimulation to tooth pulp in man.

(c) *Chemical pain*: Bradykinin, prostaglandin, or histamine solution, applied to an open blister in man produces a sharp, sustained pain.

(d) *Thermal pain*: Mice placed on a hot plate may be used as an illustration.

(e) *Ischaemic pain*: Blood flow in an arm is occluded by the application of a tourniquet in man.

(f) *Writhing pain*: Dilute acetic acid solution injected i.p. into mice causes the animals to exhibit a characteristic writhing response. This test can be used to distinguish between narcotic and non-narcotic analgesics as the latter by an anti-inflammatory action can prevent the writhing response as well as the leakage into the peritoneum of intravenously injected dye.

Quantitative estimation of pain is either by *quantal response* in which the percentage of animals in a group responding to a fixed pain stimulus, e.g. fixed temperature and time of exposure, is determined, or by *threshold response* in which the amount of stimulus, e.g. pressure, heat, electrical voltage, or chemical concentration, required to induce the characteristic response in each animal is determined. Both types of measurement can be used to determine the analgesic potency of a drug.

Note the following points of difficulty with measurement of analgesic potency:

(a) In animal experiments, e.g. the hot-plate method using mice, it is assumed that the animal responds to a pain sensation similar to that which a human would experience under the same conditions. There is no way of proving that this is so. The test is acceptable only in so far as it can be used to show empirically that some drugs which are useful in man, also decrease the pain response in these tests. The limitations in extrapolation of such tests to man are obvious.

(b) Experimentally-induced pain in humans, e.g. using ischaemia, should be preferable and these have been explored. The results obtained are subjective and are often influenced by training and motivation. Investigators have difficulty in confirming each other's results. Part of the problem is that volunteers recognise experimental pain for what it is. The response is therefore free of the psychological component so important in pathological pain.

(c) The chronic pain of cancer and postoperative pain have been used to assess analgesic potency. In this case the *double blind* technique is used. Neither the patient nor the observer knows which of two sets of preparation is the drug or placebo (an inert preparation with the same physical characteristics as the active drug). Even in these instances, up to 20% of patients report relief from pain after placebos.

19.4 ANALGESIC DRUGS

Analgesics are drugs used to relieve pain without causing unconsciousness. They are in this respect to be contrasted with general anaesthetics. Analgesics are classified as narcotic (opiates) and non-narcotic (aspirin-like) analgesics. The opiates have a greater effect on the subjective reaction to pain (see 19.2) than on the pain sensation. In contrast, most aspirin-like drugs act mainly at peripheral sites; opiates have no effect at these sites but act at all levels of the CNS.

Morphine-like drugs (opiates)

Morphine is an alkaloid of opium, the dried juice obtained from the capsules of *Papaver somniferum*. Opium contains many other alkaloids e.g. codeine and papaverine. A good grade opium may contain as much as 10% by weight of morphine, 10% papaverine and 0.5% codeine. The chemical structures of some opiate drugs and their antagonists are shown in Fig. 19.1. Morphine, codeine and heroin are phenanthrene derivatives. Papaverine is a benzylisoquinoline derivative. It has no analgesic activity. The phenanthrene structure is not necessary for analgesic action as can be seen from Fig. 19.1 for methadone and meperidine (pethidine). In three-dimensional models however

Fig. 19.1. Structures of some morphine-like drugs.

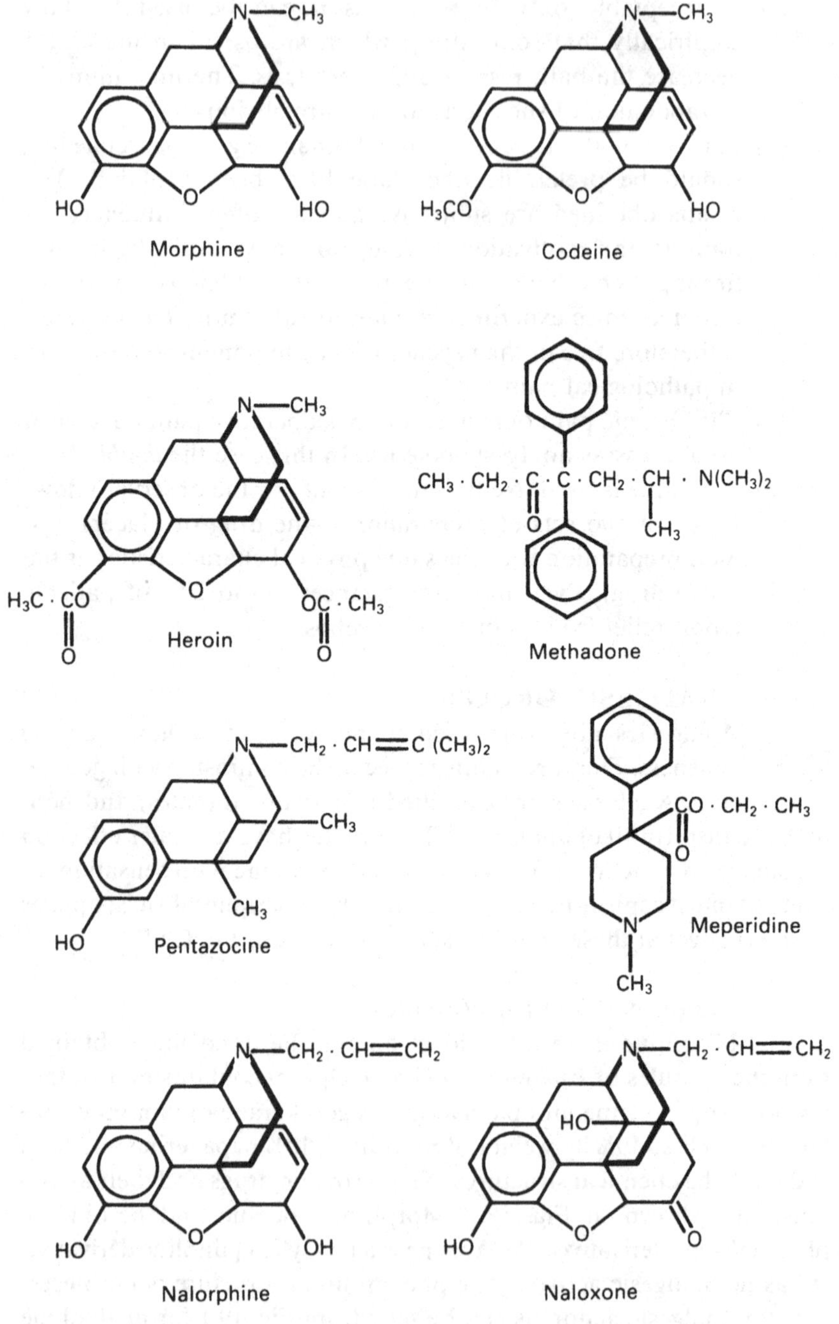

Morphine

Codeine

Heroin

Methadone

$CH_3 \cdot CH_2 \cdot C \cdot C \cdot CH_2 \cdot CH \cdot N(CH_3)_2$

Pentazocine

Meperidine

Nalorphine

Naloxone

meperidine and methadone resemble the D(−) isomer of morphine suggesting that these drugs and morphine act on the same (opiate) receptors. Substitution for an allyl group on the nitrogen as in pentazocine, nalorphine and naloxone produces compounds which are opiate antagonists. Nalorphine is a partial agonist: when given alone, it produces the effects of morphine (see below), but it counteracts the effects of morphine when given with or after morphine. Naloxone has relatively pure antagonistic properties and lacks the analgesic and depressant actions of morphine. It can be used to treat opiate overdosage, but will precipitate withdrawal symptoms (see below) in an addict. Pentazocine is also a partial agonist; it is used for its analgesic properties. It lacks the unpleasant side effects of nalorphine.

Pharmacological actions of morphine-like drugs
(1) Receptors
From the work of Kosterlitz and others there is evidence from functional and ligand binding studies that

(a) the pharmacological actions of opiates in the central nervous system are mediated by specific but multiple receptors.

(b) at least three opioid receptors have been identified:
   (i)   δ receptors have relative selectivity for methionine and leucine enkephalins (see pp. 439–50.)
   (ii) k receptors have relative selectivity for dynorphine A and pentazocine (their stimulation produces central analgesia).
   (iii) μ receptors – morphine is the prototype ligand (their stimulation produces central analgesia and euphoria).

(c) There is a great deal of overlap in receptor type and the pharmacological responses evoked by their activation. The degree of selectivity of the agonists mentioned is only relative and not enough to permit a dogmatic classification. Another problem is that in many cases, opioid receptors have been classified from binding studies which may not reflect accurately agonist potencies in producing pharmacological effects.

(d) All the receptor types are blocked by naloxone. Highly potent and selective antagonists and agonists are needed for a clear classification of opiate receptors, because this approach has the potential for the development of agonists which can produce analgesia without the numerous complications of morphine.

(2) Analgesia

This is the cardinal action for which morphine is used in therapeutics. Morphine analgesia is associated with a change in mood, giving a calming soothing effect, and euphoria – a feeling of well being and optimism. The pain may be present, but the individual's reaction to it is changed; the pain can be ignored. Most of the analgesic action of morphine in pathological states in man comes from its power to induce change in mood, detachment and relief of anxiety. Unfortunately it is this euphoria that leads to dependence which is characteristic of opiates (see page 423). Morphine is indicated for: severe pain of short duration e.g., after road traffic accident or bullet wound; severe pain of long duration as in terminal cancer; relief of anxiety in heart attack (also to reduce sympathetic activity and reduce cardiac work); and in pre-anaesthetic medication. A concomitant action of morphine is hypnosis or drowsiness. This may be a direct sedative effect, or it may be that sleep occurs as a consequence of euphoria and detachment from pain.

(3) Respiratory depression

Morphine primarily depresses the respiratory centres in the brain. The depression of respiration is observable even with small doses. In man death from morphine poisoning is nearly always due to respiratory depression and arrest. This is due to a reduction in the sensitivity of the brain stem respiratory centre to $p.CO_2$ in the arterial blood. Therefore morphine is contra-indicated in patients with respiratory insufficiency and in labour where the drug may produce a fatal respiratory depression in the foetus. In left ventricular failure (paroxysmal nocturnal dyspnoea) where the alveoli are congested, the respiratory centres react excessively to afferent impulses from the congested lungs. In this instance the depressant effect of morphine on respiration is beneficial.

(4) Cardiovascular system

Morphine in therapeutic doses has minimal effects on the cardiovascular system. It may, however, produce orthostatic hypotension due to a combination of effects: inhibition of catecholamine release; histamine release; and depression of the vasomotor centre. Care should be taken therefore when using morphine in patients with low arterial blood pressure.

(5) Smooth muscles

In the stomach, morphine causes a decrease in hydrochloric acid secretion, but a more pronounced effect is decreased motility associated with an increase in tone of the muscles of the stomach and duodenum and of sphincters which leads to a delay in the passage of stomach contents and to constipation. In the small intestine, digestion is slowed by morphine because the drug reduces biliary and pancreatic secretion. There is increase in tone of intestinal muscle as well as of ileocaecal valve. Furthermore there is decreased propulsive movement as ACH release in the organ is blocked by morphine. All this adds up to constipation which is a characteristic effect of morphine. The mechanism of the tone-increasing action of morphine is not fully understood. Only large doses of atropine block the effect; it is therefore not mediated by ACH. In any case morphine directly blocks the release of ACH from parasympathetic nerves. Possibly, it is due to increased intramural generation of a prostaglandin. Morphine is known to stimulate prostaglandin synthesis.

The delay in the passage of gut contents gives rise to increased desiccation in the large intestine; this, allied to sphincter spasm, further retards the advance of contents through the colon. Another factor which contributes to morphine-induced constipation is that centrally the drug blocks the normal defaecation reflex. In former times, morphine was used to treat diarrhoea, e.g. in mixtures containing morphine and kaolin. This application of a highly addictive drug is no longer justified.

(6) Genito-urinary system

Morphine reduces the volume of urine probably because it causes the release of antidiuretic hormone and increased sweating (due to dilatation of skin blood vessels caused peripherally by reducing noradrenaline release and centrally by an action on the vasomotor centre). On the uterus, morphine has no significant direct inhibitory effect on contractions, but overdosage may affect involuntary abdominal contractions, and so delay labour. It may also depress the respiration of the foetus. Pethidine may be used instead; note that infants born to mothers addicted to opiates are physiologically dependent on the drugs.

(7) Eye

Morphine causes a marked constriction of the pupil of the eye in man. The effect is central (cortical) in origin and can be blocked by atropine. No tolerance develops to this action of the opiates. The 'pin-point' pupil effect of the opiates is so uniform in man that it is used to evaluate opiate analgesics and to diagnose opiate usage (as by addicts). In cats (where morphine causes excitement, rather than sedation), the effect of morphine on the eye is mydriasis which is subcortical in origin.

(8) Other central actions of morphine
Antitussive action
Morphine inhibits cough by a central mechanism. This property is useful in the treatment of unproductive dry cough (where there is not much phlegm to be expectorated, and the cough is merely a nuisance, preventing the sufferer from sleeping at night). The antitussive effect is produced by both isomers of morphine whereas the D(-) isomer does not cause other CNS effects of the L(-) isomer. Thus for example, dextromethophan is a specific cough suppressant.

Nausea and vomiting
These are common effects of morphine. The emetic centre is stimulated through dopamine receptors in the chemoreceptor trigger-zone (CTZ). Another factor which contributes to nausea is that morphine causes hypotension (see above). This produces nausea more in ambulant patients than those who lie or sit still, suggesting a vestibular mechanism. Note that morphine may actually directly depress the emetic centre. This centre is activated by the nearby CTZ. Nausea is more likely after subcutaneous injection of morphine because then, the drug reaches the CTZ more rapidly; whereas with i.v. injection the drug reaches the emetic centre as rapidly as the CTZ, so then the incidence of nausea is less. Tolerance to this effect develops rapidly; it can be prevented by the simultaneous use of a dopamine receptor antagonist, e.g. chlorpromazine or cyclizine in cancer patients. This may, however, deepen the hypotension caused by morphine.

Individual opiates
There are some important differences between morphine and other commonly used opiates which should be noted (see summary Table 19.1). Codeine occurs naturally as an opium alkaloid. Its analgesic potency is about 10% that of morphine (note: about 10% of codeine is also excreted as morphine which suggests that morphine is the active metabolite). It is useful for the same range of pain as aspirin – headaches, muscle pain, backache – rather than severe pains of colic,

Table 19.1 *Properties of morphine-like drugs*

Opiate	Depression of respiration	Analgesic potency	Histamine release	Constipation	Addictive activity	Inhibition of vasomotor centre	Anti-tussive action
Morphine	+++	+++	+++	+++	+++	+++	+++
Codeine	0	+	0	+	0	0	++
Heroin	++++	++++	+++	+-	++++	+++	++++
Pethidine	++	++	0	0	++	0	+
Methadone	++	+++	+	0	+	0	+++

Intensity of action: ++++, very marked; +++, marked; ++, moderate; +, slight; 0, negligible.

trauma, and advanced malignant disease. Codeine produces little euphoria, and has minimal effects on the vasomotor centre or respiration. It rarely causes addiction, but it can be used to mitigate the withdrawal symptoms of morphine and other opiates.

Heroin (diacetylmorphine)

Is a synthetic compound. Qualitatively, heroin has similar actions to morphine, but it is more potent than morphine and possesses a greater power to induce addiction than morphine. Heroin is converted in the CNS first to monoacetylmorphine and then to morphine, but it is more rapidly acting than morphine; the acetylation of the two hydroxyl groups increases lipid solubility, hence heroin penetrates the CNS more rapidly than morphine. This is the reason why drug abusers prefer heroin to morphine. Because it is absorbed from mucous membranes addicts use it as a snuff. It is reputed to be less constipating than morphine. The therapeutic use of heroin is highly restricted to relief of pain in the terminally ill patient.

Pethidine (meperidine)

Pethidine was originally developed as an atropine-like drug. Then it was found to possess morphine-like effects. It has about one tenth of the analgesic activity of morphine and is shorter acting. Euphoria is less marked. Pethidine has no effects on cough but it may depress respiration especially if given i.v. Because it blocks muscarinic receptors, pethidine does not constrict the pupil and it tends to relax smooth muscles. In the bowel, motility is reduced, but constipation is not common. Pethidine may release histamine, but it is less likely to precipitate bronchospasm in the asthmatic. Indeed, pethidine relaxes constricted bronchial muscle. Pethidine is also preferred to morphine in labour because of its weaker depressant action on respiration. It is a drug of addiction although withdrawal symptoms are less severe than those associated with morphine dependence.

Methadone (physeptone)

Methadone is similar qualitatively to morphine and equipotent in analgesic activity. It is less sedative, and longer acting than morphine so that withdrawal symptoms are slower to develop, more protracted but less severe. For this reason, methadone is used in the treatment of morphine or heroin addiction as a replacement therapy.

Dihydrocodeine

Resembles codeine in having a relatively limited analgesic potency. For moderate analgesia, the drug has about one third the activity of morphine, but the maximum analgesic effect is much less than that which can be achieved with morphine, a situation which is reminiscent of partial agonism described in Chapter 4. Dihydrocodeine is a more potent analgesic than codeine and is useful in moderately severe pain, having less side effects in labour, being without effect on foetal respiration. It has minimal sedative effect and addictive power and is therefore useful as an antitussive agent and in the treatment of chronic pain of cancer.

Opiate antagonists

These are divided into two broad groups:

Group 1

Pure antagonists, e.g. *naloxone, naltrexone.* These compounds produce no observable morphine-like effects on their own when given in moderate doses whereas when given in quite small doses they can reverse the effects of morphine. In patients with respiratory depression due to morphine or opiate drugs there is prompt increase in respiratory rate. Sedative effects, and reduced blood pressure are reversed. It is conceptualised that these drugs have a high affinity for the opioid receptor but do not activate it. Naloxone is a more potent antagonist at the μ- than at the k- and γ- opiate receptors.

Group 2

Partial agonists, e.g. *nalorphine, pentazocine, buprenorphine.* These compounds behave somewhat like morphine in the absence of morphine. Thus, nalorphine reproduces almost all the effects of morphine when used in normal man; it lowers body temperature, causes constriction of the pupil, depresses respiration. In postoperative pain, nalorphine is almost as potent as morphine in analgesia. It can also cause sedation in a good proportion of patients but many patients also experience unpleasant reactions such as anxiety and hallucination. Because of these, the drug is not used as an analgesic on its own. The dysphoric effects of nalorphine can be antagonised by naloxone. Nalorphine can also antagonise morphine-induced CNS and gastrointestinal effects, but the antitussive and hypothermic effects are not easily antagonised probably because nalorphine is itself potent in producing these effects.

Therapeutic uses

Morphine antagonists are used in the treatment of narcotic-induced respiratory depression. In this regard it is important to bear in mind that respiratory depression caused by barbiturates is not antagonised but can be made worse by nalorphine. Pure morphine antagonists such as naloxone which produce no respiratory depression by themselves have significant advantages in situations where the aetiology of the respiratory depression is not clear. They are also used in the diagnosis of physical dependence. In addicts, a small (0.5 mg) subcutaneous dose of naloxone precipitates mild to severe withdrawal syndrome which lasts for about 2 h. This effect does not occur in non-addicts. Morphine antagonists are also used in the treatment of compulsive narcotic users, and some partial antagonists, e.g. pentazocine are used as analgesics. The duration of action of the antagonists is shorter than that of the opiates, and as the antagonism disappears, the effect of the opiate becomes re-established.

Tolerance

Tolerance is observed as a gradual increase in the dose of a drug required to produce the same effect. Tolerance should be distinguished from physical dependence. It is possible to develop tolerance to a drug without accompanying physical dependence on it. However, tolerance develops to all addictive drugs. Tolerance to opiates is attributed to opiate receptor desensitization or to down regulation of receptor density.

Drug addiction

This is a state of periodic or chronic intoxication produced by the repeated consumption of a drug, e.g. opiate, cannabis, cocaine. Its characteristics are:

(1) An overpowering desire or need (compulsion) to continue taking the drug and to obtain it by any means.
(2) A tendency to increase the dose.
(3) A psychological and generally a physical dependence on the effects of the drug.
(4) The addiction is detrimental to the individual and to society.

Drug habituation

This is a condition resulting from the repeated administration of a drug, e.g. tobacco or alcohol. Its characteristics are:

(1) A desire but not a compulsion to continue taking the drug for

the sense of improved well-being which it engenders.

(2) Little or no tendency to increase the dose.

(3) Some degree of psychological dependence on the effect of the drug but absence of physical dependence and hence of an abstinence syndrome.

(4) Habituation is detrimental, if anything, to the individual.

Drug abuse

This is the consumption of a drug apart from medical need or in unnecessarily large quantities.

Drug addiction, drug habituation or drug abuse are all instances of drug dependence, which can be psychological or physical. In psychological dependence, the individual relies on the pleasure which he derives from taking the drug, e.g. the pipe smoker who can relieve his desire simply by sucking on the stem of his pipe. Physcial dependence is more serious because withdrawal of the drug is accompanied by serious physical ailments. The WHO expert committee has suggested the use of the term *Drug Dependence* instead of *drug addiction* or *drug habituation* which then become

Addictive Drug Dependence and
Habitual Drug Dependence, respectively.

Causes of addiction are:

(a) Hospitalisation,

(b) The activities of dope peddlars.

(c) Possibly the possession of character traits associated with addicts.

The abstinence syndrome

If morphine is withdrawn abruptly from an addict, a characteristic reaction develops known as the *opiate abstinence syndrome.*

(1) Ten to twelve hours after withdrawal, little signs begin to develop, occasional yawning, mild perspiration and lachrymation.

(2) After about 36 h, the patient becomes extremely restless, getting in and out of bed, and develops severe headaches accompanied by vomiting and diarrhoea.

(3) At this stage the patient loses appetite, and rapidly loses weight. Death may soon follow, in about 72 h, from dehydration and cardiovascular collapse.

Codeine and methadone can be used as replacement drugs in the treatment of morphine addicts.

Non-narcotic analgesics

The class of analgesics to be discussed here are known as non-narcotic because unlike the opiates, they as a rule, cause no euphoria or sedation; their action is exerted predominantly at peripheral sites. They are effective against mild pain. The drugs most commonly used for this purpose are the salicylates, and p-aminophenols (Fig. 19.2). The fundamental action of these (aspirin-like) drugs is inhibition of fatty acid, cyclooxygenase. Many other potent inhibitors of this enzyme, used mainly as anti-inflammatory agents, are discussed later. There is no consistent clearcut structure–action relationship among these compounds in their inhibition of cyclooxygenase. An important point to note is that the salicylates are equally potent as anti-inflammatory, antipyretic and analgesic drugs, whereas the para-aminophenol derivatives (e.g. paracetamol) are analgesic and antipyretic, but have weak anti-inflammatory action. Some other compounds, e.g. indomethacin have powerful anti-inflammatory activity but are weak analgesics and antipyretics (see Table 19.2). The explanation of this

Fig. 19.2 Non-narcotic analgesics.

SALICYLATES

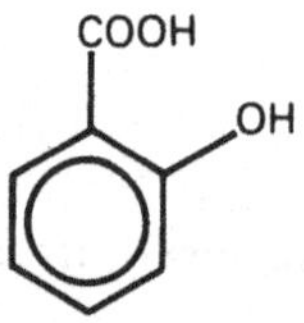

Salicylic acid

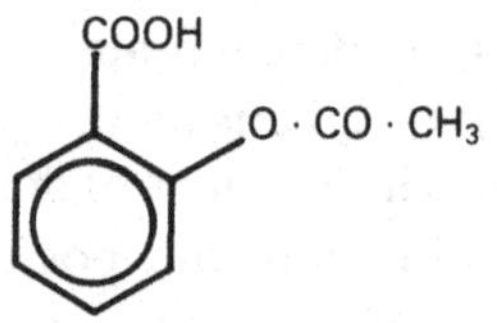

Acetylsalicylic acid
(aspirin)

p-AMINOPHENOL DERIVATIVES

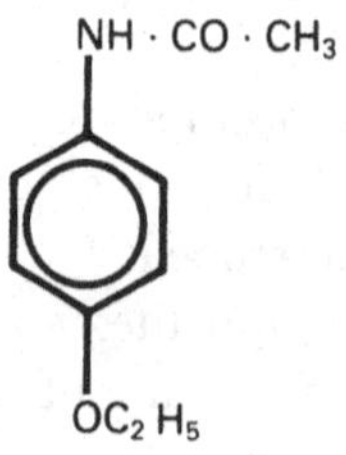

Phenacetin

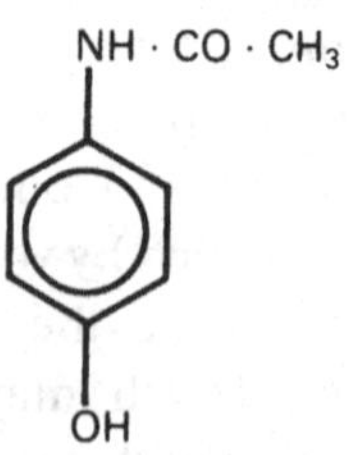

Acetaminophen
(paracetamol)

Table 19.2 *Comparative actions of some aspirin-like drugs.*

Drug	Inhibition of fatty acid cyclooxygenase			Associated pharmacological actions		
	Brain enzyme	Peripheral enzyme	Anti-inflammatory	Anti-inflammatory	Antipyretic	Analgesic
Aspirin	++	++	++		++	++
Paracetamol	++	0	0		++	++
Phenylbutazone	0	++	++		0	0
Indomethacin	0	+++	+++		0	0
Mefanamic acid	++	++	++		++	++

Intensity of action: +++, very intense; ++, intense; +, moderate; 0, weak/negligible.

discrepancy is that peripheral and CNS cyclooxygenases have different sensitivities to the inhibitors. The brain enzyme is sensitive to salicylates and paracetamol which are thus analgesic and antipyretic, whereas the peripheral enzyme is sensitive to inhibition by salicylates and indomethacin which are therefore anti-inflammatory. Peripheral and CNS enzymes are insensitive to paracetamol and indomethacin respectively. Mefenamic acid, aspirin, and paracetamol are the most useful analgesics among the aspirin-like drugs. These observations point to the likelihood that a substantial component of analgesic action of aspirin-like drugs is CNS in origin in addition to their action peripherally.

Pharmacological properties of aspirin-like drugs
Analgesia

The types of pain relieved by aspirin-like drugs are those of low intensity, particularly headache, or muscle pain. The drugs are ineffective against intensive pain of visceral origin, trauma or cancer. The maximum analgesic effect of aspirin-like drugs is much lower than that of narcotic analgesics. The main advantages of these drugs over the morphine type are:

(a) Their use does not usually lead to tolerance and physical dependence.

(b) They do not depress respiration in therapeutic doses. On the contrary in toxic doses they can stimulate respiration.

(c) Nausea and vomiting do not usually occur with the usual analgesic doses (these may be experienced with high therapeutic doses).

(d) Constipation does not usually result from the therapeutic use of aspirin-like drugs.

Antipyretic action

Aspirin-like drugs with antipyretic actions (see Table 19.2) lower temperatures rapidly in febrile patients, but *not* when the body temperature is normal. Body temperature is maintained by a delicate balance between heat production and heat loss. The thermostatic control mechanism is situated in the hypothalamus. In fever, the balance between heat production and heat loss is still maintained but the thermostat is set at a higher temperature than normal. The aspirin-like drugs act to reset the thermostat at a lower point and then increase heat loss through increased peripheral blood flow and sweating.

Mechanism of action

Aspirin-like drugs alleviate mild/moderate pain by virtue of a peripheral and most probably also a CNS action. Peripherally, aspirin-like drugs relieve pain by a modification of the cause of pain at the site of origin. Pain is usually caused in inflamed tissues by products of arachidonic acid metabolism (e.g., prostaglandins) (see Fig. 19.3) as well as other pain-producing substances. Prostaglandins sensitise the pain receptors to mechanical stimulation or to stimulation by other substances such as bradykinin; aspirin-like drugs inhibit the production of arachidonic acid metabolites, thereby preventing the amplification of mechanical and chemical stimulation. Direct CNS actions of aspirin-like drugs have been described and these suggest a hypothalamic site. The antipyretic action of aspirin-like drugs is also linked to inhibition of the formation of arachidonic acid metabolites, (prostaglandin E_1 (PGE_1), or thromboxane), which are some of the most potent fever-producing substances known. Part of the evidence is as follows:

When fever is induced in experimental animals by the injection of bacterial toxins or pyrogens, a rise in the concentration of PGE_1 in the cerebrospinal fluid (CSF) can be demonstrated. Aspirin prevents the fever and the rise in the prostaglandin content of the CSF in parallel, but has no effect on fever directly induced by the injection of prostaglandins into the cerebral ventricle. Aspirin does not affect normal body temperature which suggests that prostaglandins are probably not involved in the normal regulation of body temperature. This latter is a complex mechanism and there is evidence that it is a hypothalamic function which may involve thermogenic amines, e.g. noradrenaline, 5-HT, and ACH).

Other actions of aspirin-like drugs
Respiration

Aspirin-like drugs stimulate respiration directly and indirectly. In therapeutic doses, aspirin increases oxygen consumption and CO_2 production in skeletal muscle by uncoupling oxidative phosphorylation. The increased CO_2 production stimulates respiration. The consequent increased alveolar ventilation balances the increased CO_2 production. Thus CO_2 tension (pCO_2) does not rise. This is the indirect effect of aspirin on respiration when given in high therapeutic doses. If a barbiturate or morphine is present so that the respiratory centre is no longer responsive to raised CO_2, the pCO_2 rises quickly and respiratory acidosis can develop.

As aspirin-like drugs gain access to the medulla, they stimulate the

Fig. 19.3. Metabolism of arachidonic acid.

(1) Arachidonic acid (AA) is freed from its phospholipid binding site in the cell membrane at injury by the enzyme phospholipase A2 (1). This enzyme can be inhibited by mepacrine, chloroquine, and probably corticosteroids.

(2) Fatty acid cyclooxygenase pathway. AA is rapidly converted by cyclooxygenase (2) to the endoperoxide (PGH_2). The production of PGH_2 is accompanied by release of free radicals which are probably responsible for the tissue destruction in inflammation. What PGH_2 is converted to depends on the physiological needs of the organ. In platelets, PGH_2 is converted to thromboxane (TxA_2), a powerful stimulant of platelet aggregation and adhesion. This is to ensure that when a blood vessel is injured, clotting quickly follows. In the wall of blood vessels *in situ*, the product is prostacyclin (PGI_2), the most potent inhibitor of platelet aggregation and adhesion known. This ensures that clotting does not occur *in situ*. At sites of inflammation (joints, muscle, lungs, etc.) the products are stable prostaglandins (PGE_2 and PGF_{2a}). The corresponding one-double-bond prostaglandins (PGE_1 and PGF_{1a}) are formed from eicosatrienoic acids in the place of AA.

(3) Lipoxygenase pathway. AA is converted through intermediate products by the enzyme lipoxygenase to a mixture of leucotrienes (LTC_4, LTD_4, LTE_4). This pathway is important in lungs. Slow-reacting substance of anaphylaxis (SRSA) extensively studied in connection with bronchial asthma is now thought to be a mixture of leucotrienes. These compounds are potent bronchoconstrictors.

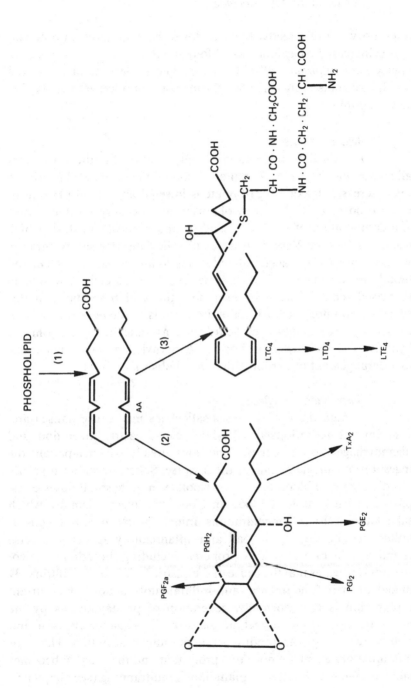

respiratory centre directly. In toxic doses the respiratory minute volume is increased by as much as 10-fold and there is a drastic reduction in pCO_2 and *respiratory alkalosis* ensues. These effects can be observed in salicylate poisoning when the plasma concentration goes up as high as 400 µg/ml.

Acid–base balance

In salicylate intoxication, compensation for the respiratory alkalosis quickly ensues. Renal excretion of bicarbonate, Na^+ and K^+ ions increases. Plasma bicarbonate is lowered and blood pH returns towards normal. At a late stage of poisoning especially in infants, there is a combination of *respiratory acidosis* and *metabolic* acidosis which occurs as follows: Very high doses of salicylates depress respiration which allows CO_2 to accumulate leading to an increase in pCO_2, and blood pH decreases. Since plasma HCO_3^- is already low due to increased renal bicarbonate excretion, the acid–base status at this stage is respiratory acidosis. Superimposed is a true *metabolic acidosis* caused by accumulation of acids such as salicylic acid (from the hydrolysis of aspirin), phosphoric acid, pyruvic, and lactic acids (due to a derangement of carbohydrate metabolism).

Gastrointestinal effects

In high therapeutic doses salicylates may cause nausea and vomiting. More seriously, salicylates cause gastric ulceration and haemorrhage and where these conditions already exist in a patient, the ingestion of salicylates makes them worse. Salicylate-induced gastric bleeding leads to blood loss in the stool; even quite small doses of aspirin can cause loss of blood in stool. The mechanism by which salicylates at high concentrations injure gastric mucosal cells is unknown. The finding that all anti-inflammatory agents of diverse chemical structure have this property (including the adrenocorticosteroids) indicates that the cause of the gastric lesion may be intimately linked to their fundamental anti-inflammatory action. One current explanation is that normally, generation of prostaglandins by the mucosal cells helps to protect the gastric mucosa against abrasion and acidity because prostaglandins stimulate mucus secretion. The anti-inflammatory agents remove this protection and the mucosa becomes more vulnerable. Another explanation is ion-trapping (see chapter 5).

Effects on blood
Ingestion of aspirin by normal individuals causes a definite prolongation of the bleeding time; a single dose of 0.65 g (two tablets) of aspirin approximately doubles the bleeding time of a normal person for a period of 4 - 7 days. There are two possible mechanisms for this effect.

(a) Effect on platelet aggregation
Clotting in injured blood vessels begins with adherence of platelets to exposed connective tissue, followed by the release of adenosine diphosphate (ADP) by platelets and platelet aggregation. In this connection, the inhibition of cyclooxygenase by aspirin is important because the cyclic endoperoxide intermediates in arachidonic acid metabolism (thromboxanes) are potent in triggering platelet aggregation. Inhibition of cyclooxygenase is irreversible; hence the prolongation of bleeding time for several days after a single dose of aspirin.

(b) Effect on plasma prothrombin
In large doses aspirin reduces the plasma prothrombin level and this effect can be antagonised by vitamin K. This suggests that aspirin competes with the vitamin for enzyme sites in the liver during synthesis of prothrombin. This effect does not account for the prolongation of bleeding time seen with moderate doses of aspirin. However, because this effect on prothrombin synthesis and the effect on platelet aggregation can synergise, aspirin should be avoided in patients with severe hepatic damage, hypoprothrombinaemia, vitamin K deficiency, haemophilia, or in patients on oral anticoagulant therapy.

19.5 INFLAMMATION

Inflammation is a fundamental response of tissue cells to injury. Rheumatoid arthritis is a common disease the underlying mechanism of which is inflammation. The following is a mechanism of inflammation associated with rheumatoid arthritis. The first stage involves the reaction of antigen with an antibody (rheumatoid factor) in the presence of complement. The antigen–antibody complexes release from cells pharmacologically active substances such as histamine, 5-HT, bradykinin, and prostaglandins. These substances have the following properties at the site of inflammation.
(1) They increase capillary permeability leading to a leakage of

water and plasma proteins from blood vessels into extravascular compartments causing swelling.

(2) They are chemotactic, that is, they attract white blood cells (leucocytes) which migrate from the lumen of blood vessels into the site of inflammation. The white blood cells phagocytose the antigen–antibody complexes. During this activity, these cells release phospholipase enzymes some of which liberate unsaturated fatty acids such as arachidonic acid for the synthesis of metabolites such as prostaglandins. The arachidonic acid metabolites attract more leucocytes and the inflammatory state is maintained. Most products of arachidonic acid metabolism play an important role in inflammation (see Fig. 19.3).

(3) The substances released are pain-producing substances which accounts for the pain of rheumatoid arthritis. Even small concentration of prostaglandins potentiate the pro-inflammatory actions of the other mediators.

Anti-inflammatory agents

There are two major groups of anti-inflammatory agents – non-steroidal anti-inflammatory agents and steroidal anti-inflammatory agents.

Non-steroidal anti-inflammatory agents
Aspirin

Despite the development of several newer agents, aspirin is still a useful drug in the treatment of rheumatoid arthritis. It reduces inflammation in joints and surrounding tissues. Doses of up to 5 g a day can be given in these conditions. But there is no fixed dose that may be applicable to all patients. The majority of patients with rheumatoid arthritis can be controlled by aspirin alone.

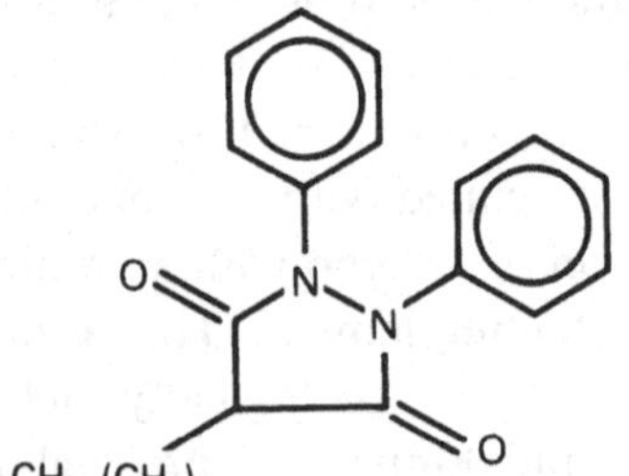

CH₃ (CH₂)₃

Phenylbutazone

Phenylbutazone

The anti-inflammatory effects of phenylbutazone are similar to those of aspirin; phenylbutazone inhibits the synthesis of prostaglandins, uncouples oxidative phosphorylation and inhibits the biosynthesis of mucopolysaccharides. For pain of nonrheumatic origin, its analgesic efficacy is inferior to that of aspirin. Because of its relatively high toxicity, phenylbutazone should not be used as a general purpose analgesic or antipyretic.

Phenylbutazone is completely absorbed from the gastrointestinal tract after oral ingestion. At therapeutic doses, phenylbutazone is 98% bound to plasma proteins, and the plasma half-life is 50 to 100 h. Biotransformation takes place in the liver. One of the products of metabolism, *oxyphenylbutazone*, has antirheumatic and sodium- and water-retaining properties similar to those of phenylbutazone; it is also extensively bound to plasma proteins with a half-life of several days and contributes to the pharamacological and toxic effects of the parent drug. Phenylbutazone and oxyphenylbutazone are excreted only slowly in urine since plasma binding limits glomerular filtration. Most of the drug is excreted as metabolites.

Phenylbutazone is poorly tolerated in many patients; 10–15% of patients discontinue treatment. Nausea, vomiting, gastric discomfort, and skin rashes are the most frequently reported side effects. More serious effects are peptic ulcer, haemorrhage, hypersensitivity reactions, nephritis, agranulocytosis, and aplastic anaemia. Patients taking phenylbutazone should be kept under close observation including examination of their blood.

Indomethacin (INDOCID)

Indomethacin is a potent anti-inflammatory drug effective in the treatment of rheumatoid arthritis and acute gout. In these diseases indomethacin is more potent than aspirin but also more toxic, so that in doses of indomethacin which most patients can tolerate, the drug is not superior to aspirin. Indomethacin does not possess analgesic properties which are distinct from its anti-inflammatory properties. The drug is too toxic to be used as a general analgesic–antipyretic.

Mechanism of action

(a) Like the salicylates, indomethacin is a potent inhibitor of prostaglandin synthesis and this may thus form the basis of its anti-inflammatory activity.

(b) It inhibits motility of polymorphonuclear leucocytes which is important in the maintenance of the inflammatory state.

(c) Like aspirin, it uncouples oxidative phosphorylation.

Indomethacin is rapidly and completely absorbed from the gastrointestinal tract, peak plasma concentrations being reached in about 3 h, is highly bound to plasma protein, and toxic. Up to 20% of patients discontinue treatment.

Toxic side effects include peptic ulceration, severe frontal headache, dizziness, mental confusion, severe depression and psychosis. Indomethacin should not be used in pregnant women, children, or patients with psychiatric disorders, epilepsy, or Parkinson's disease.

Anti-inflammatory drugs used in the therapy of gout

An acute attack of gout occurs as a result of an inflammatory reaction to crystals of monosodium urate that are deposited in the joint tissue from hyperuric acid body fluids. The inflammatory response involves local infiltration of the inflamed area by leucocytes which phagocytose the urate crystals. The phagocytosing activity of the leucocytes somehow leads to a lowering of the pH of the synovial fluid due to increased production of lactic acid. The low pH favours further deposition of urate crystals.

Colchicine

Colchicine, an alkaloid of *Colchicum autumnale*, is a unique anti-inflammatory agent that is effective only against gout arthritis. Colchicine inhibits migration of leucocytes into the inflamed area and reduces the lactic acid production associated with phagocytosis. The cycle of urate crystal deposition is thereby interrupted.

Colchicine is also antimitotic, arresting cell division in the metaphase in both plants and animals. Its anti-inflammatory action appear to be unrelated to arachidonic acid metabolism; it has been found to increase prostaglandin concentrations in inflamed tissues.

Colchicine provides quick relief in acute gout arthritis. It can also be used to prevent an attack. Nausea, vomiting, diarrhoea and abdominal pain can occur.

Allopurinol

This drug inhibits the formation of uric acid from xanthines. Uric acid in man is formed by the xanthine oxidase-catalysed oxidation of soluble hypoxanthine and xanthine. Allopurinol is a sub-

Xanthine   Allopurinol

strate for, and a competitive antagonist of, xanthine oxidase; it is converted to alloxanthine which is also an antagonist of xanthine oxidase. Allopurinol is effective in both the primary hyperuraemia of gout or in gout secondary to blood discrasias. Colchicine is recommended for use in combination during the initial stages of treatment with allopurinol.

Steroidal anti-inflammatory drugs

Adrenocorticotrophic hormone (ACTH), hydrocortisone, and synthetic analogues of cortisone, e.g. triamcinolone, betamethasone and dexamethasone, possess strong anti-inflammatory properties. They suppress the local heat, tenderness and swelling of inflammation. They inhibit the oedema, capillary dilatation, migration of leucocytes and phagocytic activity. The later stages of inflammation such as capillary proliferation, and deposition of collagen are also inhibited. Although the corticosteroids are potent anti-inflammatory drugs, they do not affect the underlying cause of the inflammation; so infections may continue to proliferate while the patient feels better or a peptic ulcer may perforate without producing clinical symptoms. They should be used with care.

Mechanism of action

There are several hypotheses to explain the mechanism of anti-inflammatory action of the corticosteroids. One point that can be accepted without much debate is that their action is a direct one on the local site of inflammation since some of them are active on local application, e.g. bethnovate ointment. One hypothesis is that the steroids stabilise lysosomes thereby preventing their rupture and the consequent release of lysosomal enzymes. One such enzyme is phospholipase A_2 (Fig. 19.3), which splits fatty acid precursors from binding sites for prostaglandin synthesis. Membrane stabilisation may explain the finding that under certain experimental conditions, the anti-inflammatory steroids prevent the release of prostaglandins from intact cells although they do not directly inhibit cyclooxygenase. There is also evidence that anti-inflammatory steroids induce the synthesis of small molecular weight proteins (e.g. macrocortin, renocortin, lipomodulin) which then act to inhibit prostaglandin release or phospholipase A_2. However, it seems likely that the anti-inflammatory action of the steroids may be due to a combination of different effects including suppression of immune reactions, stabilisation of cell membrane in blood vessels, and inhibition of fibroblasts. Cortico- steroids can be given by mouth but are usually given by injection (i.v. or i.m.) in order to achieve high concentrations in plasma rapidly. They can also be administered topically to inflamed mucous membranes or skin.

Inflammatory conditions in which corticosteroids are indicated

In all cases, it should be remembered that once steroid therapy is started, the patient may have to rely on it for many years of life, with serious consequences. Hence, steroid therapy should be attempted only after it is clear that the condition is not responding to non-steroidal anti-inflammatory drugs such as aspirin. The steroids can be used in the treatment of the following.

Rheumatoid arthritis. In this case, the steroids may be used in combination with other non-steroidal drugs in addition to physical management of the disease.

Osteoarthritis. In this the drug can be injected locally into the affected joint.

Rheumatic carditis.

Collagen diseases.

Allergic diseases such as hay fever, serum sickness, urticaria, drug hypersensitivity and anaphylaxis.

Bronchial asthma

The corticosteroids should not be used in acute or chronic asthma if the condition can be controlled by other measures. If a steroid must be used in status asthmaticus, the patient should be placed on other forms of therapy as soon as possible.

Eye problems

Corticosteroids are frequently used to suppress inflammation in the eye. They are applied topically. Prolonged therapy of this kind may precipitate increased intraoccular pressure (glaucoma). Topical application of corticosteroids to patients with bacterial, viral, or fungal conjunctivitis may mask and indeed aid the spread of the infection in the eye and lead to loss of sight. Corticosteroids should also not be used in cases of mechanical lacerations in the eye. They delay healing and promote the spread of infections.

Skin diseases

A variety of these also respond to topical corticosteroids.

Toxic effects of adrenocortical steroids

Two types of toxic effects are associated with corticosteroid therapy; those due to (1) continued use of large doses and (2) withdrawal symptoms.

If corticosteroids are suddenly withdrawn from a patient who has been on large doses of the drugs for prolonged periods, there is a characteristic withdrawal syndrome, consisting of fever, muscle pain, malaise. Corticosteroids should be withdrawn gradually. Prolonged therapy with corticosteroids results in suppression of the pituitary-adrenal function which may take months or years to return to normal. During this period, the patient has to be protected from stressful situations such as surgery or infections.

The principal complications arising from prolonged therapy include increased susceptibility to infections, peptic ulceration, myopathy, behavioural disturbances, and osteoporosis.

Other anti-inflammatory drugs

(a) *Chloroquine and hydroxychloroquine* are used for the treatment of rheumatoid arthritis. Its mechanism of action is unknown but probably involves inhibition of phospholipase A_2. For this purpose, much larger doses are employed and for longer periods than are used in the treatment of malaria; careful consideration of toxicity must therefore be taken. The commonest toxicity in such cases is retinopathy, characterised by loss of central visual acuity, granular pigmentation of the macula, blurring of vision. The visual loss does not progress after cessation of therapy, but the damage is irreversible. Chloroquine is highly concentrated in the irides of laboratory animals. Chloroquine is used when other treatments are unsuccessful.

(b) *D-Penicillamine* The main use of this chelating agent is in the treatment of copper, mercury, zinc, or lead poisoning where the drug promotes the excretion of these metals in the urine. The drug can also be used in the treatment of rheumatoid arthritis that is refractory to other treatments. The mechanism of action is unknown and unrelated to its metal-chelating properties.

(c) *Gold salts*, e.g. aurothioglucose and gold sodium thiomalate. Gold relieves the symptoms of rheumatoid arthritis. Its use is indicated when other more conventional therapies fail. The mechanism of action is not clearly understood; it is taken up by macrophages; phagocytosis and the activity of lysosomal enzymes are inhibited.

FURTHER READING

Flower, R.J. (1988). Lipocortin and the mechanism of action of the glucocorticoids (XI Gaddam Lecture). *Br. J. Pharmacol.* 94, 987–1015.
Flower, R.J., Moncada, S. & Vane, J.R. (1985). Analgesic-antipyretics and anti-inflammatory agents; drugs employed in the treatment of gout. In *Goodman and Gilman's The Pharmacological Basis of Therapeutics*, 7th edn (ed. A.G. Gilman, L.S. Goodman, T.W. Rall & F. Murad). Macmillan, London.

20

Drugs acting on the central nervous system

20.1 INTRODUCTION

Continuing advances in neuropharmacology show that disorders of movement, neuroses, psychoses and other disease of CNS origin can be traced to biochemical lesions in specific areas of the brain; specific abnormalities in transmitter function, synthesis or release can be identified and associated with certain CNS diseases. Consequently the action of many of the drugs used in the treatment of CNS diseases can now be explained in terms of interaction with specific CNS structures. A major objective in this area of study is the development of new highly selective drugs for the amelioration of very perplexing diseases such as schizophrenia, epilepsy, etc. for which there are still no satisfactory therapies. In this chapter, the mechanisms of action of some drugs currently used in the treatment of disorders of motor activity and mental illnesses are described. Also discussed are some CNS-acting drugs that are widely abused.

20.2 MOTOR ACTIVITY

The CNS control of movement of limbs is complex; it is achieved by a flow of impulses to and from different parts of the CNS. It involves coordinated contractions of some muscles and reciprocal relaxations of others, through the activation or inhibition of spinal neurones. Superimposed on this is the voluntary control involving centres in the cerebral cortex which can initiate, modulate or arrest a particular sequence of movements.

Three parts of the brain take part in the control of motor activity – the cerebellum, basal ganglia and the cerebral cortex. The cerebellum is concerned with the acquisition and learning of complex motor tasks which are then executed with precision with minimal regulation from other areas of the brain. The basal ganglia (including the caudate nucleus, substantia nigra, putamen and globus pallidus) is concerned with fine control of movement; a malfunction here is often associated with movement disorders. Many disorders in which there are involuntary or abnormal motor movements have origins in the basal ganglia. The cerebral cortex is the highest level of voluntary control over motor systems; it is intimately linked with the cerebellum and the basal ganglia functionally. The cerebral cortex is 'wired' directly to the spinal neurones through the pyramidal tracts; but the major control signals for movement and posture leave the brain by an extrapyramidal network of nerves.

Epileptic seizures

Epilepsy refers to a complex of disease conditions characterised by frequent but brief attacks of seizures (convulsions) accompanied by unconsciousness, and abnormal and excessive discharges which show on an electroencephalogram (EEG). Attacks may be accompanied by characteristic body movements and autonomic hyperactivity. Epilepsy may be caused by many factors such as infection, or trauma, but often the cause is not known. The commonest type of epilepsy is *grand mal*. This originates in the cerebral cortex; it can be symptomatic (i.e., caused by e.g. hypoglycaemia, hypocalcaemia, tumour in the brain, or drugs) or more frequently it is idiopathic. Grand mal is characterised by an initial loss of consciousness followed immediately by loss of posture (the patient falls down) and tonic contractions of all body muscles proceeding to synchronous, clonic jerking and a slow return to consciousness. There is characteristic post-seizure depression which may be prolonged.

Another form of epileptic seizures is *petit mal*: characteristic features are brief attacks of unconsciousness (a few seconds) and it is often unaccompanied by muscle movements. *Psychomotor epilepsy* is characterised by attacks of confused behaviour and a generalised EEG activity and spiking in the anterior temporal lobe. Epileptic seizures may also be *diencephalic* in which there is autonomic and behavioural hyperactivity, or it may be *focal cortical* where the convulsions are confined to specific limbs or muscles (Jacksonian epilepsy) or *myoclonic* which is characterised by isolated clonic jerks. *Status epilepticus* is characterised by frequent seizure attacks occurring at short intervals.

Mechanism of action of anti-epileptic drugs (anti-convulsants)

Seizures are caused by sudden excessive bursts of local electrical discharges in the cerebral cortex. These may excite part or the whole brain to cause localised or generalised convulsions. The seizure is maintained by a recirculation of the excitatory impulses. Posttetanic potentiation (i.e., the progressive enhancement of transmitter release and of synaptic transmission during repetitive activation) is another factor which contributes to the maintenance and spread of the seizure.

The mechanism of action of antiepileptic drugs is not unequivocally understood. Their actions may involve the following.

(a) An increase in the concentration of GABA, or a facililation of GABAergic transmission. GABA causes an increase in Cl^- ion conductance and hyperpolarisation. This raises the threshold of excitation, thereby preventing the initiation of epileptogenic discharge or its spread. Possibly there exist in the cerebral cortex endogenous anticonvulsant peptides with appropriate receptors (phenytoin receptors, c.f. with opiate receptors activated by morphine). It is suggested that these receptors may be activated by hydantoin and barbiturate anticonvulsants, and that GABAergic and benzodiazepine receptors are linked in a complex way to these phenytoin receptors.

(b) Some of the drugs have been shown to prevent *post-tetanic potentiation*, e.g. phenytoin and carbamazepine.

(c) Membrane stabilisation is another mechanism which has been suggested for phenytoin; it explains why the drug is also used in the treatment of cardiac dysrhythmias.

(d) It is possible also that the drugs may affect membrane Na^+, K^+-activated ATPase. The activity of this enzyme is vital for the maintenance of transmembrane ion gradient. Phenytoin stimulates this enzyme.

Anticonvulsants

Drugs used in the treatment of epileptic seizures (anticonvulsants) are listed in Table 20.1. Anti-epileptic drugs must usually be given prophylactically for prolonged periods and sometimes in high doses. Therefore, in addition to their anti-epileptic effects, acute and long term side effects are of particular interest. These are listed for some important drugs in Table 20.2. The usefulness of phenytoin is

Table 20.1 *Anti-epileptic drugs (anticonvulsants)*

Type of seizure	Drugs used
Grand mal (focal cortical seizures)	*Barbiturates*: phenobarbitone, mephobarbitone, primidone
	Hydantoins: phenytoin, mephenytoin, diphenylhydantoin
Psychomotor epilepsy	Primidone, phenytoin, mephenytoin
	Acetylureas: phenacemide, pheneturide
Petit mal	*Succinimides*: phensuximide ethosuximide, methsuximide
	Oxazolidinediones: trimethadione, paramethadione
Status epilepticus	*Benzodiazepine*: diazepam (i.v.), nitrazepam *Hydantoin*: phenytoin

due to both its effectiveness in the treatment of a wide range of seizures and its relative freedom from side effects.

Other points to note are:

(a) Treatment needed depends on the type of epilepsy, and accurate diagnosis is important because the wrong drug may make the condition worse rather than better.

(b) The most often used anti-epileptic drugs (e.g., phenobarbitone, phenytoin, the succinimides) contain free benzene rings in their structures. They are metabolised by hydroxylation (to increase aqueous solubility and decrease lipid solubility) which requires folic acid as a cofactor. Prolonged therapy with large doses of these drugs can set off a series of vitamin deficiencies. Folic acid deficiency may occur due to its exhaustion in the hydroxylation reaction; this can lead to folate deficiency anaemia. Also a derangement of hydroxylation (which is necessary to maintain an adequate concentration of activated vitamin D) may occur, and hence inadequate absorption of calcium from the gut leading to osteomalacia.

(c) Phenobarbitone is the basic anticonvulsant molecule; primidone and mephobarbitone are metabolised to phenobarbitone in the body. The toxicity of the barbiturates is therefore due to phenobarbitone.

Table 20.2 Some side effects of anti-epileptic drugs

Side-effects	Anti-epileptic drugs				
	Sodium valproate	Phenobarbitone	Phenytoin	Ethosuximide	Carbamazepine
Drowsiness	+	+++	+	++	+
Ataxia	0	++	++	0	++
Allergy	0	+	++	+	++
Blood dyscrasias					
folate-deficiency					
anaemia	0	++	++	++	++
leucopenia	0	0	0	++	+
Osteomalacia	0	++	++	0	+
Gingivitis	0	0	++	0	0
Teratogenicity	0	0	+	0	0

+++, frequent occurrence; ++, moderate frequency; +, occasional occurrence; 0, uncommon.

Parkinsonism

This disease was first described by James Parkinson in 1817. It is a basal ganglia defect which can arise in a number of ways, e.g., it can be drug-induced (i.e., iatrogenic), idiopathic (degenerative) or infective. The primary problem whatever the cause, is overall deficiency in dopamine function compared to ACH (muscarinic) function in the caudate nucleus. The symptoms consist of tremors, and difficulties in movement (akinesia). This includes difficulties in initiating or arresting a sequence of movements; impaired handwriting (micrographia), impaired speech; and rigidity. Mental faculties are not generally affected.

The idea that there might be a catecholamine deficiency in the brain in Parkinson's disease arose in the 1950s as a result of the following observations.

(a) Reserpine, known to deplete brain catecholamines, caused, as a side effect, akinesia in patients receiving the drug as a treatment for psychosis. These effects were counteracted by treatment with L-dopa.

(b) Dopamine was later found to be highly concentrated in the basal ganglia.

(c) Studies with fluorescent techniques in experimental animals showed the presence of dopaminergic neurones projecting from the substantia nigra to the caudate nucleus.

(d) The concentration of dopamine in the basal ganglia was very low in brains of people who died of Parkinson's disease. This was discovered at autopsy.

A simplified view is that for a balanced locomotor control in the basal ganglia, dopaminergic (inhibitory) and cholinergic (excitatory) transmissions must be in equilibrium and that Parkinsonism arises when there is failure in the dopaminergic component with consequent overwhelming cholinergic activity. This is why the therapeutic options in the treatment of the disease are antimuscarinic drugs or drugs which promote dopaminergic transmission.

Anticholinergic drugs

Belladonna alkaloids were first used in the treatment of patients with Parkinson's disease by Charcot in 1892. They were superseded by the synthetic anticholinergic drugs; the most useful synthetic muscarinic receptor antagonists are those which cross the blood–brain barrier. The structures of some are shown in Fig. 20.1.

Some general points to note about this group of drugs are:

(a) Indications for their use

Atropine-like drugs were most useful in the treatment of Parkinson's disease before the discovery of L-dopa. Now, the anticholinergics have been relegated to a supportive role; but they are still useful for various purposes, e.g. (i) in the treatment of mild symptoms, (2) as alternatives to L-dopa in patients not responding to the drug or unable to withstand its toxicity, and (3) in the treatment of Parkinsonian syndrome in patients treated with antipsychotic drugs such as chlorpromazine (see page 452).

(b) Individual drugs

Although the drugs are similar in their therapeutic profile, some are more useful in certain types of Parkinson's disease than others and the physician must consider the clinical situation, e.g. age of the patient and other medication being taken by the patient in selecting a particular anticholinergic. All the drugs can control the sialorrhoea (excessive salivation) of Parkinsonism.

Atropine and scopolamine are effective in controlling the tremor, scopolamine being 10 times more potent and more useful than atropine.

Fig. 20.1. Synthetic atropine-like drugs used in the treatment of Parkinson's disease.

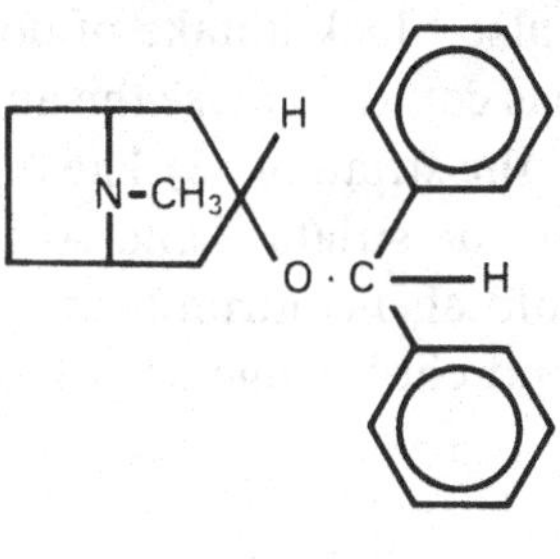

Benztropine

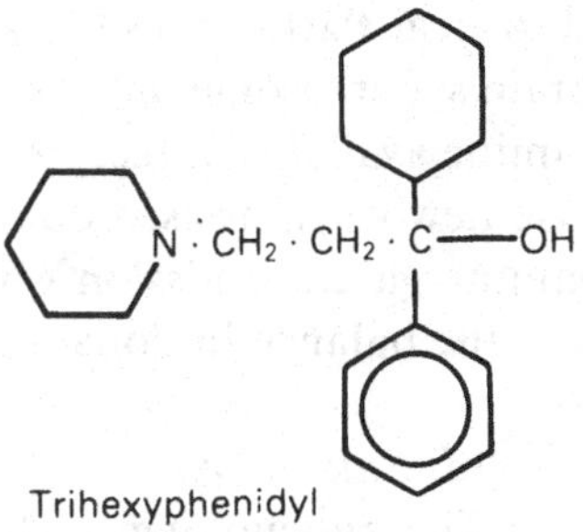

Trihexyphenidyl

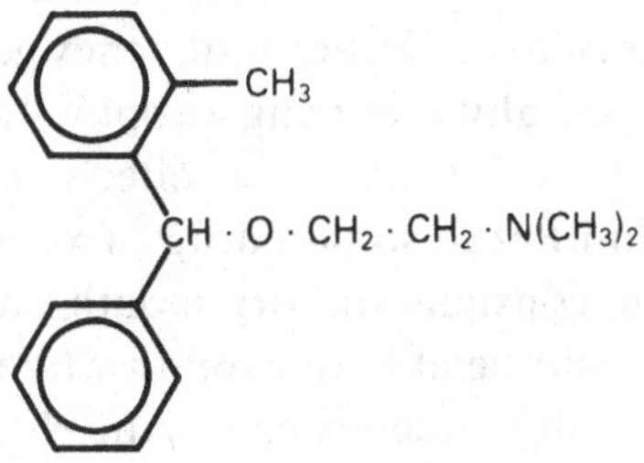

Orphenadrine

Benztropine is useful in all types of Parkinson's disease; it abolishes the tremors, rigidity and spasm, with a long duration of action. It causes sedation which may be useful in the elderly. Benztropine is also thought to inhibit dopamine uptake. *Trihexyphenidyl* relieves tremor by abolishing cholinergic activity in the striatum, but it is less effective in treating rigidity and akinesia; on the other hand, *procyclidine* controls rigidity with minimum effect on tremors. *Ethopropazine* is structurally, a phenothiazine related to the antihistamine, promethazine (not used in the treatment of Parkinsonism). Ethopropazine is an anticholinergic and also antihistamine pheniazine (note the point that a major side effect of the important antipsychotic phenothiazine, chlorpromazine, is Parkinsonian syndrome, and must not be used in patients with Parkinson's disease). Ethopropazine is effective in controlling tremors and rigidity. It is not known whether the histamine H_1-receptor blocking action of this drug is involved in its anti-Parkinsonian activity.

(c) Mechanism of action

The anticholinergic agents have a variety of pharmacological actions which may contribute to their therapeutic value. (1) The anticholinergic action *per se* may block cholinergic projections to the striatum, thereby restoring the balance between cholinergic and dopaminergic activities in this area. (2) Many of the anticholinergics used to treat Parkinson's disease can also block uptake of dopamine by brain synaptosomes *in vitro*; the drugs could increase the amount of dopamine available at receptor sites in the striatum. (3) The drugs can release newly synthesised dopamine in the striatum and so facilitate dopaminergic transmission which would also contribute to a restoration of the balance in dopaminergic and cholinergic activities.

(d) Side effects

The anticholinergic drugs now commonly used in the treatment of Parkinson's disease are preferred for two reasons: they enter the CNS more easily than, for example, anticholinergics used in the treatment of ulcer (see p. 379). Secondly, they generally have fewer side effects than the naturally occurring atropine-like alkaloids. Nevertheless atropine-like peripheral side effects commonly occur with anticholinergic anti-Parkinsonian drugs. Examples of these effects are blurring of vision, constipation, dry mouth and urinary retention (at this stage, you should be able to explain why this is the case!). These side effects are troublesome especially in elderly patients. Common CNS related side effects are mental confusion, somnolence, delirium and hallucination.

Drugs which promote dopaminergic activity

There are two approaches. One is to increase directly the concentration of dopamine in the striatum by giving L-dopa, and the other is to use drugs which stimulate the release of dopamine or directly stimulate dopamine receptors.

Levodopa

Levodopa is the L-isomer of dihydroxyphenylalanine (L-dopa); the D-isomer is toxic. The aim in using levodopa is to provide the dopaminergic neurones in the striatum with a dopamine precursor. L-dopa is there converted to dopamine whose concentration in the brain is then restored to normal, leading to a relief of Parkinsonian symptoms. Dopamine itself does not enter the CNS. In this disease, the dopamine transmission failure is not due to a degeneration of dopaminergic neurones nor to a deficiency in L-amino acid decarboxylase; neither is it due to a total absence of stored dopamine, since some drugs can relieve Parkinsonian symptoms by releasing residual dopamine from storage. The cause of reduction in striatal dopamine is not known; it is speculated that in Parkinsonism, the synthesis of dopa from tyrosine (tyrosine hydroxylase) is deficient. The striatal dopamine deficiency hypothesis does not exclude the possibility of other more complex interactions. For example, if dopa is taken up into neurones other than dopaminergic ones, e.g. 5-hyroxytryptaminergic neurones, it can be decarboxylated and released along with 5-HT. Until we can delineate more precisely, the role of different CNS neurotransmitters in the control of locomotion and the effect of interactions between them, the present hypothesis can only be regarded as a useful working model.

Levodopa produces improvement in the akinesia and rigidity with less effect on tremors. Speech is improved and sialorrhoea is controlled. Levodopa is the most successful drug now available for the treatment of all forms of Parkinson's disease.

Some further points of clinical interest to note are discussed below.

(a) Decarboxylation of L-dopa in peripheral neurones

Aromatic L-amino acid decarboxylase is widely distributed in extra-cerebral sites including noradrenergic neurones and liver. Thus levodopa undergoes extensive first pass metabolism in the liver; consequently (a) not much of administered levodopa gets into the CNS and (b) the increased amount of dopamine in peripheral noradrenergic neurones and possibly also at autonomic ganglia can give rise to complex cardiovascular side effects. To reduce peripheral decarboxylation of levodopa, drugs have been developed which inhibit peripheral dopa decarboxylase so that when used in combination with levodopa, much of the latter enters the brain. An example of such a drug is carbidopa. The structure is shown below.

HO—⬡—CH$_2$ · CH · NH$_2$ with COOH group above CH (Levodopa); HO group below ring.

HO—⬡—CH$_2$ · C–COOH with CH$_3$ above and NH · NH$_2$ below (Carbidopa); HO group below ring.

Levodopa   Carbidopa

Carbidopa prevents preferentially the peripheral decarboxylation of levodopa either because the drug has difficulty in penetrating the CNS (there is no apparent reason why this should be so) or because it has a higher affinity for the peripheral isoenzyme than the brain enzyme. The advantages of combination of carbidopa with levodopa (the combination contains 10% carbidopa) are: (i) It allows the effective dose of levodopa to be considerably reduced (by as much as 75%). (ii) Several side effects can be obviated (see below); e.g. nausea and vomiting are common side effects when levodopa is used alone. This is due to stimulation of dopamine receptors in the CTZ; with carbidopa this is reduced. (iii) The pyridoxine antagonism of levodopa action (see below) is avoided. (iv) Because dopa decarboxylase is inhibited, plasma levels of levodopa are predictable and a steady state therapeutic regimen is achieved more readily.

(b) *Interaction of levodopa with other drugs*
Low doses of *pyridoxine* (as can be found in many multivitamin preparations) can reduce the therapeutic efficacy of levodopa. This is because the vitamin powerfully increases the activity of dopa decarboxylase and therefore reduces the amount of drug reaching the brain. This action of pyridoxine is lost when levodopa is used in combination with carbidopa.

Antipsychotic drugs, e.g. reserpine, haloperidol, chlorpromazine, produce a Parkinsonian syndrome by depleting the striatum of dopamine (haloperidol, reserpine) or by blocking dopamine receptors (chlorpromazine, haloperidol). These drugs can nullify the therapeutic efficacy of levodopa. They are therefore contraindicated in Parkinson's disease and may precipitate the symptoms when the patient's condition is controlled by levodopa.

Monoamine oxidase inhibitors, e.g. phenelzine and isocarboxazide, should not be used concurrently with levodopa. These drugs inhibit monoamine oxidases present in the intestine and in the liver (MAO-A) as well as brain monoamine oxidase (MAO-B). They can therefore cause a build-up of dopamine and exaggerate the effects of levodopa centrally and peripherally. Since the peripheral effects are undesirable MAO inhibitors of this class should be avoided in patients undergoing treatment with levodopa. Selective brain enzyme (MAO-B) inhibitors, e.g. *deprenyl* can be used to enhance the effects of levodopa. This is of therapeutic value provided it is borne in mind that excessive dopamine in the striatum can cause dyskinesias similar to those of, for example, *Huntington's chorea* (this is a rare hereditary disease associated with involuntary irregular movements due to excessive dopaminergic activity and is treated with tetrabenazine which blocks dopamine storage in the striatum).

(c) *Side effects*

The side effects of levodopa are those relating to the peripheral or central actions of dopamine. Hypotension is a common side effect and may have both central and peripheral components. Its mechanism is not clear; the peripheral component may involve the hyperpolarising effect of dopamine at ganglia, complex interactions with peripheral and central adrenoceptors, and possibly a false transmitter role in tryptaminergic/noradrenergic neurones. Another important side effect is cardiac dysrrhythmias which is attributed to the action of dopamine on cardiac beta-adrenoceptors. Most patients experience nausea and vomiting. This is due partly to an action on the gastrointestinal tract (this may be minimised by taking the drug with food which also decreases the peak concentration of the drug in plasma) and partly to excessive stimulation of dopamine receptors in the chemoreceptor triggerzone in the brain: phenothiazines, e.g. chlorpromazine, should *not* be used to control the levodopa-induced nausea (see above). The most serious side effects of levodopa are abnormal involuntary movements (dyskinesias) which are experienced by up to 50% of patients on the drug; these include grimacing, head bobbing, involuntary movements of the arms, legs or trunk. No tolerance develops to these effects of levodopa; rather they tend to increase in frequency and intensity with increase in the duration of treatment. Unfortunately these is no antidote to levodopa induced dyskinesias except careful control of dosage. Patients treated with levodopa also frequently experience psychological disturbances.

Drugs which stimulate dopamine receptors or release dopamine
Amantadine
This was originally developed as an antiviral agent but was subsequently found to relieve some symptoms of Parkinson's disease. It facilitates the release of dopamine from intact dopaminergic neurones. Its therapeutic activity may be enhanced by combination with levodopa.

Bromocriptine
This drug directly stimulates dopamine receptors. It is used in combination with levodopa or levodopa with carbidopa. It is reputed to cause less dyskinesia, but can cause visual and auditory hallucinations and hypotension.

Apomorphine
This is best known for its emetic effect but has minor therapeutic uses in Parkinson's disease. The drug directly stimulates post synaptic dopamine receptors and regulates dopamine turnover by a negative feedback loop which may also involve GABA. In the striatum GABAergic transmission is inhibitory.

Other drugs
The tremors of Parkinson's disease involve activation of beta-adrenoceptors. Consequently, some patients may benefit from propranolol.

20.3   SPASTICITY
Spasticity is a muscle rigidity of CNS origin. It may cause distorted postures or movements with or without pain. It is caused by complex and extensive lesions in the brain and spinal cord. The condition may be aggravated by anxiety; many of the drugs used to treat the disease are anxiolytics. Muscle spasms of different types may have peripheral origins, e.g. arthritic spasms, migraine or trauma; treatment of these conditions is quite different from the treatment of spasticity of CNS origin. The condition may be very marked in cerebral palsy in children. This is a condition in which there is widespread brain damage resulting in mental retardation.

Many of the drugs used to treat spasticity are muscle relaxants with a central mode of action, e.g. mephenesin, baclofen, benzodiazepines, cyclobenzaprine.

Mephenesin is now little used but several newer drugs with similar actions are available, e.g. *carisoprodol, chlorphenesin*. Their mode of action is not fully understood. All types of hypertonia whether of spinal or supraspinal origin are diminished by mephenesin. Most of these drugs preferentially reduce polysynaptic reflexes leaving monosynaptic reflexes such as 'knee jerk' unaffected. They are thought to reduce transmission through chains of interneurones; the longer the chain the more effective the drug is. The drugs are therefore also referred to as *interneuronal blockers*.

The benzodiazepines, e.g. diazepam, appear to have a more selective action on reticular formation neurones that control muscle tone than on spinal interneuronal activity, whereas mephenesin type drugs show no such selectivity. Specifically diazepam facilitates transmission in GABAergic neurones.

Baclofen (*p*-chlorophenyl GABA) is a derivative of GABA. It crosses the blood–brain barrier more easily than GABA. Baclofen stimulates GABA$_B$ receptors and causes depressant actions mainly in the spinal cord. GABA$_B$ receptors are defined as those sensitive to blockade by baclofen and are insensitive to bicuculline.

Baclofen

Dantrolene

Dantrolene is different from all other drugs so far mentioned in that its action is peripheral. It reduces muscle contraction by interfering with events triggered by receptor activation. It inhibits excitation–concentration coupling by decreasing the release of calcium ions from, or by increasing their sequestration in, sarcoplasmic reticulum.

Dantrolene

20.4   TRANQUILISERS

Tranquilisers are used in the treatment of two major kinds of mental disorders. Minor tranquilisers are used in the treatment of *neuroses* (anxiety states); these are relatively mild mental disorders that are in fact normal components of behaviour that have become exaggerated so that the patient cannot cope with everyday stresses of life. Neuroses usually have definite causes of which the patient is aware (i.e., the patient has insight). Examples of minor tranquilisers are meprobamate. benzodiazepines and barbiturates. These drugs especially benzodiazepines are so widely accepted and seem to be so effective in providing escape from life's problems that they are grossly abused especially in tropical countries where they can be purchased without prescription. Major tranquilisers are used to treat *psychoses*, e.g. schizophrenia. These are severe mental disorders which in advanced stages are characterised by grossly abnormal mood, emotional behaviour, hallucinations and delusions. Psychoses usually occur without apparent cause and the patient has no insight into the problem.

Major tranquilisers used in the treatment of psychoses

Several chemically distinct classes of drugs effective in the treatment of the psychoses, e.g. schizophrenia, manic depressive illnesses, and severe anxiety, are referred to as major tranquilisers or neuroleptics. Some writers object to the word 'tranquilisers' because it suggests that the drugs produce a feeling of *tranquility* whereas the effects of the drugs are subjectively usually quite unpleasant. Examples are listed in Table 20.3. These compounds have very complex heterocyclic structures. Some are shown in Fig. 20.2. There are no easily identifiable structure–activity relationships; but in X-ray crystallography, part of the structure of chlorpromazine closely resembles one conformation of dopamine itself. This is part of the evidence associating this group of drugs with dopamine receptor blockade.

The discovery of chlorpromazine revolutionalised the treatment of schizophrenia but as the brand name *largactil* implies, chlorpromazine has a *large* number of *actions* many of them quite unpleasant. Many derivatives of phenothiazine and other heterocyclics are now available for the treatment of the psychoses. These drugs produce an array of side effects, so that the choice of drug is governed by this factor as much as by its ability to relieve psychotic symptoms.

Neuroleptics cause a type of sedation that is different from that seen with sedatives, e.g. barbiturates or anaesthetics. Even with large doses as used in schizophrenia, there is no loss of consciousness. The patient

Table 20.3 *Comparative severity of major side effects of major tranquilisers*

Drug	Extra-pyramidal	Sedation	Hypotension	Anti-muscarinic
	Side effects			
Chlorpromazine	++	+++	+++	++
Thioridazine	+	+++	++	+++
Haloperidol	+++	+	+	+
Pimozide	+	0	0	+++
Trifluoperazine	+++	+	+	+
Fluphenazine	+++	+	+	+

+++, severe; ++, moderate; +, mild; 0, insignificant.

Fig. 20.2. Structures of some major tranquilisers.

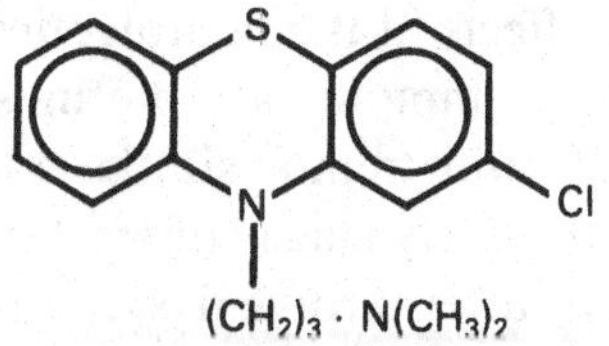

Chlorpromazine (a phenothiazine)

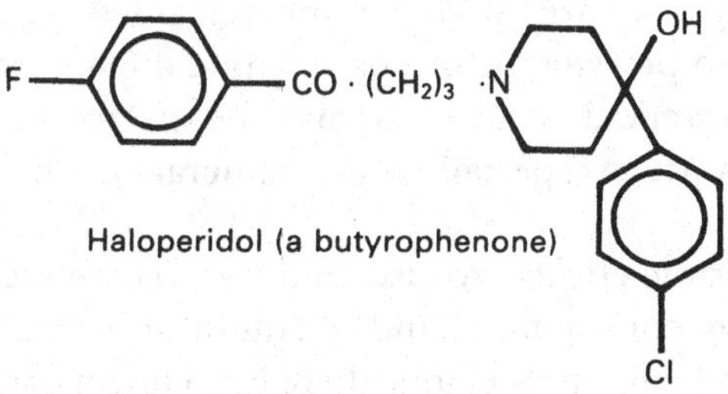

(CH₂)₃ · N(CH₃)₂

Haloperidol (a butyrophenone)

is apathetic, drowsy and indifferent but can be aroused easily. Experimentally, neuroleptics block conditioned reflexes preferentially whereas anaesthetics inhibit all reflexes to cause unconsciousness.

Mechanism of action

The antipsychotic drugs block dopamine receptors in the nigrostriatum. The first evidence for this came from observations with amphetamine which in high doses can cause toxic psychosis with symptoms resembling those of paranoid schizophrenia. This action of amphetamine can be blocked by neuroleptics and amphetamine is known to cause the release of dopamine in the brain.

The idea that neuroleptics act by blocking dopamine receptors is important not only because it is helpful in the rational design of new neuroleptic drugs but also because the idea forms the basis for scientific study of the biochemical lesions which give rise to the psychotic syndrome. That neuropleptics block dopamine receptors is supported by direct and indirect observations. All the drugs used in the treatment of psychoses inhibit the binding of 3H-haloperidol (a dopamine receptor antagonist) to brain slices. The indirect point is that neuroleptics increase dopamine turnover (i.e. increase synthesis and destruction). There is an increased production of homovanillic acid (formed from dopamine by the combined action of MAO and COMT) which is evidence of increased dopamine turnover. Increased dopamine turnover is thought to be triggered by postsynaptic dopamine receptor blockade.

Side effects

The major side effects of the neuroleptics are shown in Table 20.3. The extrapyramidal symptoms are the most troublesome. They include akinesia, rigidity and tremor similar to Parkinson's disease and they occur during the early stages of treatment. Patients on prolonged therapy may also suffer tardive dyskinesia (involuntary movements of the facial, tongue or limb muscles). The condition is attributed to dopamine overactivity in the striatum. This is thought to be a compensatory increase in dopamine release or increased receptor number due to presynaptic or postsynaptic dopamine receptor blockade. Extrapyramidal symptoms may be overcome by using anti-Parkinsonian drugs especially the cholinergic antagonists, but not L-dopa.

Antimuscarinic effects are also common. These include dry mouth, blurred vision, constipation, and retention of urine. Although all the drugs block dopamine receptors, there is no direct correlation between dopamine receptor blockade and production of extrapyramidal symptoms implying that differential affinities of the drugs for dopamine D_1- (postsynaptic) and D_2- (presynaptic) receptors are relevant factors. Another factor is the affinity of the drugs for muscarinic receptors. Those agents which have the *lowest* incidence of extrapyramidal actions also have the *greatest* affinities for cholinergic receptors in the brain. This is understandable from the dopamine versus cholinergic activity theory of Parkinsonism; compare columns 1 and 4 in Table 20.3 – antimuscarinic activity is inversely correlated with extrapyramidal activity. Sedation and hypotension on the other hand are directly correlated. This is because both are due to blockade of alpha adrenoceptors peripherally and in the CNS.

Reserpine

Another antipsychotic agent that has not been discussed so far is reserpine. This alkaloid isolated from *Rauwolfia* species was the first major tranquilisers to be used successfully in the treatment of psychosis. Its mechanism of action is inhibition of catecholamine (NA and dopamine) uptake into storage and a consequent depletion of amines and transmission failure. The Parkinsonian syndrome induced by reserpine (due to depletion of dopamine in the striatum) is particularly severe because reserpine has no antimuscarinic activity.

Reserpine

Reserpine also releases 5-hydroxytryptamine in the gut; therefore a common side effect is diarrhoea (5-HT facilitates cholinergic transmission). The most serious side effect of reserpine which has led to its discontinuation in the treatment of psychoses is severe depression accompanied by a strong urge in the patient to commit suicide. Reserpine is used in low doses in the treatment of hypertension usually in combination with other drugs.

Other side effects of major tranquilisers

Other side effects of neuroleptics arise from their blockade of dopamine receptors in hypothalamic centres involved in control of emotional behaviour as well as appetite, drinking and sexual drives. By blocking dopaminergic activity and thereby suppressing the function of the hypothalamus, neuroleptics interfere with these activities. Appetites and libido are reduced, and in the male impotence (failure of erection or if there is erection, failure of ejaculation) may occur. The ability of the individual to adjust to external temperatures is compromised – body temperature falls in a cold atmosphere and rises when it is hot.

Sedatives/hypnotics

These are used to treat minor neuroses, to relieve anxiety (.e.g., benzodiazepines, meprobamate) or as sedative/hypnotics in the treatment of insomnia or other sleep disorders (e.g., barbiturates).

Barbiturates

Previously, the most widely used sedative hypnotics were the barbiturates, but benzodiazepines, e.g. diazepam, are now preferred because of serious side effects caused by barbiturates. Some of these are (i) depression of respiration in overdose, (ii) drowsiness, (iii) physical dependence and abuse potential, and (iv) induction of hepatic microsomal enzyme. Barbiturates are still frequently used for various purposes to induce sedation, sleep or anaesthesia depending on dose or route of administration. The use of ultrashort-acting barbiturates (thiopentone) in general anaesthesia (pp. 405–6) and of long-acting barbiturates (phenobarbitone) as anticonvulsants (p. 441) have already been referred to. For the treatment of sleep disorders, a short-acting barbiturate, e.g. secobarbitone is indicated for patients who have difficulty in falling asleep; a medium-acting drug, e.g. butobarbitone is indicated for patients who have difficulty staying asleep.

Non-barbiturate sedatives

Examples are *glutethimide* (doriden); this has similar actions to phenobarbitone, but may in contrast to the latter cause convulsions. *H₁-receptor antagonists* (antihistamines), e.g. diphenhydramine, or promethazine are also used as mild sedatives. All these drugs cause depression of the ascending reticular activating system. Another drug which causes depression of brain *neurones* is *alcholol* (*ethanol*). Alcohol induces talkativeness and unrestrained and sometimes irresponsible behaviour and gives the impression of causing a stimulant effect. In fact, alcohol in moderate doses causes disinhibition (inhibits inhibitory neurones) and in large doses causes general depression and anaesthesia. Alcohol is not used as an anaesthetic because the difference between the dose producing anaesthesia and that causing fatal depression of respiration is small. Chronic compulsive alcohol consumption is consequent on physical and psychological dependence. The characteristic withdrawal syndrome is *delirium tremens* – anxiety, sweating, insomnia, restlessness, convulsions – which may be controlled by benzodiazepines, chlorpromazine or phenobarbitone. Chronic consumption may cause cirrhosis (see p. 127), alcoholic hepatitis, and malnutrition. Alcohol must be avoided in patients with renal disease, hepatic disorders or peptic ulcers. Also because of its depressant effect on brain cells, the interaction of alcohol with a wide range of drugs acting on the CNS can give rise to bizarre effects. Alcohol potentiates the action of all CNS-depressant drugs, e.g. barbiturates and benzodiazepines.

The benzodiazepines, e.g. diazepam (valium). Several hundreds of benzodiazepines (BZs) are available with broadly similar actions. Most of their effects result from actions exerted in the CNS. These are sedation, hypnosis, decreased anxiety, muscle relaxation, and anticonvulsant activity. Peripherally some BZs may produce neuromuscular blockade and coronary vasodilation when given intravenously. Exceptionally some possess significant analgesic actions, but this is not a characteristic property. Anti-anxiety and sedative effects are the properties for which the drugs are widely used. Whether these two effects arise from the same fundamental action is not known. It is clear that the BZs have effects on specific CNS functions. For example, they specifically diminish aggressive behaviour (meprobamate but not barbiturates or phenothiazines, have similar action) without effect on general CNS activity. They also specifically suppress conditioned avoidance behaviour.

Mechanism of action
BZs act on polysynaptic rather than monosynaptic pathways and the site is predominantly postsynaptic. The drugs bind to benzodiazepine receptors to facilitate GABAergic transmission. This needs some explanation. Activation of GABA receptors causes the opening of Cl^- ion channels and hyperpolarisation. Benzodiazepines bind to an allosteric site and by so doing facilitate GABA action. The

evidence is as follows: benzodiazepines potentiate GABA effects, and antagonists of GABA receptors (bicuculline and picrotoxin) prevent the CNS actions of benzodiazepines and those of GABA. Inhibitors of GABA synthesis (e.g., thiosemicarbazone) reduce, and inhibitors of GABA degradation (e.g., aminoacetic acid) potentiate, the CNS actions of benzodiazepines. BZs are inactive when the brain is depleted of GABA. These points suggest an indirect GABA-mimetic action of the BZs but this is not due to release of GABA or to a direct stimulation of GABA receptors (the ability of BZs to compete for binding with GABA correlates poorly with their CNS effects in man). Rather, the benzodiazepine receptor is thought to be a protein that normally modulates the binding of GABA to its recognition site. Blockade of the BZ receptor augments GABA binding to its receptor and GABAergic transmission.

20.5   DRUGS USED TO TREAT PSYCHOTIC DEPRESSION (ANTIDEPRESSANTS)

Common depressive states are *manic depression* and *endogenous depression*. These clinical conditions are associated with changes in the metabolism of monoamines (NA, 5-HT and dopamine) and in the level of metabolites which are detected in the CSF. It is uncertain whether these changes are the effect or the cause of depression. Be that as it may, it is clear that drugs which increase monoaminergic functions are highly successful in the treatment of depression. The two best known groups of drugs are monoamine oxidase inhibitors (MAOI) and the imipramine type of drug which block high-affinity uptake of monoamines. The overall effect of both types of drug is to increase the concentration of monoamine at receptor sites. Some new antidepressant drugs that are neither MAOI nor uptake inhibitor, e.g. *iprindole* and *mianserin*, also seem to produce beneficial effects through monoaminergic mechanisms. For example, mianserin increases NA release by blocking presynaptic alpha-adrenoceptors.

Monoamine oxidase inhibitors (MAOI)

The discovery of MAOI as antidepressants was a case of serendipity. In 1951 iproniazid was found to elevate mood in tuberculosis patients under treatment with the drug which was subsequently found to inhibit monoamine oxidase. Iproniazid is no longer used. Examples of new drugs are shown in Fig. 20.3. The drugs relieve depression without inducing mental excitement or delirium, increase synaptic concentration of monoamines (NA, 5-HT, DA), produce down regulation of beta-adrenoceptors and restore REM latency (this is shortened in depression). The important action of MAOI is to elevate mood. This effect could be due to an increased intraneuronal concentration of monoamines, but the correlation of MAO inhibition with mood-elevating activity of various drugs is not good. Also, MAO inhibition can be demonstrated shortly after the start of therapy, but mood elevation takes much longer to occur. Pharmacokinetic factors may account for the poor correlation referred to above, and clinical bnenefits may be due to other delayed adaptive CNS changes following MAO inhibition. The usefulness of MAOI is limited by side effects; the most important of these is the potentiation of the cardiovascular effects of dietary tyramine – the socalled 'cheese effect'. This has been referred to on page 362. The discovery by Johnstone in 1968 that there were two forms of the enzyme (MAO-A and MAO-B) with different substrate and inhibitor specificities, sparked the hope that it would be possible to develop MAO antidepressants which did not potentiate the cardiovascular effects of tyramine. MAO-A is selectively inhibited by *clorgylline* and 5-HT is the specific substrate. MAO-B is selectively inhibited by *deprenyl*. Both isoenzymes are found in the human brain, but the human intestinal enzyme is largely MAO-A. As would be expected, deprenyl has been found not to potentiate tyramine (after deprenyl there is enough MAO-A in the intestine to prevent the 'cheese effect'). The specificities referred to above are not absolute; there is a

Fig. 20.3. Examples of antidepressant drugs.

MAO inhibitors   Uptake inhibitors

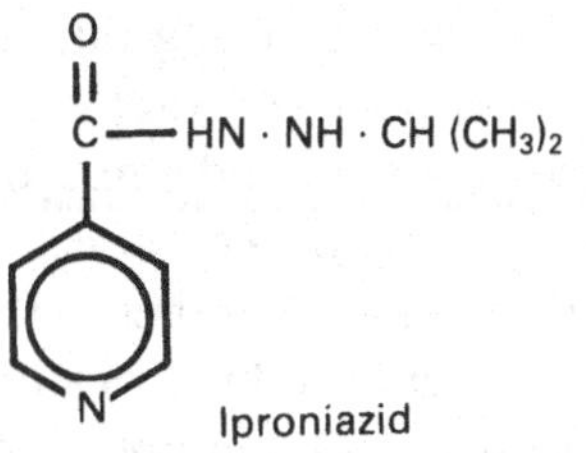

Iproniazid

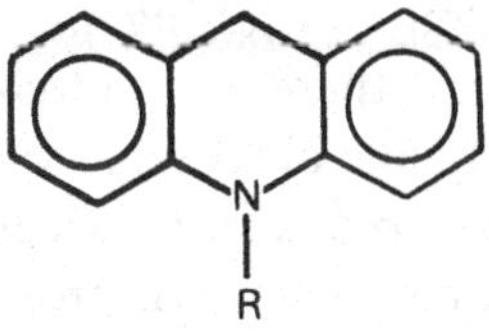

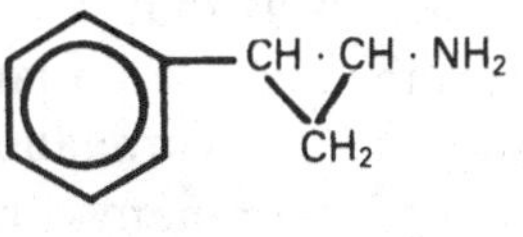

Tranylcypromine

R= —CH₂·CH₂·N(CH₃)₂ Imipramine
R= —CH₂·CH₂·NH·CH₃ Desipramine

great deal of overlap in substrate and inhibitor affinities for the isoenzymes and no MAOI is at present available that is free of cardio-vascular complications.

MAOI are of two types:

(a) *Reversible competitive antagonists*

Examples are amphetamine and ephedrine. These penetrate the blood–brain barrier, and are not deaminated by MAO, but they block its action and also release CA giving rise to a CNS-stimulant action. These drugs are not used routinely as antidepressants.

(b) *Irreversible antagonists*

Some of these, e.g. *phenelzine*, are also indirectly acting sympathomimetic amines. Some others, e.g. pargylline, block alpha-adrenoceptors as well as MAO. The irreversible inhibitors are the drugs usually referred to as MAOI.

Side effects

Several side effects are seen with the MAOI; the most important is the potentiation of the cardiovascular actions of monoamines in food and beverages (see above). Other cardiovascular actions are hypertension due to indirect sympathomimetic action of the MAOI and hypotension due to increased NA in central synapses, ganglion blockade (see Fig. 15.2), and in the case of pargylline, also alpha-adrenoceptor blockade.

Imipramine and related drugs

The term 'tricyclic' is also used to describe this group of antidepressants (see Fig 20.3). It should be born in mind that other drugs possessing three rings, e.g. phenothiazines, are not antidepressants and there are 'bicyclic' antidepressants, e.g. viloxazine. The effect of uptake blockers is to increase the concentration of monoamines at the receptor site. This leads to a reduction in amine turnover due to a stimulant action on presynaptic receptors. The drugs block the uptake of NA, and 5-HT but with different degrees of effectiveness; e.g., desipramine blocks NA uptake 100 times more effectively than 5-HT. Since it is not clear which amine, NA or 5-HT, is the more important for the antidepressant action, it is not surprising that the correlation between uptake activity and mood elevation is not good for many compounds.

Other drugs.

Chlorpromazine can be used in the manic phase of manic depression. *Lithium* is useful in the long-term management of manic depression. It is an element similar to sodium. When given as a salt (lithium carbonate) the ion enters cells by a similar mechanism to sodium, but is not efficiently extruded by the $Na^+-K^+-ATPase$ pump that removes Na^+ from the cell. Lithium therefore accumulates to give rise to secondary effects such as increased NA turnover, increased 5-HT synthesis, inhibition of choline uptake and other changes in cholinergic function. Lithium is effective in the long-term management of manic depression, but it requires accurate monitoring of plasma levels to avoid severe toxic side effects.

Before the discovery of antidepressant drugs, depression was treated by various forms of convulsive therapy such as ECT, pentylenetetrazole shock and insulin shock treatment. ECT is still used in patients resistant to available drugs.

20.6   CNS STIMULANTS

Many substances can stimulate the CNS through a wide spectrum of mechanisms to cause a range of psychedelic effects. Examples are illustrated in Fig. 20.4. These substances are widely abused as recreation drugs. Consequently their availability is highly restricted in most countries of the world. The effects they produce are psychological and usually depend on the individual, the surroundings, genetic make-up, and expectations. The range of effects is similar to those that would be seen among schizophrenics. Some of the effects are usually experienced acutely by an individual on a 'trip' but some of the drugs, e.g. amphetamine, can actually induce chronic psychosis on repeated usage. Common psychological manifestations are *hyperaesthesia* (enhanced sensory perception), synaesthesia (transposition of sensory perception, e.g. colours are *heard*, sounds are *tasted*), distortion of time and space, delusions, hallucinations, depersonalisation, euphoria, etc. Amphetamine, lysergic acid diethylamide (LSD) (the S in the abbreviation comes from the German '*Saure*' for 'acid'), mescaline, cocaine, cannabis and heroin are commonly abused for their psychological effects. There is no single hypothesis that can explain the mechanism of this array of effects elicited by psychedelic drugs. They all act centrally on monoaminergic mechanisms. Cocaine is a potent uptake inhibitor; it therefore increases the concentration of NA at receptor sites which may account for its stimulant action. Amphetamine has similar actions but it is also an MAO inhibitor. LSD and mescaline have high affinity for 5-HT receptors. Tetrahydrocannabinol, the most psychoactive component of cannabis, causes dreamlike states probably by an action on memory mechanisms.

Drug abuse

This is the consumption of pharmacologically active compounds for nonmedical purposes. *Incorrect* use of drugs even when medically indicated also constitutes abuse; but the concern in this section is with the nonmedical use of drugs with CNS activity. In some instances what constitute *abuse* may vary with the occasion and the cultural environment. Whereas a chronic alcoholic is thought of as abusing alcohol, a person who drinks an excessive amount at a party is not. In traditional African societies, colanuts (containing CNS stimulants) are eaten ceremoniously but excessive consumption simply to stay awake (e.g., by long-distance lorry drivers and students preparing for examinations) constitute abuse. Both the social drinker and the chronic alcoholic would be regarded as drug abusers by a devout religious adherent, who on the other hand, may tolerate colanuts or hashish.

Two kinds of dangers are inherent in drug abuse; these are the toxic effects of the abused substance and the problem of dependence (psychological and physical). The extensive toxicities of some commonly abused drugs, e.g. alcohol, opiate drugs, benzodiazepines, tobacco, and barbiturates, have been referred to and it has been mentioned that amphetamines can cause toxic psychoses; but the toxic effects of some drugs used traditionally are not widely appreciated. For example, colanuts cause wakefulness and overcome fatigue; excessive consumption of some varieties can cause blurring of vision, presumably due to their content of atropine-like principles. Professional drivers in Nigeria, especially long-distance lorry and bus drivers eat colanuts to stay awake; the effect on their eyes may well partly account for high accident rates particularly at narrow bridges. Dependence is, however, the most serious danger in drug abuse.

Drug abuse is at present a serious problem in Western industrialised societies and is increasing in cities in third world countries. No doubt, like everything else associated with Western technology, drug abuse will spread among the young and affluent; the impact on traditional society would be even more devastating because of the proportionately greater influence of the abusers on developing weak economies and insecure societies, and absence of effective control measures. It is thus important that third world countries should develop strategies for combating the problem before it is established as it is now in industrialised societies. One way of doing this is through education, especially of the young. Facts to disseminate are that (i) drug abuse begins with experimentation often as part of the exploratory process of adolescence; there is a desire to conform with the behaviour of peers who are taking or experimenting with drugs, (ii) induction into the habit is facilitated by availability of the drug (hence control of drugs is an important element in any strategy to combat drug abuse), and (iii) that the long-term harmful effects to the individual and to society far outweigh the temporary euphoria and excitement which the abused drugs produce. Some commonly abused drugs and their properties are listed in Table 20.4. and Fig. 20.4.

Fig. 20.4. Some commonly abused drugs.

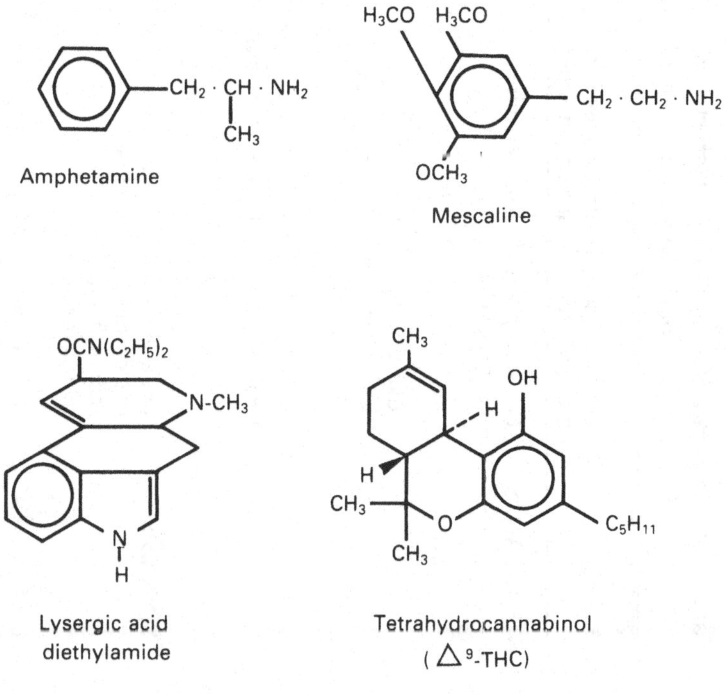
H3CO H3CO
CH2 · CH · NH2
CH3
CH2 · CH2 · NH2
Amphetamine
OCH3
Mescaline
OCN(C2H5)2
N-CH3
N
H
CH3
OH
H
H
CH3
O
C5H11
CH3
Lysergic acid diethylamide
Tetrahydrocannabinol
(Δ9-THC)

Table 20.4 Properties of some well-known drugs of abuse. The list is not exhaustive. Almost any substance with CNS actions can be abused e.g. antihistamines, and volatile organic solvents and products containing them have been abused.

Category	Common (street) name of drug	Proper name or major constituent	Source	Usual mode of consumption	Dependence/ side effects
STIMULANTS	Dolls, co-pilots, bennies, benz	Amphetamines	Synthetic	Orally, smoked or sniffed up the nose, or injected	Psychic dependence, psychoses, dry mouth, anorexia, constipation, insomnia, dizziness
	Coke, Charlie, *Lady, snow, dust*	Cocaine	*Erythroxylum coca*	Sniffing or snorting it up a tube into nose, smoked, or injected	Psychic dependence, psychoses, hallucinations, loss of appetite, impotence, sleeplessness, tremors
	Khat	Cathine, cathinone	*Catha edulis* (North East Africa)	Leaves are smoked chewed or brewed	Psychic dependence
CANNABIS	Ganja, grass, pot, hashish, Indian, hemp. marijuana	Tetrahydrocan-nabinol	*Cannabis sativa*	Leaves are smoked, brewed and drunk, or chewed	Psychic dependence, psychotic syndrome, atrophic brain damage (conflicting evidence)
HALLUCINOGENS (psychedelics, psychotomimetics)	Acid. Domes strawberry fields	LSD (lysergic acid diethylamide)	Synthetic derivative or ergot alkaloid	Orally	Characteristic rapid tolerance, psychic dependence (a minority of individuals).

	Mescaline	*Lophophora williamsii* (cactus plant)	Orally	Acute reactions to hallucinogens including mydriasis, tremor, hyperreflexia, fever. Salivation and variable effects on heart rate and blood pressure are referred to as 'bad trips'
Magic mushroom	Psilocin and psilocybin	*Psilocybe mexicana* (Fungi)	Eaten or brewed	As above
STP	DOM (dimethoxy-methylamphetamine)	Synthetic	Orally	
–	DMT (dimethyl-tryptamine)	Synthetic	Injected or smoked	*Bad trips* common
Dust	PCP (phencyclidine)	Synthetic	Sniffed, injected, eaten or smoked	*Bad trips* common
DEPRESSANTS Downers, blockers, blue angels, etc.	Barbiturates (e.g., nembutal, tuinal)	Synthetic	Orally, but can be injected	Psychic and physical dependence; overdose or co-administration with alcohol causes severe respiratory depression/coma
Downers, blockers, blue angels, etc.	Benzodiazepines	Synthetic	As above	Dependence potential is low but increases with dose. Large doses cause depression, anxiety, rebound insomnia.
OPIOIDS Dope, dragon, heavy drugs, hard stuff, etc.	Morphine, heroin (diamorphine), methadone	*Papaver somniferum* (morphine, codeine)	Orally or injected; heroin powder can be sniffed	High psychic and physical dependence liability. Severe abstinence syndrome.

FURTHER READING

Bell, C. (1984). Dopaminergic Nerves. In *IUPHAR 9th Int. Congr. Pharmacology Proc.* vol. 1, eds: W.D.M. Paton, J.R. Mitchell & P. Turner. London, Macmillan Press, pp. 231–244.

Blascko, H. (1959). The development of current concepts of catecholamine formation. *Pharmac. Rev.*, 2, 307–316.

Grundy, H.F. (1985). *Lecture Notes on Pharmacology*. Blackwell Scientific Publications, Oxford, London.Symposium 11 (1984). Phospholipase A₂ Inhibitors. In *IUPHAR 9th Int. Congr. Pharmacology Proc.* vol. 2, eds. W.D.M. Paton, J.M. Michell & P. Turner. London, Macmillan Press, pp. 31–50.

Symposium 25 (1984) GABA Receptors. In *IUPHAR 9th Int. Cong. Pharmacology Proc.* vol. 3, eds. W.D.M. Paton, J.M. Michell & P. Turner. London, Macmillan Press, pp. 153–194.

Maddock, D.H. (1987). *Drug Abuse: A Guide for Pharmacists*. London, The Pharmaceutical Press.

21

Cardiovascular and renal system

21.1 INTRODUCTION

Diseases of the cardiovascular system, e.g. ischaemic heart disease, heart failure, hypertension) constitute major causes of death in Western industrialised societies. Until recently these were not considered major health problems in developing populations, but the picture is rapidly changing as these degenerative diseases are replacing infectious diseases as major causes of death in third world countries.

After reading this chapter, the student should know the mechanism of action of cardiac glycosides and the rationale for their use in congestive heart failure; the mechanism of action of different classes of anti-arrhythmic drugs, and of the different types of drugs used in the treatment of hypertension. Diuretics are included here rather than in a separate chapter, they are important drugs in the treatment of hypertension (see also Chapter 16) and in congestive heart failure.

Features of myocardial action

The heart is innervated by both branches of the autonomic nervous system. The sympathetic drive is mediated by noradrenaline acting on beta-1 adrenoceptors and the vagal input is mediated by ACH acting on muscarinic receptors. Beta-adrenoceptor agonists increase the force (inotropy) and rate (chronotropy) of myocardial contraction, whereas muscarinic agonists cause the opposite effects. The autonomic drives are superimposed on impulses generated and conducated in cardiac pacemaker tissues (sinoatrial (SA), atrioventricular (AV) nodes, and the His-Purkinje system) independently of nervous input. To appreciate the way drugs affect cardiac action, it is necessary to define some fundamental physiological parameters.

Excitation–contraction coupling

This is the mechanism by which events provoked by a stimulus at the cell membrane (e.g., electrical impulse or receptor activation) are linked to the contractile processes. An impulse at the surface of the myocardial cell membrane causes an initial rapid change in permeability to Na^+ and K^+ (Na^+ in, K^+ out); this depolarisation is followed by complex Ca^{2+} movements resulting in contraction. Depolarisation causes an increase in Ca^{2+} influx. This *trigger* Ca^{2+} is thought to mobilise *activator* Ca^{2+} from intracellular stores. Activator Ca^{2+} then combines with troponin C; this facilitates the interaction between actin and myosin resulting in mechanical contraction (systole). Sequestration (return of Ca^{2+} to storage sites) is followed by muscle relaxation (diastole).

Repolarisation is brought on by Na^+/K^+ activated ATPase (sodium pump) which pumps Na^+ out of the cell and K^+ in. These ionic movements give rise to a complex action potential illustrated in Fig. 21.1

A beta-adrenoceptor agonist such as adrenaline intensifies all the Ca^{2+} movements resulting in a more rapid and greater contraction (positive inotropy). Sequestration is also more rapid, hence the contraction is of a shorter duration; there is also an increase in rate of contraction. The *refractory period* is the time between depolarisation and repolarisation during which an impulse arriving at the cell membrane cannot initiate excitation. Drugs which alter the effective refractory period can give rise to abnormal cardiac rhythms (*arrhythmias, dysrhythmias*). *Automaticity* is the spontaneous generation of impulses locally in the myocardium; occurrence of automaticity is favoured by conditions which shorten the effective refractory period.

Failing heart

In the failing heart (congestive heart failure, CHF), the pumping power of the myocardium is reduced; the left ventricle is not emptying completely and as the failure progresses, the heart is enlarged.

In a normal heart, an increase in the ventricular end-diastolic volume (VEDV) leads to an increase in the work done (stroke volume). This is consistent with Starling's law which can be explained by saying that stretching the cardiac muscle makes more actin and myosin combination sites available (the limit is reached when too much stretch makes the actin and myosin strands too widely separated). In CHF, the work output does not increase appreciably with increase in VEDVs. These points are illustrated in Fig. 21.2. The work output of the heart in relation to VEDV is best measured in a heart-lung preparation in

Fig. 21.1. Excitation–contraction coupling in cardiac muscle.
(a) *Ionic movements*. Depolarisation (Na$^+$ in, K$^+$ out) (1) is followed by influx of Ca^{2+} ions (trigger Ca^{2+}) which release (activator) Ca^{2+} (4) from sarco-plasmic reticulum (SR). Activator Ca^{2+} facilitates interaction of actin and myosin to cause muscle contraction (systole). Then activator calcium is stored (sequestration) to cause relaxation (diastole). Two pumps are at work. The Na$^+$/K$^+$ – activated ATPase (3) pumps Na$^+$ out and K$^+$ in. Na$^+$/K$^+$ – ATPase is blocked by digitalis causing [Na$^+$]i accumulation and [K$^+$]i loss. Pump (5) exchanges [Na$^+$]i for [Ca^{2+}]o. This is activated when pump (3) is blocked by digitalis thereby increasing [Ca^{2+}]i.
(b) *Action potential*. Phase 0 of the action potential represents the initial rapid depolarisation. 1 = rapid repolarisation to plateau level of voltage; 2 = long sustained depolarisation; 3 = rapid repolarisation (diastole); 4 = diastolic voltage trough.

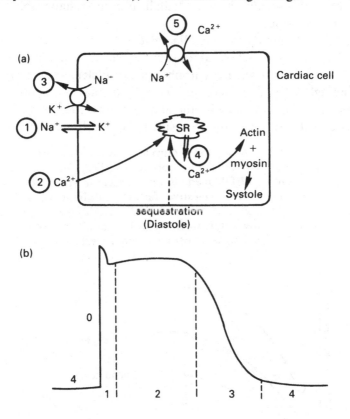

which peripheral resistance and heart rate are constant (these can profoundly affect stroke volume). A positive inotropic effect (PIE) is produced by digitoxin in a failing heart. PIE is defined as an increase in stroke volume which the cardiac muscle can be made to achieve at a given VEDV (see Fig. 21.2 and also Mechanism of action of cardiac glycosides, below).

21.2   THE CARDIAC GLYCOSIDES

The cardiac glycosides are drugs with a pronounced effect on the heart. In therapeutic concentrations all of them act to increase the contractility of the heart muscle. Since Withering's description of the use of digitalis in the treatment of dropsy in 1785, cardiac glycosides have formed the mainstay of the drug treatment of congestive heart failure. In this section the term digitalis is used exchangeably with the cardiac glycosides.

All the commonly used cardiac glycosides consist of an aglycone that has a steroid nucleus, an unsaturated lactone ring at the 17 position, and a sugar linked to carbon 3 of the nucleus (Fig. 21.3).

The aglycone of the molecule is the part that is essential for the observed action on the heart; the attached sugar increases water solubility and the ability of the glycoside to cross cell membranes.

Fig. 21.2. Work done (stroke volume) in relation to the ventricular end-diastolic volume (VEDV). In a normal heart, increase in VEDV leads to an increase in stroke volume (Starling's law). In congestive failure, minimal work output is achieved even at relatively high VEDV (V_2). After digitalis (FH + digitoxin) the same work output is now achieved at a lower VEDV (V_1). This is a positive inotropic effect.

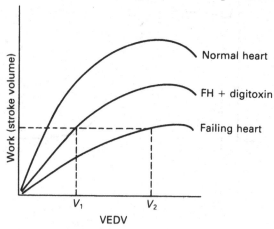

The cardiac glycosides are obtained from both animal and plant sources, e.g. white and purple foxglove (*Digitalis lanata* and *Digitalis purpurea*), Mediterranean sea onion (squill), strophanthus and many tropical and temperate zone plants.

The cardiac glycosides exhibit interesting pharmacokinetic profiles which explain the differences in their route of administration, onset and duration of action. For example, digitoxin, one of the least water-soluble and the most lipid-soluble glycosides, is well absorbed after oral administration. The more water-soluble glycosides digoxin, ouabain, and lanatoside C, are usually given parenterally.

The onset and duration of action of the cardiac glycosides is determined largely by the extent to which they are bound to plasma protein and whether they are excreted into the gut or not. About 90% of digitoxin is bound to plasma albumin; this contributes to its slow onset of action (and the need for an initial loading dose) (see page 148). Car-

Fig. 21.3. Structures of cardiac glycosides. Each contains the steroid nucleus. At C_{17} there is a lactone ring which is essential for cardioactivity. To C_3 a hydroxyl group is added; through a series of glycosidic linkages, a sequence of sugars can be inserted that determine the physical properties of the compound. The steroid–lactone structure (minus the sugars) obtained by hydrolysis is called an *aglycone* or *genin* as shown.

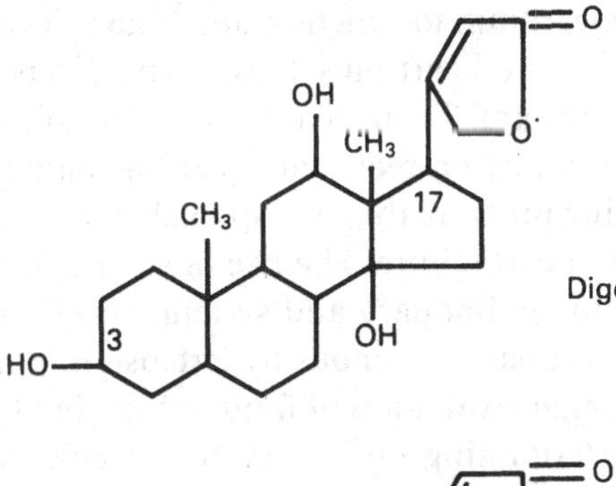

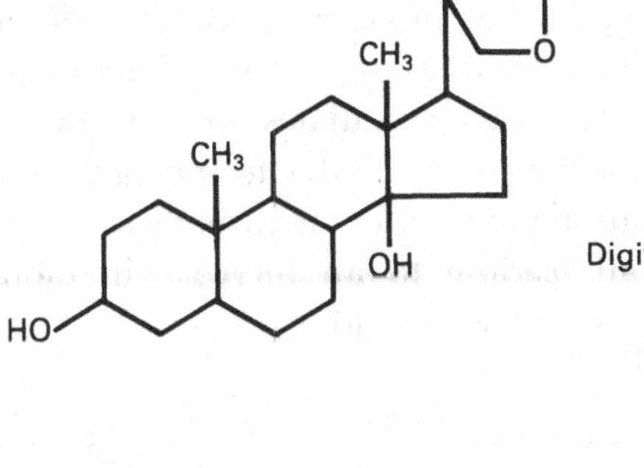

diac glycosides with an intermediate time of onset of action are proportionately less protein bound; digoxin for example is about 20% bound to plasma albumin. Ouabain, the most rapidly acting glycoside, is not bound at all.

Digitoxin is metabolised in the liver; one of the metabolites is digoxin. The metabolites and a small percentage of digitoxin are excreted into the gut via the bile. These are then reabsorbed, thus setting up an enterohepatic circulation. These are finally excreted in the urine. Digoxin, lanatoside C, and ouabain are excreted largely unchanged.

Action of digitalis in CHF

The cardiac glycosides have multiple direct and indirect cardiovascular effects with both therapeutic and toxic consequences.

The glycosides are of special value in heart failure resulting from chronic cardiac muscle malfunction or from overload of the ventricles as a result of systemic hypertension, atherosclerotic coronary artery disease, and in acute myocardial infarction. They are of lesser value in heart failure due to mechanical causes such as mitral or aortic stenosis or cardiac tumor with obstruction. In CHF the main problem is a deteriorating myocardium.

In order to compensate for its declining force of contraction, the heart rate rises; the filling pressure of the ventricles increases, thus 'pushing' the myocardium to function at a higher level of the Starling curve (Fig. 21.2). As the heart muscle is progressively stretched by an increased filling pressure, the myocardium is able to contract more forcibly and hence maintain a reasonable cardiac output. However, it is the increased filling pressure that is responsible for many of the symptoms of congestive heart failure. The rise in ventricular filling pressure is transmitted to the pulmonary and systemic capillaries, with resultant pulmonary and systemic venous hypertension. When the pressure becomes high enough, exudation of fluid occurs into the extravascular spaces. As the deteriorating myocardium worsens, the ability of the heart to increase its output is impaired. The renal blood flow is decreased resulting in the release of renin from the juxta-glomerular apparatus. The renin activates angiotensin from its plasma precursor angiotensinogen, and this stimulates the secretion of aldosterone which now acts on the renal tubules to increase the reabsorption of sodium; there is an increase in the total body sodium and a retention of body water, all leading to an increase in blood volume, and increased formation of tissue fluid.

The resultant poor circulation in the pulmonary and systemic vascular network hinders the exchange of gases both in the lungs and peripheral tissue. The resulting cyanosis promotes increased capillary permeability and further loss of fluid into the extravascular spaces resulting in oedema. This is a simplification of the pathophysiology of congestive heart failure but it serves as a sufficient basis for the explanation of the action of digitalis in the condition.

On administration, cardiac glycosides increase the cardiac output, decrease the heart size and decrease the venous pressure. They produce diuresis and relieve oedema. All these effects are a consequence of the increase in contractile force that they produce. The heart size is reduced, because the positive inotropic action of digitalis results in more complete systolic emptying. The increased cardiac output increases the blood pressure and this reflexly reduces sympathetic drive to the heart and to the blood vessels, particularly to the veins and the peripheral arterioles. As a result, the heart rate falls, the peripheral resistance and venous pressure fall, the perfusion of the kidney is improved. There is enhanced urinary excretion of fluid and oedema is relieved.

In addition to its positive inotropic effect, digitalis has several other complex effects on the heart. Digitalis directly depresses the conducting tissues responsible for carrying impulses from the sinu-auricular (SA) node. Furthermore, digitalis stimulates the vagus to release ACH and sensitizes the SA node to ACH action. In patients with heart failure, however, the most important component of digitalis action that results in a decreased heart rate is the reduction in sympathetic drive to the heart.

Mechanism of action of cardiac glycosides

The action of the cardiac glycosides is mediated by an increase in intracellular free Ca^{2+}. Cardiac glycosides inhibit the membrane Na^+/K^-–ATPase causing the intracellular accumulation of Na^+. On the arrival of an action potential, the Na^+ then competes with and displaces Ca^{2+} from intracellular stores into the intracellular labile pool, where it is available for the contractile mechanism. By enhancing inotropism, digitalis allows the myocardium to function at a lower filling pressure (Fig. 21.2), and reduced myocardial oxygen consumption.

Toxicity

The therapeutic index for the cardiac glycosides is very low (see page 56). That is, the toxic doses of the glycosides are only slightly above the therapeutically effective doses.

Loss of appetite, nausea, and vomiting are usually early signs of digitalis toxicity. Stomach cramps with pain and diarrhoea are often also present. Other toxic manifestations include cardiac dysrhythmias, fatigue, stupor, coma, amnesia, restlessness, confusion and headache. At its extreme, digitalis causes heart block as a result of its direct and indirect actions on the myocardial conducting tissues.

A decrease in potassium concentration in the plasma enhances digitalis toxicity. Thus, concurrent administration of chlorothiazide diuretics during digitalis therapy may precipitate toxic signs. Also, in the aged, whose excretion of digitalis may be slow, toxicity may be encountered more often. In hypokalaemic states, it is advisable to stop treatment with digitalis until the hypokalaemia is corrected by giving a potassium supplement. Sustained release tablets (slow K) are available. Potassium-sparing diuretics like spironolactone, amiloride or triamterene may be used if there is need for concurrent diuretic therapy.

21.3   ANTI-ARRHYTHMIC DRUGS

The term arrhythmia is used to describe disorders of heart rate or rhythm due to the origin of impulse from an ectopic focus or to abnormal conduction of a normally generated impulse. Drugs used to restore normal rhythm and rate are known as anti-arrythmic drugs. The properties of these drugs are complex; this has led to various ways of classifying this group. A clinically useful classification is that suggested by Vaughan Williams. This is based on the effects of the drug on the automaticity, conductivity, and repolarization characteristics of myocardial tissues. Using his criteria for classification, some of the commonly used anti-arrhythmic drugs are divided into five classes as shown in Table 21.1. It should be stressed, however, that drugs belonging to one class may share some electrophysiological properties with drugs in another group.

Class I anti-arrhythmic drugs

Drugs belonging to this class characteristically exert membrane-stabilising activity, including local anaesthetic activity on nerves. They decrease the maximum rate of depolarization in atria, His-Purkinje, and ventricular myocardial cells by reducing the magnitude of the inward sodium current during phase 0 of the action potential. Quinidine and procainamide are typical examples of this class of drugs.

Quinidine

This is an isomer of quinine and it shares many of its pharmacological actions. They are both cinchona alkaloids, and they are also used in the treatment of malaria infection.

Actions on the heart

Quinidine increases the threshold potential for electrical excitation of the cardiac muscle. It increases the effective refractory period of both the myocardial and conducting tissues. The functional refractory period is also slightly prolonged. In therapeutic contractions, quinidine decreases the conduction velocity in isolated atria, Purkinje fibres and ventricular muscle. It increases the action potential duration of cells of the SA node and other tissues of the heart capable of spontaneous depolarisation.

As already mentioned, the direct effect of quinidine on the heart is due to its ability to decrease membrane permeability to sodium (and possibly to potassium). Since the slow spontaneous diastolic depolarisation in the SA node is mediated by the entry of calcium rather than of sodium into the cell, quinidine and similar drugs will have little or no effect on the firing rate of the SA node. In an abnormal site of pacemaker activity (ectopic site), quinidine decreases the slope of phase 4 depolarisation. The membrane responsiveness of adjacent cells is also decreased, and accordingly premature impulses initiated before complete repolarisation (during phase 3) or after an appreciable degree of phase 4 depolarisation are not propagated.

The direct effects of quinidine on the heart are complicated by its vagal blocking action. Thus it causes an increase in heart rate in unanaesthetised animals and in man. This tachycardia is due in part to quinidine's atropine-like effect and is partly a result of a reflex increase in sympathetic discharge to the heart, following the decrease in blood pressure on quinidine administration.

Quinidine is given orally for the treatment of acute or chronic supraventricular or ventricular arrhythmias (tachyarrhythmias).

Toxic manifestations arising from quinidine therapy are an extension of its pharmacological properties; quinidine has antimuscarinic and oxytocic properties, and like quinine, antimalarial and antipyretic actions. The drug can also induce cinchonism (see page 236). Quinidine may also induce rashes, fever, hepatitis and thrombocytopenia. Quinidine increases digoxin plasma levels and may therefore precipitate digitalis toxicity in patients taking the drug. Quinidine itself can cause partial or total heart block.

Table 21.1 *Classification of anti-arrhythmic drugs*

Class	Mechanism of action	Drugs	Other anti-arrhythmic class of activity	Other therapeutic actions
I	Membrane stabilisers	Quinidine	III	Antimalarial
		Procainamide	III	–
		Lignocaine		Local anaesthetic
		Mexiletine		–
		Antazoline		Antihistaminic
		Diphenylhydantoin	II	Anti-epileptic
		ORG 6001		
		Disopyramide	III	Anti-anginal
II	Reduce adrenergic influences on the heart (beta-adrenoceptor blockade or adrenergic neurone blockade)	Propranolol	IV	Antihypertensive
		Timolol	III	Antihypertensive
		Sotalol	III	Antihypertensive
		Atenolol	III	Antihypertensive
		Oxprenolol	III	Antihypertensive
		Alprenolol		Antihypertensive
		Bretylium	III	Anti-anginal
		Metoprolol		
III	Prolong the cardial action potential	Amiodarone	I & II slight β-adrenoceptor stimulant activity	Anti-anginal
		Oxyfedrine		Anti-anginal
IV	Calcium channel blockers	Verapamil	I activity in high doses	Anti-anginal, vasodilator

		I activity in high doses	
	Nifedipine		Anti-anginal, vasodilator
	Diltiazem		Anti-anginal, vasodilator
	D 600 (Gallopamil)	?	?
	Prenylamine	?	?
V	Increase vagal tone		
	Cardiac glycoside		Stimulates the failing heart
	Edrophonium		Anticholinesterase
	Phenylephrine		Vasoconstrictor
	Methoxamine		Vasoconstrictor

Procainamide

This is the amide analogue of procaine. Its actions on the heart are similar to those of quinidine; cardiac excitability is depressed, conduction is slowed and the effective refractory period is lengthened. Unlike procaine, procainamide is not hydrolysed by plasma esterase and it is less lipid-soluble. It is therefore less able to penetrate the blood–brain barrier after systemic administration and so lacks CNS effects.

The drug is rapidly and almost completely absorbed after oral administration. Plasma concentration becomes maximal in about 60 min. It can also be administered intramuscularly or intravenously. Since about 60% of the administered dose is excreted unchanged via the kidney, considerable care should be taken in patients with impairment of renal function.

Procainamide is used in paroxysmal ventricular or atrial tachycardia as an alternative to quinidine. Toxic manifestations include occasional paroxysmal tachycardia, flushing, diarrhoea, weakness, mental depression, giddiness and, rarely, psychosis with hallucinations. Granulocytopenia and various blood disorders have also been reported.

Lignocaine

This is widely used as a local anaesthetic (see page 403). It is also an anti-arrhythmic agent now commonly used in the emergency treatment of ventricular arrhythmias encountered during cardiac surgery or resulting from myocardial infarction.

The electrophysiological effects of lignocaine on the heart are similar to those of quinidine except that it has little or no effect on the action potentials in atrial conducting fibres. It also increases the rate of repolarisation of the ventricular action potential. It therefore reduces the duration of the action potential. Lignocaine lacks vagolytic properties.

The observation that lignocaine shortens the duration of the action potential has led to a subclassification of the Class I group of drugs into 3 subgroups. Class IA drugs depress phase 0 and prolong the duration of the action potential. Examples are quinidine, procainamide and disopyramide. Class ID drugs depress phase 0 and reduce the duration of the action potential. This group is typified by lignocaine, mexiletine and tocainide. Class IC drugs depress phase 0 but have little or no effects on repolarisation and the duration of action potential. Examples are ecainide, flecainide and lorcainide.

Lignocaine has become the most widely used drug in the intensive care unit for the emergency treatment of ventricular arrhythmias resulting from myocardial ischaemia. It is usually administered by the intravenous route but it may be given intramuscularly.

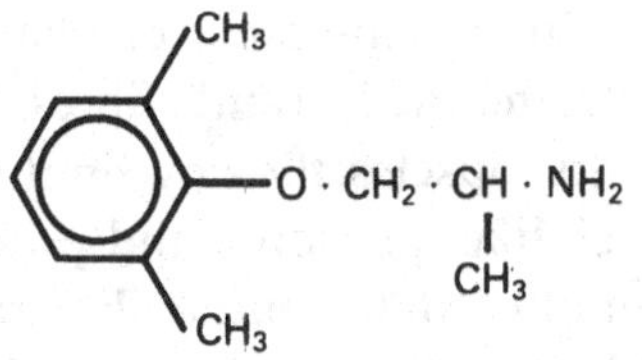

$$
\begin{array}{c}
CH_3 \\
\text{(benzene ring)}—O \cdot CH_2 \cdot CH \cdot NH_2 \\
| \\
CH_3 \\
CH_3
\end{array}
$$

Mexiletine

Mexiletine is a Class I anti-arrhythmic agent with properties closely resembling those of lignocaine. It decreases the spontaneous firing rate of ventricular pacemakers by shifting threshold voltage in a manner similar to quinidine.

Mexiletine is active following oral administration; but it can be given i.v. and is used in the treatment of ventricular arrythmias associated with myocardial infarction and recurrent ventricular tachycardia.

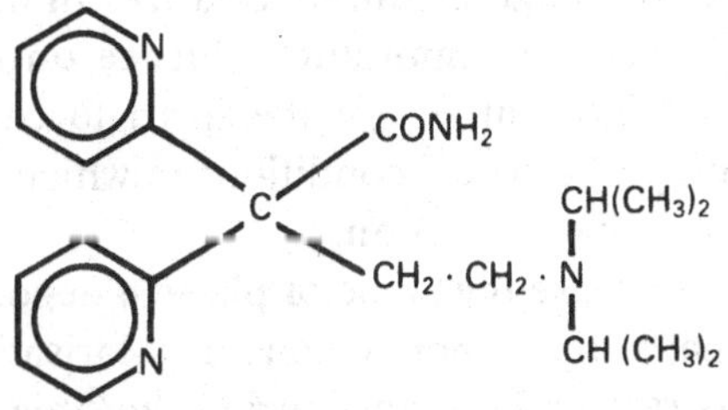

$$
\begin{array}{c}
CONH_2 \\
(pyridyl)—C \\
CH_2 \cdot CH_2 \cdot N—CH(CH_3)_2 \\
(pyridyl) \qquad CH(CH_3)_2
\end{array}
$$

Disopyramide

Disopyramide, 4-diisopropylamin-2 phenyl-2-(2-pyridyl) butyramide, has a pharmacological profile of action similar to quinidine and procainamide. It increases atrial and ventricular refractoriness, decreases sinus automaticity, and increases atrio-ventricular conduction time. Like quinidine it has atropine-like effects on the heart. The drug can be administered orally as well as i.v. in the treatment of atrial and ventricular arrhythmias.

The commonest side effects of the drug are those resulting from its anticholinergic activity; these include dry mouth, difficulty in urination, and paralysis of accommodation; heart block has been reported.

Diphenylhydantoin (phenytoin)

Phenytoin is used mainly in the treatment of epilepsy (see p. 441). However, it has some anti-arrhythmic properties. Like quinidine, phenytoin stabilises membranes of cardiac muscles. Phenytoin depresses the brain and hence reduces the sympathetic drive to the heart. This may be an additional factor in its anti-arrhythmic action.

Phenytoin causes a direct depression of phase 4 depolarization of the cells of the SA node and the Purkinje fibres. It increases the rate of conduction of the heart muscles thereby limiting the chances of re-entrant arrhythmias. Unlike quinidine and procainamide, phenytoin causes less depression of cardiac contractility and blood pressure.

Phenytoin is highly effective against atrial and ventricular arrhythmias produced by digitalis. The toxic manifestation of phenytoin depends on the route, dosage and duration of exposure to the drug. When administered i.v. as in the emergency treatment of cardiac arrhythmias, the most noticeable effects are cardiovascular collapse and/or CNS depression.

Class II anti-arrhythmic drugs

The drugs belonging to this class inhibit the adrenergic influences on the heart, either by blocking the cardiac beta-adrenoceptors or by blocking the adrenergic neurone. Changes in the activity of the autonomic system exert an important influence on cardiac rhythm. More importantly, the sensitivity of the heart to catecholamines is enhanced in certain pathological conditions in which arrhythmias are produced, e.g. myocardial infarction.

Catecholamines increase the slope of phase 4 depolarization in tissues of the heart capable of spontaneous depolarisation. They therefore increase sinus rate and enhance atrial, Purkinje and ventricular automaticity. In tissues like the Purkinje and mitral valve fibres, abnormal automaticity due to slow channel calcium current may be produced by high potassium and catecholamine levels. Drugs that block the effect of catecholamines in enhancing this abnormal automaticity would be anti-arrhythmic.

Beta-adrenoceptor antagonists

The beta-adrenoceptor blocking agents owe their anti-arrhythmic activity to receptor blockade. In addition, many of the beta blockers exhibit a membrane-depressant effect; this local anaesthetic or quinidine-like effect has occasioned much debate about the anti-arrhythmic mechanism of the β-blockers. The quinidine-like effect may not be the main mechanism of anti-arrhythmic action of the class of drugs: some β-adrenoceptor blockers (e.g., practolol and antenolol) lack quinidine-like activity yet are effective anti-arrhythmic drugs. Also dextropropranolol shares the same membrane-stabilising activity as the laevo isomer; but the former has less than one hundredth of the β-adrenoceptor blocking potency, and is a less effective anti-arrhythmic drug than racemic propranolol.

Propranolol has been shown to inhibit the ability of cell membranes and sarcoplasmic reticulum to bind and store calcium ions.

Beta-blockers increase the refractory period of the AV node and thus slow transmission of impulses from the atria to the ventricles; they are useful in controlling ventricular rate in cases of supraventricular tachycardia and fibrillation.

Patients whose cardiac status is compromised by an arrhythmia may be particularly vulnerable to the adverse effects of the β-blockers. Thus cardiac failure may result from the decrease in myocardial contractility produced by β-blockers. This is of particular importance in patients in whom myocardial contractile performance is heavily dependent on sympathetic drive. Since the β-blockers increase the AV conduction time, AV block may be produced. This is more noticeable with β-blockers lacking partial agonist activity but which have potent membrane-stabilising activity.

Bretylium

Bretylium is an adrenergic neurone blocker. It produces a prolongation of phase 2 of the action potential in ventricular muscle and Purkinje fibres. It also prolongs the effective refractory period in this tissue. This effect is believed to be independent of endogeneous catecholamines. Thus bretylium exhibits some Class III properties.

Class III anti-arrhythmic drugs

Drugs belonging to this class have the ability to prolong the refractory period and hence the action potential duration. A typical example is amiodarone.

Amiodarone

This is a benzofuran derivative which was initially introduced as an anti-angina drug but is now widely used as an anti-arrhythmic drug. Its principal mechanism of action is the prolongation of the duration of cardiac action potential and the refractory period in both atria and ventricles. In animals, amiodarone increases the ventricular fibrillation threshold and this effect has been attributed to a noncompetitive block of cardiac β-adrenoceptors.

Amiodarone may take several weeks to produce maximum therapeutic response, after chronic daily administration. On the other hand, amiodarone effect takes several weeks to wear off after discontinuation of therapy. The sustained action of the drug allows a once-daily dosing. Amiodarone is usually administered orally in doses ranging from 200 mg to 800 mg per day given 5 to 7 days per week. It could also be given intravenously for acute effects. Used acutely, amiodarone protects against arrhythmias induced by cardiac glycosides, coronary artery ligation and acetylcholine. This acute anti-arrhythmic efficacy of amiodarone has been attributed to a class I and II effects exhibited by the drug.

Amiodarone is used in the treatment of supraventricular and ventricular arrhythmias.

Class IV anti-arrhythmic drugs

The feature distinguishing this class of drugs is their ability to inhibit calcium transport across the myocardial membrane. Their most striking electrophysiological effects are in tissues in which the upstroke velocity of phase 0 is slow-channel dependent, namely the sinoatrial and atrioventricular nodes.

Verapamil

Verapamil is a synthetic papaverine derivative having significant anti-arrythmic properties. Verapamil selectively inhibits transmembrane fluxes of calcium ions in different excitable tissues. This mechanism of action accounts for the anti-anginal, anti-arrythmic and vasodilatory properties of the drug.

Verapamil is used in the termination of acute paroxysmal supraventricular tachycardia, atrial fibrillation and flutter; refractory cardiac failure, pulmonary oedema and cardiac infarction.

The adverse effects of verapamil are extensions of its known pharmocological properties. These are a transient fall in blood pressure, persistent hypotension, bradycardia and heart block.

Precautions are necessary when verapamil is co-administered with digoxin, as a marked increase in plasma digoxin concentrations may occur. Also care needs to be taken when verapamil or other calcium blockers are combined with drugs like quinidine or the β-blockers as the effects of these drugs on the heart may be additive.

Nifedipine

Nifedipine is a dihydropyridine which is readily oxidised to biologically inactive pyridine derivatives in the presence of light. Its effects on the heart are similar to those of verapamil except that nifedipine has a more selective action on the slow calcium channels while verapamil and diltiazem, at least in higher doses, also inhibit currents in the fast channels.

Nifedipine dilates the peripheral arterioles bringing about a marked decrease in peripheral resistance and a simultaneous increase in cardiac output. The reflex sympathetic response to its peripheral vasodilator effect explains the significant tachycardia usually seen on nifedipine administration. Nifedipine is used in the control of ventricular tachyarrhythmias complicating coronary artery spasm (see Table 21.1 for other class IV drugs).

Class V anti-arrhythmic drugs

This class of anti-arrhythmic drugs is typified by the caridac glycosides. Though their main use is in improving cardiac contractility in congestive heart failure, cardiac glycosides are also useful in the therapy of atrial fibrillation and flutter, and in some cases of supraventricular paroxysmal tachycardia. At first glance this is a paradoxical fact since it is known, for example, that various arrhythmias may appear on administration of large doses of the cardiac glycosides.

The cardiac glycosides impede atrioventricular conduction by prolonging the refractory period of the AV node; there is thus a reduction in the number of impulses that reach the ventricles during atrial fibrillation. The prolongation of the refractory period of the AV node by the cardiac glycosides is due partly to the direct action of the glycosides, the reflex reduction in the sympathetic drive, and the increase in vagal drive to the AV node. The cardiac glycosides are used in the treatment of atrial flutter. The ACH released by the vagus shortens the refractory period of the atria and converts the flutter into fibrillation.

Parasympathomimetic drugs like methacholine were formerly used to mimick the action of the vagus on the heart but widespread side effects have led to their use becoming obsolete. Other drugs like the anticholinesterase, edrophomium are well tolerated. The specific α-adrenoceptor agonists (phenylephrine and methoxamine) can increase the blood pressure and hence reflexly increase vagal activity just like the cardiac glycosides.

21.4   ANGINA PECTORIS AND ANTI-ANGINA DRUGS

Angina pectoris is one of the most common manifestations of ischaemic heart disease. This section discusses first the normal coronary circulation and then the pathophysiology and treatment of angina pectoris.

Coronary blood flow

The normal coronary circulation receives about 4% of the total cardiac output, while the resting myocardial oxygen consumption is about 12% of the total body oxygen consumption. To achieve this high oxygen consumption, the myocardium extracts more oxygen from the blood passing through it than any other tissue in the body. Thus the oxygen saturation of blood leaving the heart (in the coronary sinus) is about 30 to 40% while the venous blood from the rest of the body has an oxygen saturation of about 75%. Therefore, when the myocardium requires a greater oxygen supply, this must be achieved by an increase in coronary blood flow since, unlike the skeletal muscle, the cardiac muscle has a limited capacity to increase its oxygen uptake by further extraction of oxygen.

Another major difference between the coronary and skeletal muscle is that myocardial blood flow is determined almost entirely by metabolic factors. A low oxygen tension, an increase in pCO_2, a fall in pH, or the production of adenine nucleosides by the myocardium induce vasodilatation of the coronary arteries and an increased blood flow.

In normal circumstance, the coronary blood flow can increase by about five times the resting value if the situation demands it. Though coronary vessels are innervated by adrenergic nerves and are capable of vasoconstrictor response to the noradrenaline released from these nerves, the adrenergic influence is always almost overridden by the metabolic influences listed earlier.

Also unlike the skeletal muscle, cardiac muscle has an extremely limited capacity for anaerobic metabolism. The skeletal muscle can incur an oxygen debt which can be repaid at a later time while the myocardium cannot. Thus in situations requiring an increase in cardiac oxygen supply, the only means by which this requirement can be met is through an increase in blood flow. In situations where there is an imbalance in the oxygen requirement and oxygen availability of the myocardium, then the symptoms of angina are manifested.

Angina may be a secondary manifestation of disorders such as systemic hypertension, anaemia, thyrotoxicosis, obesity, syphilis, and the action of drugs, e.g. sympathomimetic amines. Angina pectoris is recognised by a steady, continuous pain with a characteristic choking quality, usually felt in the midline, anywhere from throat to the xiphisternum and this may spread to either side or the front of the chest. It may radiate to the throat, lower jaw, an the inner or outer border of the arms as far as the fingers, or to the interscapular region.

Anti-angina drugs

The main aims of anti-anginal drug therapy are to increase the oxygen supply to the myocardium or to reduce the demand for oxygen so that the heart's requirements are met by the available supply. Examples of anti-angina drugs are: the nitrites and organic nitrates, the beta-blocking drugs, the calcium channel blockers, amiodarone, and lidoflazine.

The organic nitrates and nitrites

These agents are simple nitric and nitrous esters of polyalcohols. Some of these compounds are used in angina therapy; their properties are summarised in Table 21.1. The actions of the organic nitrates and nitrites are due to their conversion to nitrite ion in target tissues. They relax all smooth muscles of the body. The smooth muscle of the blood vessels (arteries and veins) and of the intestine, biliary tree, and ureter are all relaxed. All blood vessels are affected but vasodilation is marked in the coronary arteries, cerebral, splanchnic, and cutaneous vessels. Dilatation of small post-capillary vessels leads to venous pooling of blood.

The anti-anginal effects of these drugs may not be due to their direct effects on the heart. Though the drugs are capable of increasing coronary blood flow in the normal heart, they do not improve blood flow in ischaemic regions of the myocardium. The anti-angina effects have been postulated to be due to their action on the peripheral circulation. They dilate the systemic veins to produce peripheral venous pooling and diminished left ventricular size. The left ventricular end diastolic pressure falls. Furthermore the nitrates dilate the systemic arterioles, thus lowering the peripheral vascular resistance and systolic blood pressure. These reductions in left ventricular volume and systemic pressure result in improved endocardial blood flow, diminished intramyocardial wall tension, and diminished external cardiac work. The myocardial oxygen demand is diminished and angina is ameliorated. The fall in blood pressure caused by the nitrites may induce reflex tachycardia. However in most cases, this reflex increase in heart rate does not offset the beneficial effect of the drugs.

Table 21.2   *Organic nitrates and nitrites used as anti-angina drugs*

Drug	Route of administration	Onset of action	Duration of action
Amyl nitrite	Inhalation	10–20 s	5 min
Erythrityl tetranitrate	Sublingual	5–10 min	2–4 h
	Swallowed	20–25 min	2–4 h
Propatyl nitrate	Sublingual	1 min	15 min
Sorbide nitrate	Sublingual	5–10 min	2 h
Glyceryl trinitrate	Sublingual	2–3 min	30 min
	Ointment	15 min	5 h
Octyl nitrite	Inhalation	30 s	6 min

The use of organic nitrates and nitrites is strongly influenced by the existence of a high-capacity nitrate reductase in the liver. Thus bioavailability of orally administered organic nitrates is very low. Consequently, the sublingual route is preferred and nitroglycerine and isosorbide dinitrate are well absorbed by this route. Other routes of administration include transdermal absorption when the compound is applied to the skin as an ointment, buccal absorption from slow-release preparations, and inhalation as with amyl nitrite. Once absorbed, the nitrites have half lives of about 2–8 mins. The denitrated metabolites have much longer half lives but they are less active vasodilators. Glucuronide derivatives of the metabolites are excreted through the kidney. A number of organic nitrates with much longer half lives have been synthesised and they are used as prophylactics in angina pectoris. Apart from their application in angina pectoris, the nitrites are also useful in relieving spasm in biliary and urinary tracts.

Calcium channel blockers

Verapamil, nifedipine, and diltiazem have been used in treating angina pectoris. They all competitively block the cell membrane slow channels, resulting in a decreased influx of calcium into the cell. In angina pectoris, they relieve and prevent coronary artery spasm by increasing coronary blood flow and oxygen delivery. They reduce myocardial oxygen demand by lowering the blood pressure, heart rate and cardiac contractility.

Amotriphene group

Drugs belonging to this group include amotriphene, perhexiline, and lidoflazine. They cause a generalised depression of membrane ionic fluxes, smooth muscle tone, and Purkinje fibre automaticity; atrio-ventricular and ventricular conduction velocities are decreased. They also decrease response to a variety of agents, e.g. catecholamines, histamine and calcium.

They reduce exercise-induced tachycardia, and they decrease the peripheral resistance.

Dipyridamole
Dipyridamole is a dipiperidino-dipyrimidine. Its mechanism of action is similar to that of papaverine. In therapeutic doses, it generally decreases coronary blood flow without significantly altering the blood pressure. It is well absorbed after oral administration and it is excreted mainly via the bile in the faeces. Solutions are also available for intramuscular injections. Dipyridamole is useful in patients suffering from acute myocardial infarction and angina pectoris. Side effects include nausea, vomiting, diarrhoea, headache and vertigo.

21.5 ESSENTIAL HYPERTENSION
The aetiology and pathogenesis of essential hypertension constitute a complex phenomenon in which changes in peripheral resistance, cardiac output, vascular reactivity, vascular wall elasticity, blood viscosity, and the autonomic and central nervous systems are believed to be involved. Also implicated are hereditary, ethnic, environmental, constitutional, age, and other factors.

Irrespective of the factors which may contribute to the disease, the main marker of its existence is an elevated blood pressure. The mean arterial pressure is determined by cardiac output and peripheral resistance. An increased pressure may be induced by increases in one or both of these determinants. The main determinants of cardiac output are heart rate and stroke volume. The heart rate is controlled by sympathetic and vagal impulses which act on the basal rhythmicity of the heart muscle cells. Stroke volume is regulated mainly by alterations in sympathetic activity. In established hypertension, increased peripheral resistance is the major factor. This is attributed to increased length of resistance vessels, or increased wall thickness, i.e. decreased diameter of resistance vessels. The increased vascular resistance in hypertension due to decreased radius has been attributed to increase in vascular smooth muscle activity. This in turn may be due to hormonal influences, e.g. in secondary types of hypertension such as renal hypertension, Conn's syndrome, Cushing's disease, and phaechromocytoma. However, changes in hormonal levels have not been convincingly demonstrated in uncomplicated primary hypertension.

Another factor implicated in the genesis of the increased smooth muscle activity is an 'altered' ionic composition of the vascular smooth muscle. The offending ion is sodium.

The evidence for this is indirect, but is of particular interest in relation to the aetiology of hypertension in people of African descent (see p. 178). Arteries from hypertensive subjects respond significantly more to noradrenaline than those of normal subjects and patients with essential hypertension appear to have a greater salt-appetite than normotensive subjects. Several hypotheses have been put forward to explain how excessive salt intake or derangement in salt handling by the body can lead to elevation in blood pressure. In the 'Unified Hypothesis' put forward by Blaustein in 1977, the sodium ion balance in vascular tissue is linked with calcium ion flux and with alterations in blood pressure. It is proposed that high concentrations of sodium ion, caused by either the ingestion of salt or derangement in the excretion or retention of salt, through a range of intermediate steps, cause a decrease in the ratio of extracellular to intracellular sodium ion concentration. This in turn alters the intracellular calcium ion concentration to produce an increase in vascular resistance and a rise in blood pressure. This hypothesis is interesting in view of the high prevalence of hypertension in peoples of African descent and the reported greater sensitivity of this group to diuretic therapy than Caucasians (pp.178, 192). Could sodium retention be a genetic adaptation to life in a tropical environment where the adaptation could compensate for sodium loss through sweat?

Complications of hypertension

A sustained high arterial pressure produces changes in the various vascular beds. There is hypertrophy of the arteriolar walls in the kidney, intestine, skeletal muscle, pia mater and the skin. With respect to the myocardium, the heart work is proportional to the increase in arterial blood pressure. It therefore follows that ventricular hypertrophy is the response of the myocardium to greater work demand.

Pathological changes are also seen in the cerebral, renal and coronary circulations. Increase of blood pressure leads to elevations of resistance to blood flow in the cerebrovascular systems. Cerebral ischaemia and its consequential cerebral infarction are common complications in hypertensive diseases. Hypertensive cerebral haemorrhage is a common manifestation in essential hypertension. One of the aetiological factors in coronary heart disease or coronary insufficiency as well as impairment of renal function is hypertension.

Antihypertensive drugs

Antihypertensive drugs are used in conditions of high blood pressure requiring medication. The mere finding of blood pressure values slightly higher than normal does not in itself imply the need for therapy. The arterial blood pressure frequently returns to the normal level with rest, reassurance, and diet. In situations which do not respond satisfactorily to these measures, then the need for therapy becomes real.

It is generally believed that the best treatment of a disease is to eliminate the cause. In hypertension, however, there is generally an uncertainty about the aetiology of this disease and this has made the drug therapy of hypertension that much more empirical. A brief discussion of antihypertensive drugs and their side effects follows with particular reference to putative mechanisms of action.

Direct vasodilators

This group of drugs dilate the blood vessels directly and not through any interaction with the autonomic or central nervous systems. Examples are dipyridamole, hydrallazine, diazoxide, and minoxidil.

Hydrallazine

The fall in blood pressure caused by hydrallazine activates the baroreceptor reflexes causing an increase in heart rate, stroke volume and cardiac output. Hydrallazine decreases the diastolic pressure to a greater extent than the systolic blood pressure. Renal and coronary blood flows are usually increased by hydrallazine. For this reason, hydrallazine has a theoretical advantage for hypertensive individuals with impaired renal function. However, in patients with ischaemic heart disease, anginal symptoms may be worsened.

Hydrallazine may be given orally, intramuscularly or intravenously. Side effects include headache, palpitations, nausea, vomiting, tachycardia, unpleasant taste and anxiety. More serious side effects which may require discontinuance of the drug include exacerbation of coronary insufficiency, dependent oedema, toxic psychosis, and a drug-induced lupus erythematosus. (See chapter 8 for consequences of fast or slow acetylation.)

Diazoxide

Diazoxide is a nondiuretic benzothiadiazine derivative with a potent direct relaxant action on arteries and arterioles but little or no effect on the venous capacitance vessels. The sudden reduction in blood pressure when diazoxide is given intravenously as in hypertensive emergencies, is accompanied by a reflex increase in heart rate, stroke volume and cardiac output. There is also a reflex increase in renin release and chronic treatment with diazoxide usually produces salt and water retention and hence an increase in circulating fluid volume.

Diazoxide is used in the treatment of hypertensive crises in patients with malignant hypertension, cerebral haemorrhage, encephalopathy or eclampsia. Like the thiazide diuretics, diazoxide has hyperuricaemic and diabetogenic effects (see Chapter 23). So care should be taken when it is administered to diabetic patients already on hypoglycaemic drugs.

Sodium nitroprusside

For intravenous infusion, sodium nitroprusside is dissolved in 5% dextrose solution in a concentration of 50–100 mg/l. The drug must be given under close supervision; the solution is unstable, so fresh solution is usually prepared every four hours or as soon as the sign of reduction of the ferric ion appears.

Sodium nitroprusside is ideal in the managment of most hypertensive crises. On infusion, the drug produces an immediate dose-dependent fall in blood pressure by dilating the arterioles and veins; there is a decrease in venous pressure and cardiac output. The resultant reflex activation of the sympathetic nervous system leads to reflex tachycardia and increased renin release. The mechanism of the relaxant effect of nitroprusside on the blood vessels may involve an increase in the efflux of Ca^{2+} from vascular smooth vessels.

Minoxidil

This is a potent orally effective direct vasodilator of arterioles with little effect on the venous capacitance vessels; the reduction in blood pressure by minoxidil is usually accompanied by an increase in heart rate, stroke volume and cardiac output, and an increase in plasma renin level. Minoxidil seems to promote hair growth.

Drugs that act on the renin–angiotensin system

There is evidence that in some cases of hypertension, the renin–angiotensin system is stimulated and angiotensin II, the potent vasoactive metabolite of angiotensin I, is produced and this plays an active role in maintaining an elevated systemic vascular resistance. Thus inhibition of the conversion of angiotensin I to angiotensin II is the mechanism of the antihypertensive action of a class of drugs. Similarly, competitive antagonists of angiotensin II at the receptor site have antihypertensive activity.

$$HS \cdot CH_2 \cdot \underset{\underset{CH_3}{|}}{CH} \cdot CO-N \overbrace{\qquad\qquad}-COOH$$

Captopril

Captopril is an orally active inhibitor of angiotensin-converting enzyme (ACE). It is this enzyme (peptidyl dipeptidase) that is responsible for the conversion of inactive angiotensin I to the active angiotensin II.

On oral administration, the drug is well absorbed and peak plasma concentration is attained within one hour. About 30% of the absorbed drug is bound to plasma protein.

Captopril causes both arterial and venous dilation and hence a reduction in systemic vascular resistance. Vasodilation with captopril appears to be most prominent in the renovascular bed. Renal vascular resistance falls and there is an increase in renal blood flow. Captopril increases plasma renin activity and decreases plasma aldosterone level; with decreased aldosterone production, plasma potassium concentration is increased. Experience with captopril is limited, hence the incidence and nature of its side effects are not fully known.

Drugs which impair the function of the peripheral sympathetic nervous system

Many drugs which block sympathetic outflow cause a fall in arterial blood pressure. These mechanisms have been discussed in detail in the chapter on Noradrenergic mechanisms. The clinically useful drugs are summarised in Table 21.3.

Beta-adrenoceptor antagonists (beta-blockers)

These are among the most widely prescribed drugs for the treatment of hypertension. As pointed out in Chapter 8, clinical experience indicates that the beta-blockers are useful in black hypertensives only in combination with diuretics. Their mechanism of action is not known. Five hypotheses are listed in the Table 21.3.

Table 21.3 *Antihypertensive drugs and their major sites of action*

Type of drug	Examples	Major site of action	Notable side effects
(1) Direct vasodilators	Hydrallazine, dipyridamole diazoxide, minoxidil, sodium nitroprusside	Dilation of precapillary resistance vessels	Reflex stimulation of the sympathetic nervous system and tachycardia. Minoxidil promotes hair growth on chronic use.
(2) Angiotensin antagonists	Captopril teprotide	ACE inhibitor	Increased renin and decreased aldosterone production
	Saralasin	Angiotensin II receptor antagonist	?
(3) Inhibitors of peripheral sympathetic nerve function:			
(a) Ganglion blockers	Pemipidine, mecamylamine, pentolinium	Sympathetic and parasympathetic ganglia	Constipation, urinary retention, blurred vision, impotence
(b) Adrenergic neurone depleters	*Rauvolfia* alkaloids, e.g. reserpine, syrosingopine	Blockade of uptake of amines (catecholamine, 5HT, and dopamine) into storage sites	Depression, Parkinsonian syndrome
(c) Adrenergic neurone blockers	Debrisoquine, guanethidine, bethanidine	Are taken up into noradrenergic nerves and prevent the release of NA	Postural hypotension, failure of ejaculation

(d) Alpha-adrenoceptor antagonists	Phenoxybenzamine, phentolamine (for diagnosis and management of secondary hypertension, e.g. phaeochromocytoma)	Pre- and postjunctional alpha-adrenoceptors	Reflex tachycardia, palpitations, postural hypotension
	Prazosin	Postjunctional alpha-adrenoceptor antagonist; phosphodiesterase inhibitor leading to accumulation of cGMP	Headache, palpitations
	Labetolol	Antagonist at both alpha- and beta-adrenoceptors	Postural hypotension
(4) Beta-adrenoceptor antagonists	Propranolol, timolol (see page 372)	(a) decrease cardiac output (b) central action (c) stimulate prejunctional beta-adrenoceptors (d) suppress renin release (e) block alpha-adrenoceptors	Bronchospasm in asthmatics, hypoglycaemia, may raise plasma urate to precipitate gout, impotence in the male
(5) Drugs with a central mode of action	Alpha-methyldopa	(a) converted to alphamethyl NA in the CNS to depress adrenergic brain stem neurones	Extrapyramidal disorders, loss of libido, allergic reaction with positive Coombs test

Table 21.3 (*cont.*)

Type of drug	Examples	Major site of action	Notable side effects
		(b) depress plasma renin activity	
	Clonidine	Stimulate alpha-2 adrenoceptors in nucleus tractus satorius to depress sympathetic outflow	Sedation, fluid retention, dryness of the mouth, hyperglycaemia, rebound hypertension
	Veratrum alkaloids	Sensitise the baroreceptor reflex to reduce sympathetic and increase parasympathetic drive to the heart	Afferent receptors to the vomiting centre are also sensitised, therefore nausea and vomiting are frequent side effects

Drugs with a CNS mode of action

Many drugs with CNS-depressant action (e.g., sedative/hypnotics) are beneficial in hypertension. Some other drugs developed for the treatment of hypertension, e.g. alphamethyldopa (αMD) and clonidine, seem to produce a peripheral hypotensive action by acting on CNS structures. The original 'false transmitter' mechanism proposed for alphamethyldopa (i.e., that this precursor was taken up into noradrenergic neurones where, after conversion to alphamethylnoradrenaline, it was released on nerve stimulation instead of, or in addition to the 'true' transmitter NA) has been superseded by one which assumes a CNS mode of action. In this, ∝MD is taken into noradrenergic neurones in the brain stem (nucleus tractus solitarius) where it is converted to alphamethyl NA. On release this causes a powerful stimulation of prejunctional alpha-2 adrenoceptors in the brain stem, a depression of brain stem noradrenergic neurones, and a fall in peripheral arterial pressure. Clonidine has similar actions, but acts directly on CNS alpha adrenoceptors to reduce sympathetic drive to the heart and blood vessels thereby lowering arterial pressure.

The veratrum alkaloids sensitise the baroreceptors and afferent fibres particularly in the heart and carotid sinus so that a given level of blood pressure rise results in a larger amount of afferent nerve traffic to the vasomotor centre. This then produces a reduction in sympathetic and an increase in vagal tone to the heart.

Diuretics

Diuretics are drugs used to increase urine flow. They act mainly by increasing the amount of sodium in the urine. This they achieve either by increasing the amount of sodium filtered in the glomeruli or by inhibiting the tubular reabsorption of sodium either by a direct or an indirect action. The increase in sodium in the urine is accompanied by an increase in water in order to maintain the osmotic balance.

Diuretics are classified according to their mechanism as well as their site of action in the kidney. (See also figure 21.4.)

The xanthines

The methylated xanthine alkaloids, caffeine, theobromine, and theophylline produce their diuretic effects by inhibiting the reabsorption of sodium and chloride in the proximal tubules. This effect increases the sodium load delivered to the distal convoluted tubules; xanthine alkaloids may increase the number of functioning glomeruli. The xanthines may also improve renal blood flow through their stimulant action on the heart.

Osmotic diuretics

The presence in the glomerular filtrate of any poorly absorbed material, e.g. sorbitol, mannitol, or sucrose, increases the osmotic equivalent of the urine and thus reduces the reabsorption of water and sodium by the tubules.

Osmotic diuretics given orally or i.v. may be useful in cerebral oedema.

Fig. 21.4. Diagrammatic representation of sodium, chloride and water transport in different segments of the kidney nephron. The most important mechanisms in relation to diuresis are: reabsorption of sodium chloride and water, secretion of H^+ ions, and reabsorption and secretion of K^+. These critical events occur as shown.
(1) Proximal convoluted tubule. This region is highly permeable to H_2O. Na^+Cl^- is actively reabsorbed and water diffuses along the osmotic gradient.
(2) Ascending loop of Henle; this region is relatively impermeable to water; Na^+ and Cl^- are actively reabsorbed.
(3) Collecting duct is where the hormones aldosterone (ALDO) and antidiuretic hormone (ADH) exert influence. Aldosterone causes reabsorption of Na^+ and secretion of K^+.

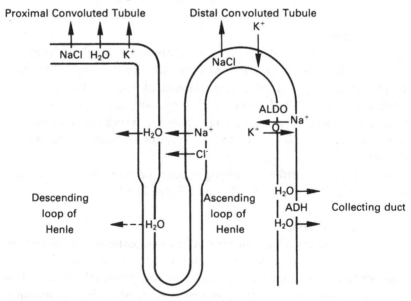

Table 21.4 *Diuretics and their major sites of action*

Class of diuretic	Examples	Major site of action	Notable side effect
Xanthine	Caffeine, theophylline theobromine	Inhibit Na^+ reabsorption in *proximal convoluted tubule*	Tolerance
Osmotic	Sorbitol, mannitol, sucrose	Increase in urinary osmotic pressure	Renal damage
Mercurial	Mercumatilin, chlormerodrin	Block $-SH-$ containing enzymes responsible for Na^+ reabsorption	Renal damage, cardiac toxicity
Carbonic anhydrase inhibitors	Acetazolamide, ethoxolamide	*Distal convoluted tubule* Inhibition of carbonic acid formation; hence lack of H^+ to exchange for Na^+	Anorexia, fatigue, agranulocytosis
Thiazide	Chlorothiazide, hydroxychlorothiazide hydroflumethiazide	*Proximal and distal tubules* Inhibition of Na^+ Cl^- ions	Due to K^+ loss – weakness, cramps, increased blood sugar
Loop (high ceiling)	Frusemide, ethacrynic acid, bumetanide	*Ascending loop of Henle* Inhibition of active reabsorption of chloride and sodium ions	Dehydration hypothermic alkalosis
Potassium-sparing	Spironolactone, triamterene, amiloride	*Distal and collecting tubules* Spironolactone is aldosterone antagonist, triamterene and amiloride act directly	Renal damage

Mercurial diuretics

The organic mercurial diuretics produce their effects by inhibiting enzymes involved in the reabsorption of sodium thoughout the nephron. They inhibit —SH-containing enzymes at this site to prevent the reabsorption of sodium and chloride; the amount of chloride lost far exceeds that of sodium lost. The mean diuretic effect of the mercurials may thus be due to increased chloride excretion.

The mercurial diuretics are probably the most potent diuretics, but their use has largely been replaced by the thiazides because of the convenience of effective oral preparations of the latter and because the thiazides are less toxic. They may be used in oedema arising from cardiac decompensation and in ascites due to liver disease.

The thiazides and related diuretics

Chlorothiazide   Hydroflumethiazide

The thiazides inhibit the active transport of sodium from the tubules into the blood but the precise mechanism and site of action of this effect is unknown. They inhibit the reabsorption of the sodium and chloride in the proximal and distal tubules.

The thiazides induce potassium loss from the distal tubule partly by increasing the amount of sodium delivered to this ion-exchange site. In addition, the thiazides have a direct potassium-depleting action (kaliuretic effect). Furthermore, the decrease in blood sodium induced by the thiazide promotes the release of aldosterone which further enhances potassium loss. The potassium drain may be such as to warrant the administration of potassium supplements.

The thiazides are usually the first drug of choice in the treatment of hypertension and they are very useful in cardiac oedema and other oedematous conditions. They can be used to reduce the volume of urine elaborated by a patient with pituitary diabetes inspidus (deficiency of ADH) and in nephrogenic diabetes inspidus (insensitivity of the kidney tubules to ADH). The mechanism of their antidiuretic effect in these conditions is not known.

The mechanism by which the thiazides lower the blood pressure in hypertensives is not clearly understood. Initially there is a loss of fluid from the body. The extracellular and plasma fluid volumes are decreased and the cardiac output is reduced. These initial effects of the thiazides are, however, transient as pretreatment levels are again attained several weeks after the institution of therapy. At this stage, tolerance to their diuretic action is also noted but the blood pressure remains lower than the pretreatment level. The observation that the hypotensive effect of the thiazides is still maintained despite a gradual loss of their diuretic activity indicates that the antihypertensive mechanism of action of the thiazides may involve effects other than their diuretic action.

Possibly the thiazides render the vascular smooth muscle less reactive to the effect of the sympathetic drive, by altering the ratio of intracellular to extracellular sodium; or the antihypertensive action is due to their ability to inhibit cyclic nucleotide phosphodiesterase and increasing vascular smooth muscle cyclic AMP and hence producing vasodilatation. Some thiazides without diuretic action are potent vasodilators, e.g. diazoxide.

The main toxic effects of the thiazides are those due to excessive potassium loss. Weakness, fatigability, nausea, cramps and epigastric discomfort are common. The potassium depletion may increase the risk of digitalis toxicity. Thiazides increase the fasting blood sugar level and decrease glucose tolerance, and can precipitate diabetes mellitus. They also induce hyperuricaemia by decreasing the excretion of uric acid and are therefore contra-indicated in patients with acute gout.

The loop diuretics

Frusemide, ethacrynic acid, and bumetanide are all together referred to as the loop diuretics to denote their site of diuretic action Also called 'high ceiling' because the maxium diuretic effect cannot be matched by even high doses of other diuretics.

Frusemide

Frusemide is a sulphonamide with pharmocological properties and adverse effects similar to those of the thiazides. It inhibits the active reabsorption of chloride ion (and hence sodium) in the ascending limb of the loop of Henle. On administration, its onset of action is very rapid (within 30 min) and it has a very potent diuretic effect. It causes depletion of sodium, and potassium, and dehydration. The potency, the rapid onset of action, and the availability of an injectable dosage form have led to the wide use of frusemide. The drug is useful for the immediate treatment of congestive heart failure, acute pulmonary oedema and hypertension. Frusemide is a much more effective diuretic against oedema associated with chronic renal failure.

Ethacrynic acid

Ethacrynic acid is chemically unrelated to the suphonamides. It is remarkable for its potent diuretic action. Ethacrynic acid inhibits the active transport of sodium in the proximal tubule and of chloride throughout the loop of Henle. Potassium and hydrogen ion excretion are also increased, presumably because of the increased amount of sodium reaching the distal tubules.

Ethacrynic acid has been of great use in patients with refractory oedema of various causes. The urine elaborated may be so voluminous as to induce fright in patients. The powerful diuretic action of ethacrynic acid and other similar loop diuretics may lead to serious electrolyte imbalance; hence the use of this class of drug is usually reserved for patients who are under close supervision.

Potassium-sparing diuretics

One of the shortcomings of the thiazide diuretics is their potassium-depleting activity. Thus if a diuretic is able to conserve potassium, then such a drug should be the diuretic of choice for the chronic treatment of patients with mild to moderate hypertension. Spironolactone, triamterene, and amiloride are drugs that produce diuresis without an accompanying potassium loss.

Spironolactone is a synthetic steroid similar in structure to aldosterone. In the kidney, aldosterone acts on the distal and collecting tubules to enhance the sodium–potassium exchange mechanism. Thus aldosterone causes sodium retention and potassium loss. Spironolactone competitively antagonises the effect of aldosterone on the kidney tubule. Thus after aldosterone administration, there is an increase in sodium and chloride excretion while the excretion of potassium and hydrogen are decreased (see also Fig. 23.3).

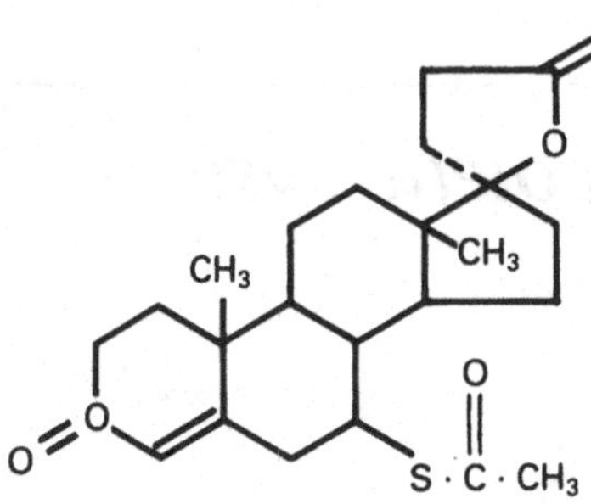

Spironolactone

Spironolactone is a weak diuretic and is usually given in combination with the benzothiadiazide derivatives to minimize thiazide-induced kaliuresis. The adverse effects of spironolactone include mental confusion, sedation, rashes, hirsuitism, and gynecomastia. Spironolactone and other potassium-sparing diuretics are contraindicated in severe renal insufficiency because of the danger of severe hyperkalemia.

Triamterene and amiloride

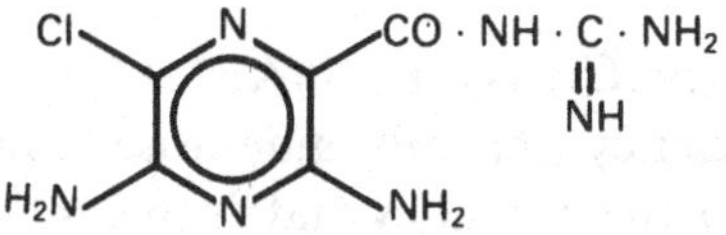

Amiloride

These two compounds have diuretic actions similar to that of spironolactone. However they act directly on the distal tubule to decrease the reabsorption of sodium. Like spironolactone, they are usually used in combination with a thiazide.

Triamterene and amiloride increase the secretion of uric acid in contrast to the effect of the thiazides, frusemide and ethacrynic acid; they may produce uric acid retention and precipitate gout. Triamterene is a pteridine derivative and it may therefore interfere with the action of folic acid.

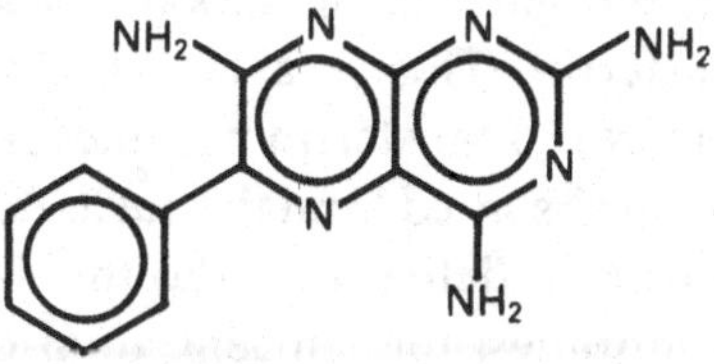

Triamterene

22

Haemopoietic system

22.1 INTRODUCTION

In this chapter information is given about iron deficiency and megaloblastic anaemias; clotting mechanisms and the properties of drugs used in the treatment of diseases caused by thrombosis are described.

22.2 IRON-DEFICIENCY ANAEMIA

Iron-deficiency anaemia may arise from various causes (see legend to Fig. 22.1). In pregnancy and during menstruation (a menstruating woman may lose up to 80 mg iron per period) and in patients suffering from chronic blood loss, the risk of iron-deficiency anaemia is particularly high. The treatment is to give iron.

Absorption and storage of iron in the body

Iron is absorbed in the ferrous form in the upper small intestine after combining with a carrier protein called apoferritin to form ferritin (see Fig. 22.1). Apoferritin has 24 polypeptide residues and a molecular weight of about 450000; it has a high capacity for combining with ferrous iron which becomes oxidised to the ferric state in ferritin.

More than one-third of the weight of ferritin is iron. The transfer of iron from ferritin in the gut wall to blood is accomplished by the plasma protein, transferrin. This is a beta-1 glycoprotein with two binding sites for ferric iron. Transferrin becomes saturated in the presence of excess iron being absorbed from the gut as occurs in iron poisoning (see below). Transferrin delivers iron to the tissues by binding to receptors on cell membranes; the concentration of receptors reflects the tissue's need for iron.

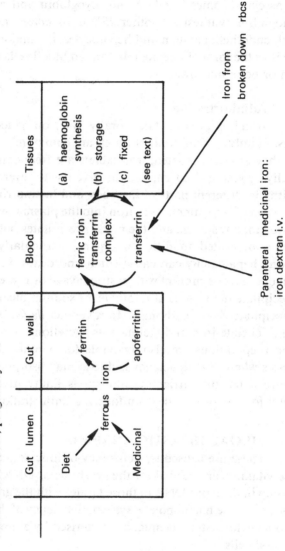

Fig. 22.1. Absorption and disposition of iron in the body. Deficiency can arise from: (1) dietary lack; (2) malabsorption, e.g. failure of the apoferritin–ferritin transport system or gut disease; (3) inadequate utilisation, e.g. failure of the transferrin transport system; (4) not indicated, increased demand, e.g. failure of the transferrin transport system; (4) not indicated, increased demand, e.g. menstruation, chronic blood loss, pregnancy.

The total body iron is about 50 mg kg^{-1} (male) and 35 mg kg^{-1} (female). Of this amount, about 5% is *fixed*, that is, present in enzymes such as cytochromes, catalase and myoglobin and not available for haemoglobin synthesis. Another 25% is in *storage* as ferritin in the reticuloendothelial system and hepatocytes; the major part of the iron (70%) is in the form of haemoglobin in red blood cells in general circulation or bone marrow.

Administration

Iron is commonly taken orally as ferrous gluconate. Mild side effects, mainly gastrointestinal upset, are common.

As they are sugar coated, iron tablets are frequently ingested accidentally by young children; this can give rise to severe posioning with bleeding in different parts of the body and haemorrhagic shock. The absorption of large amounts of iron into the plasma overloads the storage protein, transferrin, and the metal precipitates out of solution and becomes deposited in different organs, particularly the liver. The resulting hepatoxicity can cause coma and death. In iron poisoning, treatment must be prompt with gastric lavage or raw egg administered to precipitate the iron as albuminate, or sodium bicarbonate solution to precipitate ferric carbonate. Intravenous *desferrioxamine* may be given to chelate iron and facilitate its excretion.

Iron preparations are also available for parenteral administration for cases where iron deficiency is due to malabsorption, i.e. where the apoferritin–ferritin carrier mechanism is faulty. Examples are iron sorbitol for i.m. or iron dextran for i.v. administration.

22.3   MEGALOBLASTIC ANAEMIAS

These are caused by deficiency of folic acid and vitamin B$_{12}$. These vitamins are needed for the synthesis of DNA; their deficiency shows up in defective DNA in those tissues with the greatest rate of cell turnover, e.g. the haemopoietic system; deficiency of the vitamins gives rise to megaloblastic anaemia, characterised by abnormal macrocytic red blood cells.

Folic acid deficiencies

The normal diet (including green vegetables) is an adequate source of folic acid. Deficiency can occur in malnutrition; in chronic haemolytic anaemia such as may be caused by drugs (primaquine in G6PD deficiency), there is increased demand for the vitamin. Even when dietary folic acid is adequate, dihydrofolate reductase inhibitors used in the treatment of bacterial or parasitic infections (trimethoprim, pyrimethamine) or cancer (methotrexate), can cause megaloblastic anaemias by preventing the conversion of folic acid to folinic acid; this latter is the form in which folic acid can act as a coenzyme for one-carbon transfers in the synthesis of purines and nucleotides. To correct blood disorders caused by such drugs, give folinic acid (5-formyltetra-hydrofolic acid) rather than folic acid which would nullify the chemotherapeutic action of the drug (see section 12.6). Another point which was made previously (section 20.2) is that folic acid is required as a cofactor in the hydroxylation reaction for the inactivation of many drugs. Such drugs, e.g. phenytoin, debrisoquine, when used in large doses for prolonged periods can cause folic acid depletion and folate deficiency anaemias.

Vitamin B_{12} deficiencies

The main source of vitamin B_{12} is animal byproducts in the diet, and synthesis of the vitamin by bacteria in the intestinal lumen. The bacterial source is probably the reason vegetarians do not always suffer from vitamin B_{12} deficiency.

Vitamin B_{12} (cyanocobalamin) functions as a coenzyme in the complex biochemical processes involved in erythropoiesis. This vitamin, also referred to as the *extrinsic factor*, cannot be absorbed from the gut unless an *intrinsic factor*, a mucoprotein made by the parietal cells of the stomach mucosa, is present. In pernicious anaemia, the intrinsic factor is lacking, hence there is failure of vitamin B_{12} absorption even when the dietary content of the vitamin is adequate. In the intestinal lumen, vitamin B_{12} combines with intrinsic factor to form a complex from which B_{12} is translocated into the bloodstream. Here the vitamin binds to a plasma β-globulin for transportation to the liver and other tissues (see legend to Fig. 22.2 for details of defects which can give rise to B_{12} deficiency).

Treatment of pernicious anaemia

In classical pernicious anameia, B_{12} deficiency is due to impairment in the production of intrinsic factor by gastric mucosa. Associated with this is gastric achlorhydria which is an indirect diagnosis of pernicious anaemia (achlorhydria, the inability of the parietal cells of the gastric mucosa to secret hydrochloric acid, is diagnosed by the augmented Kays test, see section 24.7). The Schilling test is a direct method for assessing the ability of the gut to absorb vitamin B_{12}. Radiolabelled B_{12} is given orally, followed immediately by parenteral non-radioactive vitamin to encourage excretion; lack of radioactivity in the urine indicates defective intestinal absorption.

To treat pernicious anaemia or vitamin B_{12} deficiencies caused by other forms of malabsorption, give parenteral cyanocobalamin or hydroxocobalamin (this is more highly bound to plasma protein and longer acting).

Vitamin B_{12} deficiency can result in irreversible damage to the nervous system manifesting in a *subacute combined degeneration of the spinal cord*; this involves demyelination and cell death in the spinal column causing a whole range of neurological disorders. Parenteral hydroxocobalamin will correct this syndrome, but it should not be given with folic acid. Although this latter vitamin and B_{12} act synergistically to correct the haematological manifestations due to vitamin B_{12} deficiency, they are antagonistic when it comes to the formation of myelin.

Fig. 22.2. Absorption and distribution of vitamin B_{12} in man. Deficiency of the vitamin can occur as a result of: (1) dietary deficiency; (2) inadequate formation of intrinsic factor (Int.F); (3) bowel diseases which may prevent Int.F-B_{12} complex from attaching to suitable sites for the translocation of B_{12} to blood; (4) deficiency of the carrier protein, transcobalamin (TeII) for the transfer of B_{12} to liver stores and other tissues; (5) enterohepatic circulation involving 5 μg B_{12} daily may be affected by intestinal disease causing a depletion of hepatic stores; (6) folic acid deficiency can affect B_{12} uptake into tissue cells and its conversion to methyl B_{12} and utilisation.

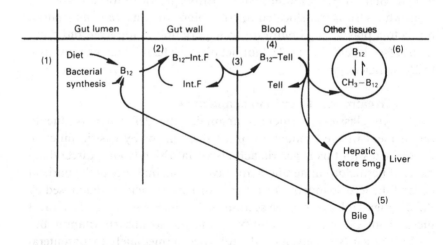

22.4 BLOOD COAGULATION

Blood coagulation is the spontaneous clotting of blood which arrests bleeding from damaged blood vessels. It involves platelet adhesion to exposed collagen in the damaged vessel wall, and platelet aggregation. The platelet plug so formed plus fibrin prevent further bleeding. Haemostasis (thrombogenesis) is the occlusion of a blood vessel by a clot (thrombus) under pathological conditions. The formation of a thrombus and the pathological conditions associated with haemostasis are of such clinical significance that it is important to understand the salient features in the mechanism of blood coagulation and the drugs used to prevent it. The events leading to blood coagulation consist of processes involving platelets and those involving blood coagulation factors.

Platelet aggregation

The adhesion of platelet to a damaged vessel wall or its interaction with collagen, thrombin, PAF (platelet aggregating factor) or ADP can set off the *release action*, i.e. the platelet releases the following pharmacologically active substances:

(a) ADP (adenosine diphosphate) induces other platelets to aggregate and to release ADP.

(b) 5-Hydroxytryptamine (5-HT) induces further aggregation.

(c) Thromboxane synthetase converts products of arachidonic acid metabolism to thromboxane A_2 (TxA_2) (see also Chapter 24). TxA_2 is a potent inducer of platelet aggregation and vasoconstriction. Stable prostaglandins (PGE_2 or PGE_1) are also formed but these may not be important in the aggregation process. *In situ*, platelets do not adhere to blood vessels and clotting does not normally occur because healthy vascular endothelium contains the enzyme prostacylin synthetase which makes prostacyclin (PGI_2) from arachidonic acid. PGI_2 is a powerful inhibitor of platelet aggregation and vasodilator.

Knowledge of the specific pathways in the metabolism of arachidonic acid is being exploited to develop anti-aggregatory agents. Aspirin is being promoted as an antithrombotic agent. In low doses, aspirin inhibits cyclooxygenase in platelets, but not in vascular endothelium; thus TxA_2 but not PGI_2, formation is reduced. Aspirin may also inhibit the release process described above. Dazoxiben, a specific inhibitor of thromboxane synthetase, is also being tested clinically as an antithrombotic agent. Prostacyclin (epoprostenol) and its more stable derivatives are also undergoing clinical trials for the treatment of thromboembolic conditions.

Blood coagulation factors

Several factors in blood that are required for coagulation to occur are formed in the liver from vitamin K. Examples of these are:

Factor I (fibrinogen), II (prothrombin), IX (Christmas factor), X (Stuart factor), XI (plasma thromboplastin antecedent), and XII (Hageman factor). All these factors play specific but interrelated roles in blood coagulation; drugs have been developed which owe their anticoagulant actions to interference with the actions of these factors. A critical step in coagulation is the conversion of prothrombin (factor II) to thrombin which then converts soluble fibrinogen (factor I) to insoluble fibrin (factors I' and I") which forms the meshwork of the clot. Calcium ion (factor IV) is required for this reaction.

Anticoagulants

Some of these act only on blood factors; herapin (prevents the conversion of prothrombin to thrombin as well as the action of thrombin in converting fibrinogen to insoluble fibrin) and calcium ion chelators, e.g. sodium citrate, sodium edetate (prevent the above reactions by removing calcium).

Herapin is a mucopolysaccharide containing negatively charged acidic groups. In nature, heparin is stored in mast cells complexed to histamine. Heparin in clinical use is extracted from animal sources and is given parenterally in the treatment of thrombotic conditions. It can also be used *in vitro* in extracorporal circuits such as heart–lung machines and in animal experimentation. The onset of action of heparin is virtually instantaneous; its action also is brief because of rapid breakdown. If an antidote is required, protamine, a strongly positively charged protein can be given.

The calcium chelators are used only *in vitro* to prevent blood coagulation as in blood stored for transfusion and for preservation of laboratory blood specimens.

Oral anticoagulants

The typical example of this class of drugs is warfarin (see Fig. 22.3). The discovery of warfarin came from the observation in the USA that cattle fed on spoiled clover (a sort of fodder) suffered a haemorrhagic disease. The disease was due to a reduction in plasma prothrombin concentration and the causative agent was ultimately identified as dicoumarol.

Warfarin is a coumarin derivative and structurally related to vitamin K which it antagonises in the production of prothrombin *in the liver*. Another group of oral anticoagulants derived from indan1,3-dione, e.g. phenindione (shown in Fig. 22.3) are more toxic than the coumarin derivatives and are now virtually obsolete for human use. Warfarin depresses the formation of Factors II, VII, IX, and X; but as Factor II (prothrombin) has the longest half life its reduction is the most significant for practical purposes. The prothrombin level is monitored as the indicator of warfarin action; this is important as warfarin has a low therapeutic index and overdosage can give rise to fatal haemorrhage.

There are two important points to note about warfarin:

(1) The drug acts only in the liver to block the formation of coagulation factors; consequently, its onset of action is delayed for 8–12 h after oral or intravenous administration. This is the time required for coagulation factors in circulation to be used up. It may take a further 3 days for the peak effect of a given dose to be reached. On the other hand, after cessation of therapy, the prothrombin levels and clotting time may take several days to return to normal. Thus anticoagulant therapy is particularly complex and should be undertaken only where facilities for monitoring prothrombin time can be assured.

(2) Many drugs can interact with the oral anticoagulants adversely to increase or decrease the effect of a given dose. This comes from the fact that the safety margin for the drug is relatively low so that its plasma

Fig. 22.3. Structures of some oral anticoagulants.

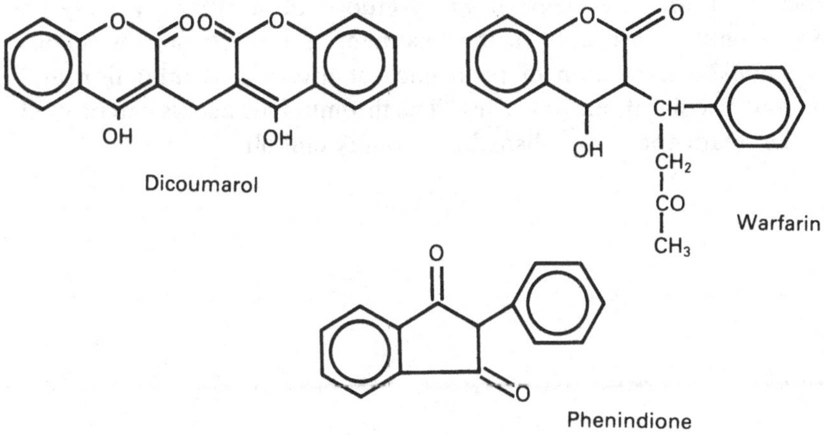

Dicoumarol

Warfarin

Phenindione

concentration must be closely controlled. Examples of drug–warfarin interactions are:

(a) Tetracyclines decrease the synthesis of vitamin K, and liquid paraffin decreases the absorption of vitamin K from the gut; both can *increase* the effect of warfarin. On the other hand cholestyramine *decreases* the absorption of warfarin and its effects.

(b) Rifampicin and barbiturates induce liver microsomal enzyme metabolism of warfarin and *decrease* its effects, whereas allopurinol and cimetidine by decreasing liver enzyme activity *increase* its effects.

(c) Ninety-nine per cent of warfarin is bound to plasma protein. Many commonly used drugs, by displacing warfarin from binding sites, can *increase* its effective plasma concentration several-fold and cause haemorrhage. Examples of such drugs are aspirin, indomethacin, clofibrate and phenylbutazone.

(d) Aspirin and clofibrate can *increase* the anticoagulant effects of warfarin by two other mechanisms; by an additive effect in inhibiting liver production of clotting factors and, peripherally, by inhibiting platelet aggregation (see above).

Thrombolytic drugs

These are used to promote the dissolution of a thrombus; their mode of action is to stimulate the conversion of plasminogen to the proteolytic enzyme plasmin, which hydrolyses fibrin. Examples are *streptokinase* and *urokinase*. These drugs are also known as fibrinolytic agents. Their main indication is in the treatment of pulmonary embolism. They are expensive and toxic. *Aminocaproic acid* is an antidote used for treatment of an overdose of a fibrinolytic agent. Anticoagulants are used in the treatment and prevention of venous thrombosis, prevention of recurrence of myocardial infarction and cerebrovascular disease (strokes). The thrombolytic agents can be used in the treatment of established pulmonary emboli.

23

Endocrine system

Section 23.1, 23.2, 23.4, parts of 23.6 and 23.8 originated from drafts kindly provided by Dr Ebere Nduka, Postgraduate Institute for Medical Research, College of Medicine, University of Ibadan.

23.1 INTRODUCTION

Endocrine glands are ductless and their secretions are delivered internally into the bloodstream. A hormone is defined as a chemical substance that is released by an endocrine gland into the blood in minute amounts and which can elicit a typical physiological response in other cells (local hormones are discussed in Chapter 24). The endocrine glands have been developed to produce an integration of regulatory mechanisms which ensure a coordinated operation of the body as a unit, for example in the control of energy production, of the digestive tract and its component parts, growth and development, composition and volume of body fluids, reproduction, and adaptation to the environment.

Hormones can be classified in terms of their chemical nature, e.g. hormones derived from aminoacids (polypeptides, catecholamines and thyroid hormones) and hormones derived from the steroid nucleus (corticosteroids). Alternatively, they may be classified in terms of physiological function, e.g. control of intermediary metabolism and growth (insulin, glucagon, cortisol, growth hormone); trophic hormones (adrenocorticotrophic hormones, thyroid-stimulating hormone); or hormones that regulate mineral and water metabolism (aldosterone).

23.2 CONTROL OF HORMONE SECRETION

Hormone release may be controlled by one or more of the following mechanisms; (a) feedback controls – the amount of hormone in circulation determines the secretory activity of the gland (Fig. 23.1); (b) Circadian rhythms; (c) other stimuli, e.g. glucose, temperature; (d) other hormones – trophic (stimulatory or inhibitory).

Feedback control of hormone secretion

Under normal circumstances, once a hormone has carried out its physiological function, its rate of secretion begins to diminish. This is due to the operation of a system (see also noradrenergic mechanisms) whereby, once the normal physiological effect of the hormone has been achieved, information is sent back to the producing gland to check further secretion. If on the other hand, the gland undersecretes, the physiological effect of the hormone is reduced; then the inhibitory feedback control decreases, causing the gland to secrete more of the hormone. Thus the feedback system helps to control the rate of secretion of each hormone in accordance with physiological needs for it (the principle is illustrated in Fig. 23.1).

23.3   MECHANISM OF HORMONE ACTION

Hormones act through receptors which are either membrane-bound (cell-surface receptors, e.g. insulin, growth hormone) or bound

Fig. 23.1. Diagrammatic representation of the principle of a feedback control in hormone release. An endocrine gland (E) produces a hormone (b) which acts on a peripheral cell (C) to influence its activity e.g. the secretion of another hormone. This in turn acts on the endocrine gland (E) to inhibit its production of the hormone (b). In some cases (e.g., secretion of antidiuretic hormone) involving the hypothalamus (HPT), the feedback mechanism includes a hormone release–stimulating or inhibiting factor (a) produced by the hypothalamus whose concentration in plasma determines whether the gland shall release more or less (b). The dashed line represents the feedback mechanism to the hypothalamus. The feedback can be negative (−) or positive (+).

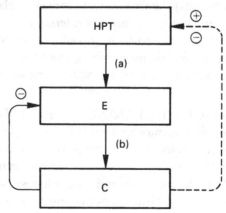

to intracellular structures (i.e., cytosolic receptors, e.g. thyroxine, steroid hormones).

Interaction of hormone with membrane or subcellular receptor may be by two mechanisms: (i) alter membrane permeability or activate transport mechanisms across the membrane. For example, insulin promotes entry of glucose into muscle cells. (ii) it may induce the formation of second messengers which in turn may lead to a cascade of reactions. A number of second messengers have been identified. For example; (a) hormone–receptor combination may activate *adenylate cyclase*. This leads to the production of cyclic AMP and once formed, the cyclic AMP triggers the hormonal effect in the cell. Thus cyclic AMP is an intercellular hormonal mediator and second messenger. (b) the combination may activate *phosphoinositol hydrolysis*. The key reaction of this transducing mechanism is a receptor-mediated hydrolysis of the phosphoinositides to give two products – diacylglycerol and inositol triphosphate both of which may function as second messengers to initiate suitable signals. Inositol triphosphate seems to act by mobilising intracellular calcium, whereas diacylglycerol stimulates protein phosphorylation.

23.4   MEASUREMENT OF HORMONES

Hormone concentrations in plasma are often needed to be known to establish a diagnosis as well as in establishing the role of a particular hormone in a given physiological process. Hormone concentrations can be determined by bioassay, chemical assay, or immunoassay.

(1) Bioassay (see Chapter 3)

An example of this type of assay is the rat uterine weight bioassay for estradiol. The increase in weight of the immature rat uterus in response to injections given subcutaneously twice daily for 4 or 5 days is proportional to the amount of estradiol injected. The advantage of the bioassay method is that it measures the biological activity of the hormone, while its disadvantage is that it is cumbersome, expensive, and less sensitive than radioimmunoassay.

(2) Radioimmunoassay (RIA)

The principle of radioimmunoassay is based on the reaction between antigen and its specific antibodies. A sample which contains an unknown amount of the hormone to be assayed (antigenic substance) is incubated with a known amount of the radioactively-labelled hormone and a constant amount of antiserum (antibody) specific to the hormone. The amount of the antiserum (antibody) is chosen so that there is sufficient to bind some but not all of the radioactive hormone. The unlabelled and labelled hormone (antigens) compete for antibody-binding sites so that the greater the amount of unlabelled hormone the less is the amount of tracer bound to the antiserum (antibody). The amount of radioactivity precipitated will be proportional to the concentration of the hormone in the test samples. The concentration of the hormone in the unknown samples is obtained by comparing the amount of tracer bound to the antiserum with the values obtained for standard solutions of the hormone.

Radioimmunoassay is a precise, specific, and exquisitely sensitive measurement of heretofore unmeasurable hormone levels. This has been made possible by the sensitivity element introduced through radiochemistry and the specificity element introduced through immunology.

23.5   PHARMACOLOGICAL ASPECTS OF INDIVIDUAL ENDOCRINE SYSTEMS

Hypofunction (i.e., undersecretion as in Addison's disease) and hyperfunction (i.e., oversecretion of hormones as in Cushing's syndrome) of endocrine glands give rise to characteristic diseases. Drug treatment entails either replacement of the undersecreted hormone (replacement therapy) or in the case of hyperfunction, the use of drugs which block the action of the secreted hormone or which reduce the secretory activity of the gland. An understanding of the biological activity of the hormones secreted by the major endocrine glands is therefore essential. Pharmacological properties of synthetic compounds used in the treatment of diseases arising from malfunction of the endocrine systems are also described in the following sections.

23.6   ADRENOCORTICOID HORMONES (ADRENOCORTICOSTEROIDS)

The major adrenocorticosteroids secreted by the adrenal cortex are cortisol, corticosterone and aldosterone (Fig. 23.2). The synthesis of these hormones is stimulated by adrenocorticotrophic hormone (ACTH) secreted by the adenohypophysis. A number of weakly androgenic hormones are also secreted by the adrenal cortex. The corticosteroids in turn exert an inhibitory effect on the ACTH secretory activity of the adenohypophysis. This feedback loop thus ensures a fine control on the level of adrenocorticosteroids in circulation and on the activity of the adrenal cortex. A persistently high level of steroids in circulation (e.g., when used in the treatment of inflammation) can cause the adrenal cortex to atrophy due to inhibition of ACTH secretion.

ACTH itself is a peptide with 39 aminoacid residues. The various pharmacological actions of ACTH are due to corticosteroids induced by it. Therefore, in the sections that follow, the pharmacological properties of only the natural and some synthetic corticosteroids are described. The drugs are classified in terms of their effects on the metabolism of carbohydrate, fat and protein (glucocorticoids) or electrolyte and water (mineralocorticoids). There is much overlap in the glucocorticoid and mineralocorticoid components of the different drugs. Therefore drugs classified as glucocorticoids are those possessing this kind of activity at a high level relative to mineralocorticoid

Fig. 23.2. Structures for cortisol (hydrocortisone), corticosterone and aldosterone.

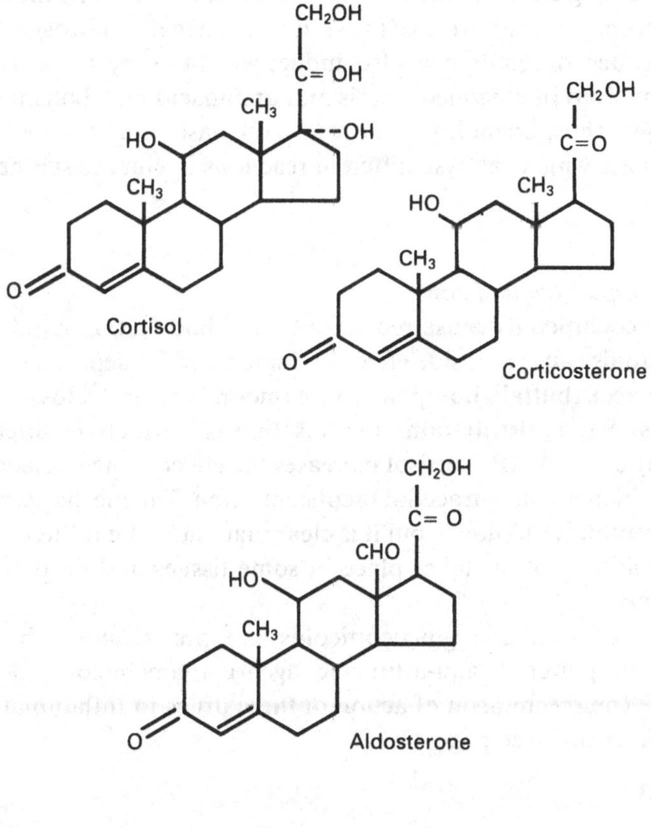

activity and vice versa. Table 23.1 shows the potencies of different corticosteroids relative to hydrocortisone on some selected parameters.

Glucocorticoids

The type substance with glucocorticoid activity secreted by the adrenal cortex is hydrocortisone (cortisol) (see Table 23.1). The following are typical glucocorticoid actions. Note the consequent unwanted effects that accompany the therapeutic use of this group of drugs.

(1) Carbohydrate and protein metabolism

Glucocorticoids promote *gluconeogenesis*; this is the formation of glucose from aminoacids. They do this in two ways. (i) The hormones mobilise aminoacids from a number of tissues such as lymphatic, muscle and skin. These are used by the liver to form glucose and glycogen; glucocorticoids also stimulate the deposition of glycogen in the liver, reduce peripheral usage of glucose, and reduce glucose uptake; hence they may raise blood sugar. One effect of long-term large-dose glucocorticoids therapy therefore is reduced mass of muscle, osteoporosis, thinning of the skin, and a negative nitrogen balance. (ii) Glucocorticoids can also induce synthesis by the liver of enzymes involved in gluconeogenesis and aminoacid metabolism, e.g. the enzymes phosphoenolpyruvate carboxykinase, and fructose-1,6-diphosphatase, which catalyse different reactions in glucose synthesis, are induced.

(2) Lipid metabolism

Glucocorticoids cause redistribution of body fat. Large doses of these steroids cause as a side effect, an increase in fat deposits in the back of the neck (buffalo hump) and face (moon face) and a loss of fat from limbs. Fat redistribution involves lipolysis which is directly mediated by cyclic AMP. Cortisol increases the effect of the nucleotide rather than increase its intracellular concentration. The mechanism of fat redistribution is unknown, but it is clear that under the influence of glucocorticoids, lypolysis takes place in some tissues and fat deposition in others.

Examples of synthetic glucocorticoids are prednisolone, beclomethasone (a powerful anti-asthmatic agent), triamcinolone, dexamethasone. The mechanism of action of these drugs in inflammation has been described (see page 436).

Table 23.1 *Relative activities of some corticosteroids*

Corticosteroids	Sodium retention (a)	Liver glycogen deposition (b)	Anti-inflammatory effect
Natural products			
Hydrocortisone	+	+	+
Cortisone	+	+	+
Corticosterone	++	0	0
Aldosterone	+++	0	0
Synthetic products			
Prednisolone	0	+++	+++
Triamicinolone	0	+++	+++

Key: +++, extremely active; ++, very active; +, active; 0, moderate to insignificant activity.

(a) Mineralocorticoid, and (b) glucocorticoid parameters.

Important uses of glucocorticoids

The use of glucocorticoids is indicated in the following instances:

(i) Topically in, e.g. allergic conjunctivitis and local inflammatory conditions. Note that when used in the eye, glucocorticoids may aid the spread of infections and cause increased intraocular pressure.

(ii) In replacement therapy (glucocorticoids plus mineralocorticoids) of acute or chronic adrenal insufficiency (Addison's disease).

(iii) In bronchial asthma (see Chapter 24).

(iv) In inflammatory conditions, e.g. rheumatoid arthritis.

(v) As immunosuppressant, e.g. in autoimmune conditions and transplantation reactions.

(vi) In cancer (see page 288).

Mineralocorticoids

The classical mineralocorticoids secreted by the adrenal cortex are *aldosterone* and *deoxycorticosterone*. These corticosteroids are virtually devoid of any glucocorticoid activity. They act on the distal tubules of the kidney to enhance the reabsorption of Na^+, and increase the urinary excretion of K^+ and H^+. Consequently, characteristic features of adrenal cortex hyperfunction include increase in weight and arterial blood pressure due to Na^+ and water retention (the blood pressure effect is also enhanced by increased sensitivity of blood vessels to circulating catecholamines due to their blockade of uptake₂ by corticosteroids), hypokalaemia, and alkalosis. Another effect of overactivity of mineralocorticoids is that K^+ loss from the body can give rise to decreased insulin release which may then exacerbate an incipient diabetic condition, made worse by the action of glucocorticoids (see above).

In contrast, in adrenocortical insufficiency (Addison's disease), the reverse conditions prevail. There are excessive sodium loss (hyponatraemia), hyperkalaemia and contraction of the extracellular fluid volume. In Addison's disease, more sodium is lost than water from the extracellular fluid through the kidney. Therefore the extracellular fluid becomes hypoosmotic. Water moves from the extracellular to the intracellular compartment. The red blood cells are hydrated. This, plus the loss of water in the kidney, results in a marked reduction in the volume of the extracellular fluid. This may lead to circulatory collapse, renal failure and death. Treatment of Addison's disease involves the use of mineralocorticoids.

Mechanism of action of mineralocorticoids in stimulating Na^+ reabsorption

Aldosterone is the most potent mineralocorticoid secreted by the adrenal cortex. Its actions in transporting epithelia (toad bladder and frog skin) have been studied extensively using the short circuit current preparation of Hans Ussing. It is proposed that aldosterone, after combining with a membrane receptor, induces the synthesis of a protein which then facilitates the transport of sodium ions. Morphologically and functionally, the epithelial cells of the distal tubule are asymmetric (Fig. 23.3), that is, they have two distinct membrane domains – apical (the cell membrane facing the tubular lumen) and basolateral or serosal (the cell membrane in contact with extracellular fluid). The epithelial cell is described as asymmetric because the enzymes, ion pumps, ion channels, and drug receptors located in the apical membrane are quite different from those in the serosal surfaces of the membrane. Part of the evidence for asymmetry is the 'sidedness' of the response to drugs in transporting epithelia. For example, in amphibian urinary bladder or skin short circuit current preparations, the sodium channel blocker, amiloride rapidly blocks sodium transport when applied to the apical membrane, but is ineffective on the basolateral side. During sodium reabsorption, sodium ions in the tubular filtrate enter the cells of the tubular epithelium down a concentration gradient through the apical domain. At the interface between the serosal surface and the extracellular fluid compartment, the sodium ions are pumped out of the cell against a concentration gradient by an energy-requiring pump similar to Na^+/K^+–ATPase. Two theories are used to explain the action of mineralocorticoids on this model. The 'permease' theory holds that the drugs increase the permeability of the apical membrane to sodium ions, while according to the 'pump' theory the action of aldosterone is at the basolateral side where the drug activates or increases the pump activity by providing additional energy to drive it.

The mechanism by which aldosterone enhances the excretion of potassium and hydrogen ions is not known, but probably involves exchange with sodium.

Fig. 23.3. Diagrammatic representation of tubular epithelial cells separated by tight junctions, tj : (a), apical, and (b), basolateral, domains. Na^+ ions enter the cells through (i) down a concentration gradient--➤, and are pumped out through (ii) by ATPase, ———➤. Aldosterone increases – – –➤ (permease theory) or ———➤ (pump theory) (see text).

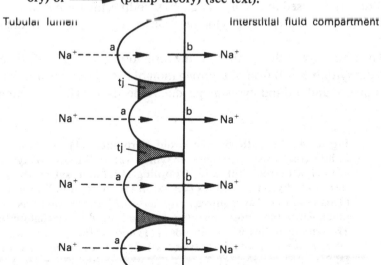

Thyroid hormones and antithyroid drugs

The main function of the thyroid gland is the maintenance of optimal metabolic activity in all tissues; this it does through the activity of the hormones it secretes.

Biosynthesis of thyroid hormones

The thyroid gland is unique in having a large quantity of the precursor material for the synthesis of its hormones stored in the gland in the form of a complex glycoprotein called *thyroglobulin* (TG). Iodinated tyrosine residues of TG constitute the thyroid hormones which are made as shown in Fig. 23.4. The following points should be noted.

Uptake of iodide

Thyroid gland takes up iodide from plasma against a concentration gradient; thyroid to plasma iodide ratios of up to 100 are possible. Ability to concentrate iodide however is not unique to the thyroid gland. Other glands, e.g. salivary gland, gut mucosa, mammary gland, or placenta can also concentrate the ion (the latter two for the benefit of the foetus). Iodide uptake by the thyroid gland is inhibited by perchlorate and thiocyanate (note the point that dietary cyanide in cassava meals raises plasma thiocyanate and hence affects thyroid function) and by certain drugs as side effects, e.g. phenylbutazone. Uptake is stimulated by TSH and controlled by an autoregulatory mechanism.

Iodide is oxidised in the thyroid gland to iodine, the form in which it is used to iodinate tyrosine. This reaction is catalysed by peroxidase enzyme.

The next stage in the synthesis is the formation of *thyroxine* (T4) and triiodothyronine (T3) from the conjugation of two diiodotyrosines or a monoiodo- and a diiodotyrosine residue respectively. These reactions

Fig. 23.4. Biosynthesis of thyroid hormones. (1) Oxidation of iodide (requires peroxidase enzyme). (2) Iodination of tyrosyl groups of thyroglobulin. (3) Coupling of iodotyrosyl residues to form iodothyronyl residues (T3, T4) in the thyroglobulin protein. (This reaction also requires peroxidase.) All these reactions take place while the tyrosyl residues remain bound to thyroglobulin. The release of the thyroid hormones (T3 and T4) from thyroglobulin takes place by proteolysis (see text). MIT = monoiodotyrosine; DIT = diiodotyrosine; T3 = triiodothyronine; rT3 = 3, 3, 5-triiodothyronine; T4 = tetraiodothyronine (thyroxine).

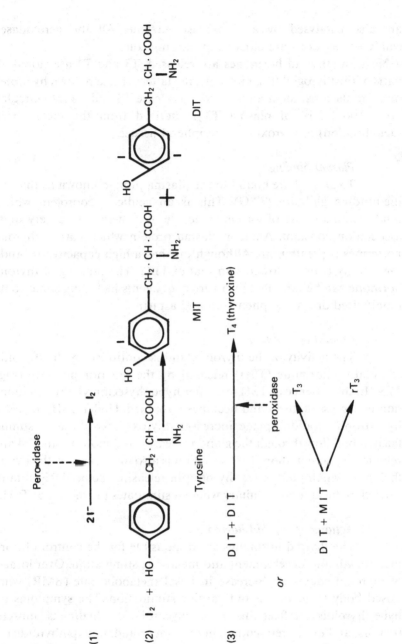

(1) $2I^- \xrightarrow{\text{Peroxidase}} I_2$

(2) $I_2 + $ Tyrosine $\longrightarrow$ MIT $+$ DIT

(3) $DIT + DIT \xrightarrow{\text{peroxidase}} T_4 \text{ (thyroxine)}$

or

$DIT + MIT \longrightarrow T_3 \quad rT_3$

are also catalysed by a peroxidase enzyme. All the peroxidase-catalysed reactions are blocked by carbimazole.

Next, the thyroid hormones are released. T3 and T4 are stored as parts of the thyroglobulin molecule; the latter is broken down by proteolysis to its constituent aminoacids to release T3 and T4 into circulation. About 30% of plasma T3 is derived from the metabolism (deiodination) of thyroxine in peripheral tissues.

Plasma binding

T3 and T4 are bound to the plasma protein known as thyroxine-binding globulin (TBG). This is an acidic glycoprotein which binds one molecule of T4 per molecule of protein with a very high association constant. Another plasma protein which carries thyroid hormones is prealbumin. Although this has a high capacity, its binding affinity is much lower than that of TBG. The binding of thyroid hormone can be inhibited by a variety of agents including some commonly used drugs, e.g. phenytoin and aspirin.

Control of secretion

The activity of the thyroid gland is controlled by the thyroid-stimulating hormone (TSH) released by the anterior pituitary (Fig. 23.5). In the absence of TSH (e.g. after hypophysectomy), thyroid function is depressed; the gland becomes atrophied. Under TSH, the cells hypertrophy, iodide uptake increases, thyroxine synthesis is stimulated, blood flow through the gland increases, and more T3 and T4 are released into circulation. TSH secretion is also influenced by the hypothalamus which produces a thyrotropin-releasing factor (TRF) that is carried to the anterior pituitary where it stimulates the release of TSH.

Actions of thyroid hormones

The thyroid hormones are responsible for the control of normal growth and development and metabolic stimulation. Overdosage of thyroxin causes an increase in basal metabolic rate (BMR) with raised body temperature and cardiac stimulation. The symptoms of hyperthyroidism reflect this, i.e. tachycardia, dysrhythmias, muscle tremors, and eyelid retraction. On the other hand, in hypothyroidism, there is bradycardia and a prolongation of cardiac action potential. There is evidence that these effects involve adrenoceptors. The cardiac symptoms and muscle tremors of hyperthyroidism can be controlled by beta-adrenoceptor blockers and the lid retraction by guanethidine. There is also the pharmacologically interesting suggestion that in hypothyroidism there is interconversion of beta₁-to alpha-adreno-ceptors in the myocardium. Propanolol and other beta-blockers can prevent the conversion of T4 to T3 in peripheral tissue.

The role of the sympathetic function in hyperthyroidism is contro-versial; for instance, diarrhoea is a characteristic feature of hyper-thyroidism, but diarrhoea also accompanies sympathetic blockade with, e.g. guanethidine. T3 is about 4 times as active as T4, but the latter is longer-acting. T4 (L-thyroxine) is the usual form of thyroid hormone therapy.

Disorders of thyroid function and their treatment
(a) *Hypothyroidism*

may result from a variety of congenital disorders such as athyrotic cretinism (failure of the gland to develop) and defects in hor-mone synthesis.

(1) *Cretinism* When deficiency occurs at birth, it produces cretinism; early signs are puffy expressionless face, short extremities, poor appetite, low body temperature, and slow pulse rate. If untreated,

Fig. 23.5. Negative feedback control of thyroid function – hypo-thalamopituitary axis. Thyroid hormones (T₃, T₄) exert a direct negative feedback on the anterior pituitary (AP) to diminish the secretion of thyroid stimulting hormone (TSH). Thyroid hor-mones also exert a negative feedback inhibition on the hypothal-amus (HPT) to reduce secretion of thyrotropin-releasing factor (TRF). (−) = inhibition; (+) = stimulation.

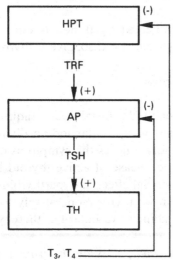

there is retardation in growth and development. Treatment consists in replacement therapy with L-thyroxine (give the highest possible dose without the symptoms of hyperthyroidism). Cretinism can be successfully treated if detected early.

(2) *Myxoedema.* In the adult, severe thyroid hypofunction gives rise to myxoedema characterised by marked retardation of mental and physical activity. Treat with L-thyroxine (give lowest dose which relieves the symptoms).

(b) *Hyperthyroidism*

This results from the excessive production of thyroid hormones; the commonest type is thyrotoxic goitre (Graves' disease). The cause is not known; but the hyperfunction of the gland is associated with the presence of thyroid-stimulating immunoglobulins such as LATS (long-acting thyroid-stimulating substance), LATS protector, and human thyroid stimulator.

The paradox that there is goitre *and* a hyperfunctioning gland is resolved by the fact that LATS is produced by lymphoid tissue and not subject to negative feedback mechanisms. There is in fact low plasma TSH concentration in Graves' disease. Symptoms include weight loss, increased appetite, heat intolerance, perspiration, tachycardia, dysrhythmias, skeletal muscle tremors, muscle weakness, and eyelid retraction. As already pointed out, beta-adrenoceptor blockers and guanethidine can be used as supporting therapy.

Treatment of hyperthyroidism
Surgery
This may be indicated, e.g. if there is a neoplasm. Surgery may be followed by hypothyroidism; if so, give L-thyroxine.

Antithyroid drugs
Iodide
The preparation used is *Lugol's Iodine* (aqueous iodine solution) given orally. It consists of molecular iodine dissolved in potassium iodide solution. It rapidly relieves the symptoms of hyperthyroidism. Iodide ions prevent the release of active thyroid hormones (T3, T4) into the blood. Its beneficial effect in hyperthyroidism is short-lasting (about 2 weeks). It can be used preoperatively to reduce thyrotoxic symptoms and the gland's vascularity, thereby making surgery safer.

Potassium perchlorate and potassium thiocyanate prevent iodide ion uptake by the gland, but they are too toxic to be of therapeutic value. The more active perchlorate causes aplastic anaemia.

Carbimazole

This is a thiourea derivative and the most widely used antithyroid drug. It inhibits the synthesis of T3 and T4 by blocking the peroxidase enzyme. By reducing plasma levels of T3 and T4, carbimazole decreases the negative feedback of thyroid hormones on the hypothalamo–pituitary axis. This increases the secretion of TSH and can result in an enlarged gland (goitre). This effect can be prevented by the concomitant administration of a small dose of L-thyroxine. Carbimazole crosses the placental barrier and is excreted in milk and can produce goitre in the foetus or infant.

Radioactive iodine (I^{131})

I^{131}, with a half like of 8 days, is the most useful iodine isotope. It is taken up by the thyroid gland where it irradiates the secretory cells with mainly beta-rays (penetration of only 2 mm) and a small amount of gamma-rays (with greater penetration). This leads to inhibition of thyroid glandular activity. Treatment with I^{131} can cause hypothyroidism which may be corrected with L-thyroxine. The use of I^{131} should be avoided in men and women of reproductive age because of the possibility of germ cell mutagenicity.

23.7 HORMONAL CONTROL OF GLUCOSE METABOLISM AND ANTIDIABETIC DRUGS

Insulin and glucagon and other peptide substances are secreted by the islets of Langerhans in the pancreas. There are about 10^6 islets per pancreas and when extracted, they contain about 8 mg of insulin. There are at least 4 types of cells in the islets: alpha (A) cells secrete glucagon, beta (B) cells secrete insulin, delta (D) and PP (F) cells secrete respectively somatostatin and a pancreatic polypeptide of unknown physiological function. A constant supply of glucose is vital for the energy needs of all tissues in the body. The various actions of insulin (hypoglycaemic) and glucagon and adrenaline (hyperglycaemic) ensure that glucose is present in plasma at the right amount constantly.

Actions of insulin and glucagon

The important actions of insulin in this respect are stimulation of:

(1) Tissue uptake of glucose:
(2) Tissue utilisation of glucose;
(3) Conversion of glucose to glycogen and its storage in the liver (liver glycogenesis);
(4) A similar action to (3) in skeletal muscle;
(5) Anti-gluconeogenesis;
(6) Lipogenesis (formation of fat from free fatty acids).

These actions of insulin tend to reduce blood sugar level.

On the other hand, glucagon acts as follows:
(1) It decreases liver and muscle glycogenesis;
(2) Stimulates glycogenolysis;
(3) Stimulates gluconeogenesis;
(4) Decreases lipogenesis.

These actions of glucagon tend to raise the blood sugar level.

Together these two functionally opposite hormones plus others, e.g., adrenaline, exert a fine control on blood sugar level.

Effect of glucose on insulin release

The concentration of insulin in plasma is controlled by the concentration of glucose in the plasma perfusing the pancreas. Glucose directly stimulates the release of insulin; there can be up to a 10-fold increase in plasma concentration of insulin after eating food (this can be blocked by dinitrophenol, but not puromycin which inhibits insulin synthesis). If glucose levels remain high, insulin synthesis is also stimulated.

Mechanisms of action

Insulin influences metabolism in a wide variety of tissues; it plays key roles in metabolism of adipose tissue, muscle, and liver. It is taken up by most tissues in the body (except red blood cells). Insulin produces its various effects (see above) by binding to insulin receptors which are present on the cell membrane of most cells. A unique aspect of insulin receptors is that their numbers can decrease rapidly in the presence of high concentrations of insulin; this is known as *down regulation*; it is attributed to less synthesis or faster breakdown of receptor protein. Down regulation is present in e.g., obesity, and diabetes (decrease in response to insulin) (see below). Diminished response to insulin (insulin resistance) can also occur as a result of diminished insulin affinity for the receptor; this can be caused by glucocorticoid therapy. Another characteristic of the insulin receptor is *negative cooperativity*, i.e. as its concentration rises, the binding of insulin to its receptors diminishes, resulting in decreased sensitivity of target cells to the hormone. These two properties ensure that insulin acts at low concentrations; and overstimulation at high concentrations is prevented.

Glucagon also acts through receptors situated on the cell membrane, but the mechanism of receptor activation is different from that of insulin. While insulin can activate its receptor on the 'lock and key' principle, glucagon needs to combine with a number of sites in series (like a zip fastener). Glucagon increases intracellular cyclic AMP in liver cells and in myocardium. In the liver this results in activation of phosphorylase *a* and inactivation of glycogen synthetase. Insulin produces the opposite effects by (a) blocking glucagon production of cyclic AMP, (b) antagonising the effects of cyclic AMP, or (c) by acting through its own intermediate messengers (e.g., cyclic GMP or Ca^{2+} ions).

Diabetes mellitus

Deficiency in the production of insulin results in *diabetes mellitus* (in Nigeria this is sometimes referred to as the sugar disease; this is wrong as it gives the impression that the disease is caused by sugar in the diet of normal people). The possible causes of insulin lack are many, for example:

Production of abnormal insulin (rare);

anti-insulin receptor antibodies;

toxic effects of drugs and xenobiotics (e.g., alloxan);

destruction of the pancreas by viral infections or an auto-immune process; or

a combination of these factors.

Diabetes can also occur in Cushing's syndrome or following glucocorticoid therapy.

The effects of insulin deficiency and their consequences are listed in Table 23.2. These major metabolic problems in diabetes may progress to serious cardiovascular complications, e.g. atherosclerosis, hypertension, ischaemic heart disease, and vascular disease.

Types of diabetes

The disease is classified as (a) *juvenile onset* or (b) *maturity onset diabetes*. Juvenile onset diabetes is the more severe type, and is due to a deficiency of pancreatic beta-cell function; it is encountered in childhood.

Maturity onset diabetes develops in later life. A majority of the

Table 23.2 *Effects of insulin deficiency (or glucagon excess)*

Effect	Consequences	Remarks
(1) Decreased glucose uptake	Hyperglycaemia (high blood sugar), glycosuria (sugar in the urine), osmotic diuresis; electrolyte depletion	Dehydration
(2) Increased protein catabolism	Increased plasma amino-acids; nitrogen loss in urine	Use of these in gluconeogenesis adds to the consequences of (1)
(3) Increased lipolysis	Increased plasma free fatty acid (FFA) causing ketogenesis, ketonuria, and ketonaemia	Acidosis

patients are obese. The most probable cause is diminishing sensitivity of tissues to insulin. Presumably exposure of insulin receptors to high concentrations of insulin over a period of time causes down regulation of these receptors (see above). Secondly, the response of the beta cells to glucose is reduced. In juvenile onset diabetes, treatment consists in giving insulin and careful regulation of the carbohydrate content of food for life. In maturity onset, treatment consists of diet control, oral hypoglycaemic drugs and insulin.

Insulin preparations
Insulin for human use is obtained from pig or horse. The main disadvantage with insulin is that it must be given by injection. The following types of insulin preparations (Table 23.3) are given by s.c. injection. They are gouped as short, intermediate and long acting. Soluble insulin has the shortest onset of action of about 0.5h. In emergencies, e.g. diabetic coma, soluble insulin may be used in combination with longer-acting preparations. Other disadvantages of insulin are the following:

(a) *Hypersensitivity reactions*
These are due to antibodies to the insulin (being derived from pig/horse) or to other animal protein contaminants in the preparation.

Table 23.3 *Insulin preparations*

Type of preparation	Description	Approximate time of action (h)	
		peak	duration
Short-acting			
Soluble insulin	Crystalline insulin in aqueous solution	2	16
Insulin zinc suspension	Suspension of amorphous zinc insulin (semi-lente)	2	14
Intermediate-acting			
Globin zinc insulin	Solution of an insulin-globin complex	6	18
Isophane insulin suspension	Suspension of insulin with a protamine-zinc complex	10	24
Insulin zinc suspension	Suspension of crystalline zinc insulin (lente)	10	24
Long-acting			
Protamine zinc insulin suspension (PZI)	Suspension of an insulin-protamine zinc complex	12	36
Insulin zinc suspension (extended)	Suspension of crystalline zinc insulin (ultra-lente)	12	36

Highly purified but expensive porcine insulin may be substituted.

(b) *Hypoglycaemia*

This can occur with an overdose of insulin or in conditions which enhance the action of insulin, e.g. alcohol enhances endogenous insulin release by glucose. Hence a patient maintained on antidiabetic drugs should avoid drinking. Beta-adrenoceptor antagonists block liver and muscle glycogenolysis induced by adrenaline. This would enhance the effect of a standard treatment with insulin. Also beta-blockers prevent the tachycardia and muscle tremor which are early warning of hypoglycaemia, so the patient is unaware of impending danger. The use of beta-blockers should be avoided in the diabetic. Treatment for hypoglycaemia is glucose orally or i.v. or glucagon s.c.

(c) *Insulin resistance*

This occurs as a result of (i) antibodies formed to it , or (ii) down regulation of insulin receptors. The incidence of (a) and (c) above have reduced since the introduction of human insulin made through genetic engineering.

(d) *Hyperglycaemia*

A general point about the management of diabetes is that hyperglycaemia can occur in spite of drug treatment. This can be caused by drugs (iatrogenic), e.g. corticosteroids raise blood sugar; thiazide diuretics (also the antihypertensive thiazide diazoxide) can cause hyperglycaemia by decreasing insulin release through potassium loss.

Oral hypoglycaemic drugs

Many compounds can cause a reduction in blood glucose; the ones used in the treatment of diabetes are either sulphonylurea or biguanide derivatives. Some structures are shown in Fig. 23.6.

Sulphonylureas

These act by: (i) Releasing insulin from the beta-cells of the islet. Following administration, plasma insulin concentration rises and its content of the gland falls. Therefore the drugs must release preformed insulin, not stimulate fresh synthesis. And (ii), by increasing the sensitivity of tissues to insulin presumably by *up* regulation of insulin receptors or increasing the binding of insulin to these receptors.

Tolbutamide is short-acting with half life of about 5 h; it is bound to plasma protein and metabolised by acetylation. ·

Chlorpropamide is long-acting with a half life of about 36 h. The effect of a single dose lasts for days; it is excreted almost unchanged by the kidney. It is a difficult drug to use since plateau plasma levels take several days to establish and hypoglycaemic effects are present several days after cessation of drug. The drug causes increase in appetite and body weight.

Glibenclamide is probably the most potent sulphonylurea derivative. Plasma glucose levels remain depressed for more than 15 h after a single dose. It is likely to cause hypoglycaemia. In addition to the actions described above, this drug seems also to stimulate insulin synthesis by a mechanism similar to glucose.

Biguanides

These lower blood sugar by complex mechanisms which may include (i) decreased glucose absorption from the gut, (ii) decreased

Fig. 23.6. Structures of some oral hypoglycaemic drugs.

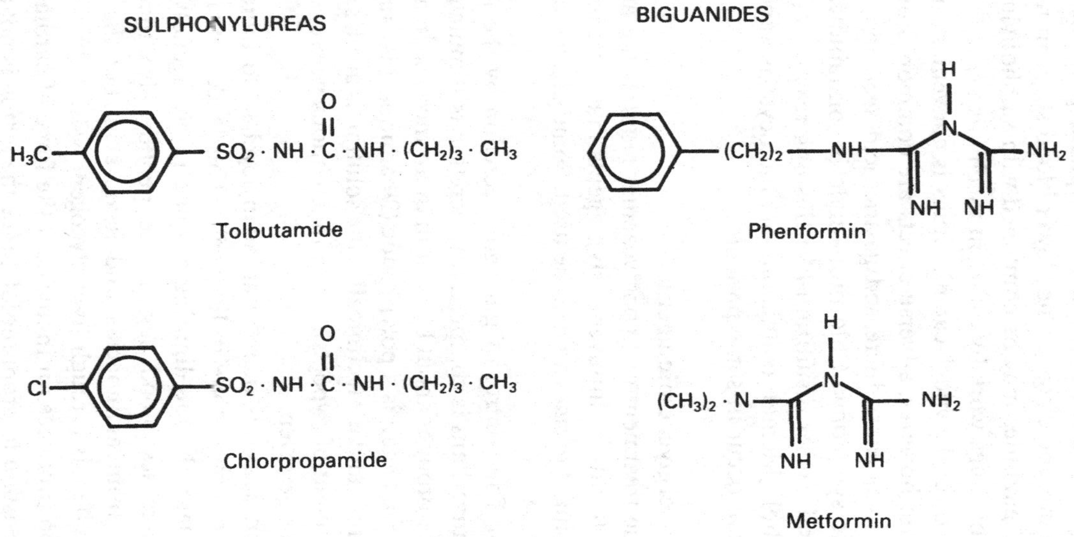

gluconeogenesis, and (iii) increased peripheral glucose utilisation. It is of interest that the drugs do not lower blood sugar in normal human subjects. Biguanides may be combined with sulphonylureas since the two types of drugs work by different mechanisms.

The use of oral hypoglycaemic drugs is convenient in comparison with insulin; however, adverse effects are common. For example the sulphonylureas cause increased gastric acid secretion, giving rise to ulcerogenic symptoms. Chlorpropamide is contraindicated in obese patients and causes disulfiram-like flushing reactions (see page 183) with alcohol. Mental confusion, agranulocytosis, and haemolytic anaemia can occur in some patients.

Hyperglycaemic agents

The treatment of hypoglycaemia requires the administration of glucose (orally or intravenously); agents that increase blood sugar by mobilising it *in situ* can also be used. Some of such agents are discussed below.

Glucagon The control of glucagon secretion by the A cells of the islets of Langerhans is complex; the secretion is stimulated by a fall in blood sugar brought about by insulin or an increase in aminoacids in the blood. Glucagon is a polypeptide (29 aminoacids) and is extracted from pancreas and used clinically (the solution is given s.c., i.m., or i.v.) in the treatment of hypoglycaemia in situations where oral or i.v. glucose cannot be given.

Glucagon activates membrane adenylcyclase to increase the concentration of cyclic AMP in liver cells. This leads to the activation of phosphorylase, the rate-limiting enzyme in glycogenolysis; glucagon thereby increases blood sugar. The peptide also increases gluconeogenesis from aminoacids and lactic acid, but the main hyperglycaemic effect is through liver glycogenolysis.

Glucagon produces an increase in the force of cardiac contraction which is resistant to propranolol. Since the action is not accompanied by dysrhythmias the drug has been used in the treatment of cardiogenic shock and congestive heart failure.

Diazoxide is chemically related to the thiazide diuretics; it was formerly developed for its antihypertensive action. It can increase blood sugar by several mechanisms: e.g. (i) release of adrenaline from the adrenal medulla; (ii) inhibition of the release of insulin; (iii) increase in the release of glucose from liver cells; and (iv) inhibition of peripheral glucose utilisation. The clinical indication for the use of diazoxide is in the treatment of hypoglycaemia due to insulin-producing tumors.

Alloxan This selectively destroys the B cells of the islets in the pancreas; it has been used extensively to produce insulin deficiency (diabetes) in laboratory animals for experimental purposes.

Streptozocin is an antibiotic produced by *Streptomyces*; it causes a highly specific and irreversible destruction of pancreatic B cells giving rise to permanent hyperglycaemia 24 h after a single dose of about 50 mg kg^{-1}. The drug has been tried in the treatment of hypoglycaemia due to insulin-producing tumors; its usefulness is limited by severe toxicity. It is an important experimental drug.

23.8 SEX HORMONES AND THE CONTROL OF FERTILITY

This section will assume previous familiarity with reproductive physiology and concentrate on the pharmacological actions of major sex hormones and the rationale for their therapeutic uses.

Gonadotrophic hormones (gonadotrophins)

The hormones secreted by the anterior pituitary which regulate ovarian and testicular (gonadal) functions are called gonadotrophic hormones. They are glycoproteins. Their secretion is under the control of the hypothalamus acting through the agency of specific gonadotrophin- releasing factors (Fig. 23.7.)

Follicle -stimulating hormone (FSH)

FSH stimulates the growth of the Graafian follicles and secretion of oestrogen in the female. In the male, FSH stimulates spermatogenesis.

Luteinising hormone (LH)

LH, also called interstitial cell-stimulating hormone (ICSH), stimulates ovulation in women. Secretion of LH reaches a peak at ovulation. In the male, LH stimulates the Leydig cells to produce testosterone while in the female, LH also stimulates the interstitial cells of the ovary to produce androgens and the corpus luteum to produce oestrogens and progesterone.

Human chorionic gonadotrophin (HCG)

HCG is secreted by the syncytiotrophoblasts of the placenta shortly after implantation of the blastocyst, to maintain the corpus luteum and stimulate it to produce oestrogen and progesterone. These hormones are necessary for the maintenance of pregnancy (they prevent menstruation and ovulation) until the foeto–placental unit can take over this function 6–8 weeks later. HCG in maternal blood is a major diagnostic confirmatory evidence of pregnancy even before the first missed period. Its presence in urine is routinely employed as evi-

Fig. 23.7. Hypothalamic releasing factors and their actions on anterior pituitary gland. The diagram also shows the actions of gonadotrophins released by the anterior pituitary on gonads and adrenal cortex (AC). HPT, hypothalamus; CRF, corticotrophin-releasing factor (causes anterior pituitary (AP) to release adreno-corticotrophic hormone (ACTH); FSHRF, follicle stimulating hormone-releasing factor; FSH, follicle stimulating hormone; GF, Graafian follicle; LHRF, luteinising hormone-releasing factor; LH, luteinising hormone; O, male Leydig cells and female interstitial ovarian cells; PRF, prolactin-releasing factor; B, breast.

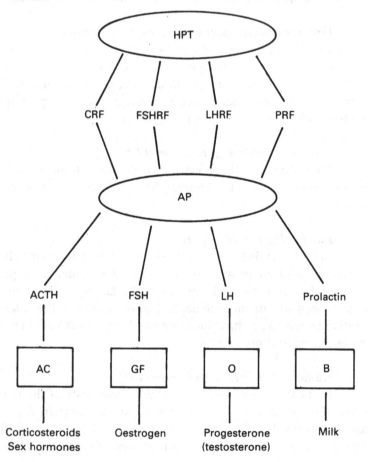

dence of pregnancy. HCG is extracted from the urine of pregnant women for clinical use (may be combined with FSH or clomiphene) to stimulate ovulation in women with amenorrhoea. Another gonadotrophin, human menopausal gonadotrophin (HMG) is present in the urine of menopausal women in whom diminished ovarian function results in reduced negative feedback on the hypothalamo–pituitary axis; the pituitary now secretes excess chorionic gonadotrophin. HMG is extracted for clinical uses similar to HCG.

Human placental lactogen (HPL)

HPL is another hormone secreted after ovulation. This is a polypeptide similar to growth hormone secreted by syncytiotrophoblast. Its level in plasma rises steadily to a plateau at term. It has lipolytic, lactogenic and growth promoting effects.

Prolactin (lactogenic hormone)

Prolactin is secreted by the anterior pituitary but unlike the gonadotrophins, its major site of action is the breast. Prolactin is the most active lactation-promoting substance known. It stimulates mammary gland maturity, and synthesis and secretion of milk constituents. The secretion of prolactin is under the control of the hypothalamus; there is evidence that the prolactin release-inhibiting hormone (found in the medium eminence) is dopamine. This explains why drugs which block dopamine receptors or reduce its concentration in the brain (e.g. chlorpromazine, haloperidol, benzodiazepines, and reserpine) can cause increase in prolactin secretion and galactorrhoea. On the other hand, prolactin release is inhibited by L-dopa, dopamine and dopamine-receptor agonists, e.g. bromocriptine (used in the treatment of Parkinson's disease). Bromocriptine can be used to control lactation *post partum* and in the treatment of galactorrhoea associated with high secretion of prolactin.

Ovarian hormones

These are mainly oestrogens and progestogens with small amounts of androgens. They play an important role in preparing the human reproductive tract for the reception of sperm and implantation of the fertilised ovum.

Oestrogens and *steroid hormones* produced by the ovarian follicle and after ovulation and during early pregnancy by the corpus luteum; later in pregnancy the foeto–placental unit takes over the production of oestrogens. The major oestrogen steroids produced by women are oestradiol, oestrone and oestriol; examples of synthetic oestrogens are stilboestrol and quinestrol. The main functions of oestrogens are to stimulate the development of the vagina, uterus, secondary sex characteristics, and general maturity of the female. Oestrogen preparations are used:

> In replacement therapy in patients with primary failure of development of ovaries, in menopause or castration.
>
> In osteoporosis for their anabolic action.
>
> With progestrogens (in the contraceptive pill) to suppress ovulation.
>
> To suppress excessive uterine bleeding due to endometrial hyperplasma, and in the treatment of cancers.

Important serious side effects are thrombophlebitis and cerebral and retinal thrombosis. Hence, they should be used with great care.

Progestogens

Progesterone is the most important progestogen in humans. It is synthesised in the ovary, testis and adrenal cortex from cholesterol, acetate and pregnenolone. Large amounts are also synthesised and released from the placenta during pregnancy. Progesterone decreases the sensitivity of the uterus to contractile agents. It plays a crucial role in pregnancy. Its production by the corpus luteum during the second half of the menstrual cycle and early pregnancy (if this occurs) and later from the placenta minimises the chances of accidental abortion. Secondly progesterone prevents ovulation by a negative feedback mechanism on the hypothalamus–pituitary system. This is to prevent a superfetation (a second conception). Prevention of ovulation is the main mechanism of action when progesterone is used with oestrogens in contraceptive pills; an additonal point is that progesterone renders the cervical mucus more acid and more viscid than normal and therefore harmful to spermatozoa.

The main clinical uses of progesterone are in contraception, ovarian hypofunction or in the treatment of osteoporosis of old age.

Testicular hormone

These are *steroid hormones* with androgen and anabolic activities. The testis produces spermatozoa and secretes testicular hormones. These activities are under the control of FSH secreted by the anterior pituitary. The most important androgen in man is testosterone. Important androgenic actions of testosterone are: normal development and maintenance of male sex characteristics e.g., penile and scrotal growth, appearance of pubic hair and beard, vocal cord changes, and virility.

Androgens are mainly used in replacement therapy in man with hypogonadism. When used in the treatment of male sterility, androgens are combined with HCG or HMG to achieve satisfactory spermatogenesis and testicular androgen production.

By its anabolic effects (nitrogen retention, increased protein synthesis), testosterone increases muscle mass; hence anabolic steroids are abused by athletes (weight lifters, wrestlers, discus and hammer throwers) to enhance muscle development and performance.

Anabolic steroids are used to treat osteoporosis in the elderly male, and oestrogen-dependent mammary carcinoma; and to improve lean meat weight in livestock. The problem with the latter use is that enough sex hormone may be retained in the animal produce (e.g. meat, milk) to cause unwanted effects in people who consume them.

An important toxic effect is cholestatic jaundice caused by derivatives of testosterone which have an alkyl substitution in the 17-position (see Fig. 23.8.). Note that testosterone itself and nandrolone are without an alkyl substitution in this position and lack this side effect.

Fig. 23.8. Structures of some androgens.

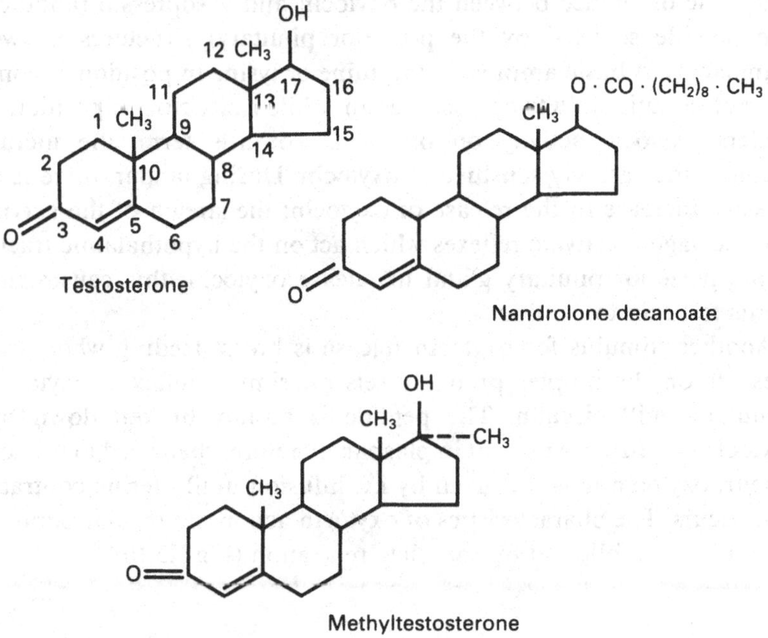

Testosterone

Nandrolone decanoate

Methyltestosterone

Drugs acting on the uterus

The activity of the uterine smooth muscle is controlled by the balance of female sex hormones (oestrogen and progesterone). Unlike most other smooth muscles, the influence of the autonomic nervous system on the uterus is negligible.

The organ is most sensitive to contractile agents when exposed to high plasma concentrations of oestrogen (oestrogen-dominated). When under the influence of progesterone on the other hand, uterine muscle tends to be unresponsive to contractile stimulation. Hence when the uterus needs to be actively contracting as in (i) menstruation to expel discarded endometrial layers, and (ii) labour to deliver the foetus and placenta, the levels of progesterone are low relative to those of oestrogen. Progesterone levels remain high throughout pregnancy until term when the sensitivity of the uterine muscle to contractile stimulants is at its highest.

Substances which contract uterine muscle

These are termed *oxytocic agents* due to the fact that a hormone, oxytocin, secreted by the posterior pituitary produces a powerful contraction of the uterus.

Oxytocin is a peptide with nine aminoacids (nonapeptide) in which two cystine residues form a bridge between positions 1 and 6 (see Fig. 23.9). The difference between the oxytocin and vasopressin (another nonapeptide secreted by the posterior pituitary) structures is two animoacids. A basic aminoacid (arginine or lysine in position 8) confers antidiuretic activity on vasopressin, while isoleucine in position 3 confers oxytocic activity on oxytocin. Towards term, the uterus becomes increasingly sensitive to oxytocin. During labour, there is a massive increase in the release of oxytocin; the stretch of the cervix and the vagina activate reflexes which act on the hypothalamic tracts to the posterior pituitary gland to release oxytocin; this causes the uterus to begin to contract.

Another stimulus for oxytocin release is breast feeding where the pressure on the nipples probably sets off similar reflexes; oxytocin stimulates milk-ejection. The peptide is rapidly broken down by oxytocinase enzymes present in plasma; therefore when used to induce labour, oxytocin must be given by i.v. infusion until uterine contraction occurs. The characteristics of oxytocin action are regular periods of contraction followed by complete relaxation (Fig. 23.10).

Ergometrine

This is an ergot alkaloid with a powerful oxytocic action. Another ergot alkaloid similar in structure is ergotamine. Both are derivatives of lysergic acid. These two compounds are probably responsible for the poisonous symptoms (ergotism, St. Anthony's fire) caused by the consumption of wheat contaminated by the fungus (*Claviceps purpurea*).

The characteristic response of the uterus to ergometrine is a sustained tonic spasm; this would be lethal to the foetus *in utero*. Therefore ergometrine is *not* used to induce labour but for the treatment of *post-partum* haemorrhage, when it is given orally, i.m. (with or without hyaluronidase), or i.v. In contrast, the main use of ergotamine is in the treatment of migraine, as it is a more powerful vasoconstrictor than ergometrine.

Mechanism of action of oxytocin

A prostaglandin may be the direct mediator of the action of oxytocin: (i) prostaglandins $F_{2\alpha}$ and E_2 are powerful oxytocic agents;

Fig. 23.9. Chemical structures of native peptides (oxytocin and vasopressin) secreted by the posterior pituitary, and their relative potencies as antidiuretic, vasopressor and oxytocic agents. Phe, phenylalanine; Leu, leucine; Ile, isoleucine; Arg, arginine.

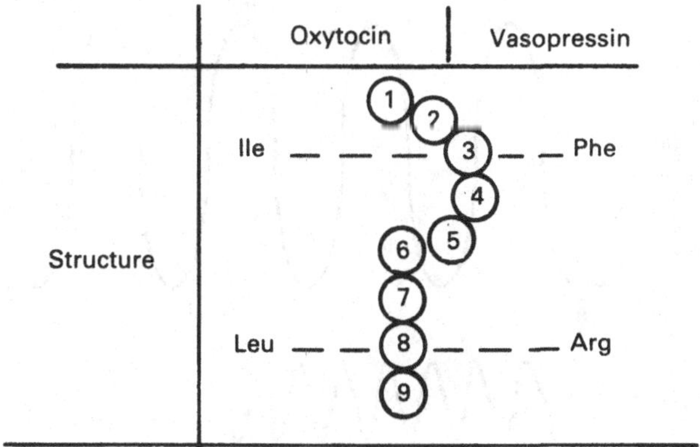

	Oxytocin	Vasopressin
Structure	Ile — — — — 3 — — Phe (residues 1, ?, 3, 4, 6, 5, 7, 8, 9) Leu — — 8 — — — Arg	
Relative activities		
Antidiuretic	1	100
Pressor	1	100
Oxytocic	100	1

(ii) the action of oxytocin on uterine muscle *in vitro* is reduced by cyclooxygenase inhibitors; and (iii) parturition is delayed in rats (and women) given aspirin during gestation.

Prostaglandins (PGF_{2a} and PGE_2) have been used in the treatment of therapeutic abortion usually after the first 12 weeks of pregnancy and for induction of labour. High doses are required with consequent numerous side effects. For induction of labour oxytocin is preferred, but if a prostaglandin is used, it may be injected directly into the amniotic sac.

Substances which relax uterine smooth muscle

The uterus is relaxed by beta-adrenoceptor agonists (beta-2). Salbutamol is used in the management of threatened abortion.

Family planning and control of fertility

It used to be said that family planning (a conscious effort to limit the number of children and to space the intervals at which they are born) is alien and unacceptable in traditional African societies. What is alien are the modern methods. Some traditional practices

Fig. 23.10. **Diagrammatic representation of patterns of uterine contractions induced by (a) oxytocin, and (b) ergometrine, administered at arrows.**

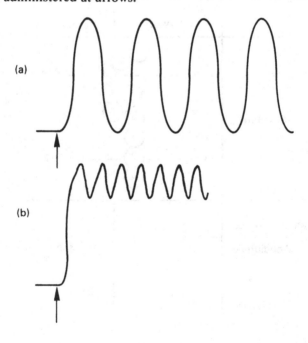

Table 23.4 *Oral contraceptives*

Composition of contraceptive	Mode of action	Remarks
Oestrogen and progestogen combination	(a) Prevention of ovulation. High concentrations of these in plasma exert a feedback inhibition on hypothalamo–pituitary axis to prevent release of FSH and LH. (b) Failure of implantation. The above gonadotrophin deficiencies lead to failure of maturation of the endometrium. Hence successful implantation cannot occur.	The oestrogen is usually ethinyloestradiol, and the progestogen is norethisterone. This is the most widely used form and known as the 'pill'. Side effects are common. The most serious of these are thromboembolism due to decreased antithrombin, increased platelet aggregation and a sustained rise in blood pressure. These are more common in older women or diabetics.
Progestogen	Prevention of passage of spermatozoa into the uterine cavity. When given throughout the menstrual cycle progestogen thickens the cervical mucus and makes it more acid and hostile to spermatozoa.	Can be taken orally (the minipill) or as a depot i.m. injection. Fewer side effects than the pill.
Oestrogen/ PGF_{2a}	Increased Fallopian tube activity. These substances cause increased Fallopian tube movements to expel a fertilised egg before implantation can occur.	This is the so-called *post coitus* contraceptive or 'morning after pill'. High doses are required, therefore toxic effects are prominent.

including taboos which forbade sexual intercourse for women while they breastfed, and breastfeeding itself (and this could go on for up to 3 years) were forms of birth control. Traditional lifestyles have been seriously affected by the pressures of modern living and baby milk formulae. So, improvements in the quality of life, reduction in infant mortality and high birth rates are pushing up populations in poor countries beyond the resources available for a reasonable standard of living. Therefore, the adoption of modern birth control methods has become imperative.

Conception can be prevented by restricting sexual intercourse to the *safe period*; the fertile period occurs around the time of ovulation which is usually midway in the menstrual cycle. This socalled *rhythm method* has a high failure rate and is unacceptable to couples who favour a spontaneous relationship. Modern reliable methods of reversible contraceptions employ mechanical barriers, e.g. condoms used by the male or sponge, diaphragms, cervical caps or intrauterine devices (IUD) inserted in the vagina. The aim of a mechanical barrier is to prevent the sperm from getting into contact with the ovum. Alternatively oral contraceptives are used (Table 23.4). The oral contraceptives presently in use are those which prevent conception by acting in the female. Others which reversibly inhibit spermatogenesis in the male are under investigation as alternatives to vasectomy.

24

Local hormones (autocoids)

24.1 INTRODUCTION

Several pharmacologically active substances are described as local hormones or autocoids because they are released/produced in response to a local stimulus and their effects are usually limited to the site of release/production. Examples are histamine, 5-hydroxytryptamine, substance P, bradykinin, prostaglandins, and slow-reacting substance of anaphylaxis (SRSA). The term *local hormone* or *autocoid* is useful in distinguishing this group of substances from hormones released by endocrine glands and which are carried in the bloodstream to act at distant sites. However, difficulties may arise with these terminologies. For one thing, there is increasing evidence that some of these substances, e.g. 5-HT, and histamine, may be neurotransmitters. For another, is a neurotransmitter by this definition a local hormone?

Our concern with these substances in this chapter is that they are thought to be involved in the local reactions which give rise to inflammation and allergic reactions such as asthma. The pharmacological properties of some local hormones are first described; this is followed by a description of the clinical conditions in which they are presumed to play a role; and then the mechanism of action of the drugs used in the treatment of these conditions are described.

24.2 HISTAMINE

Histamine is found in nearly all mammalian tissues. It is formed from the amino acid histidine by the enzyme histidine decarboxylase and deaminated by a diamine oxidase present in, e.g. the kidney, liver, and intestine (Fig. 24.1).

Histamine is stored in intracellular granules complexed to ATP and heparin, the concentrations of histamine being particularly high in mast cells and basophils. In the stored complexed form, histamine is inactive. Histamine is of clinical interest mainly because it can be liberated from storage to produce a variety of pharmacological actions. It can be liberated by organic bases, e.g. compound 48/80 and important drugs such as tubocurarine and morphine, and in allergic reactions, e.g. anaphylaxis and allergic asthma. Histamine is present in nervous tissue and in the brain.

Pharmacological actions of histamine
The actions of histamine are varied within and between species.

Smooth muscle
In general histamine contracts smooth muscles of the bronchioles in man and guinea-pigs. In horse and bovine lungs, the tracheal

Fig. 24.1. Biosynthesis and catabolism of histamine. The enzymes are: (a) L-histidine decarboxylase; (b) diamine oxidase; (c) N-methyl transferase. The major metabolite is N-methyl imidazole acetic acid.

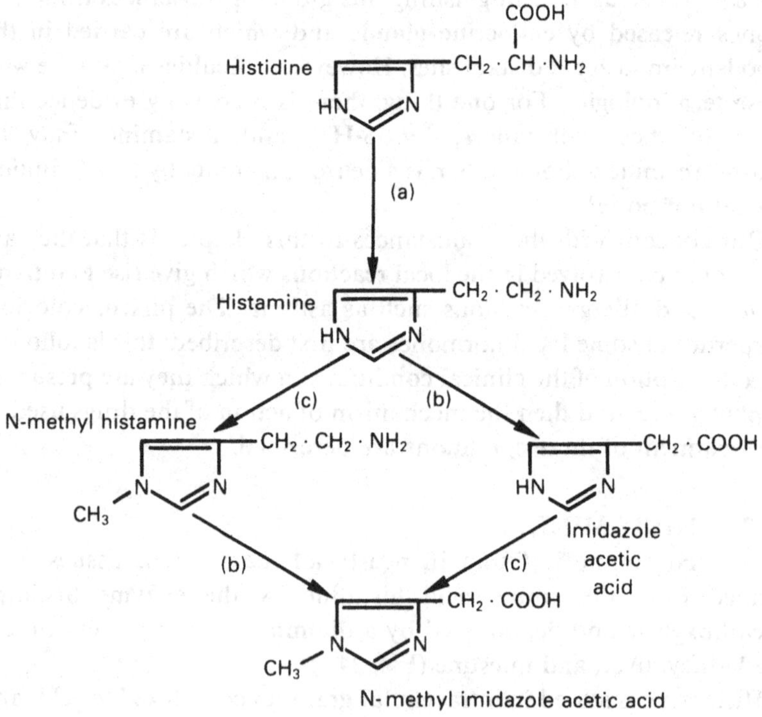

muscles are contracted, but the bronchioles are relaxed. Smooth muscles of the gastrointestinal tract are contracted in man and guinea-pigs, but rabbit and rat are insensitive.

Cardiovascular system

In general, histamine contracts large arteries and dilates arterioles. In man, i.v. injection of a small dose of histamine causes a sharp transient fall in blood pressure and an increase in heart rate and cardiac output. The cardiac action is a direct H_2-receptor mediated effect on the myocardium. In large doses the cardiovascular effect may include the actions of catecholamines released by histamine from the adrenal medulla. Histamine dilates capillaries and increases their permeability to plasma proteins. The capillary action of histamine is seen in the *Lewis triple response.* If histamine is injected intradermally in a light-coloured skin, a local *redness* is immediately produced (due to capillary dilatation) followed a little later by a *wheal* (a swelling due to leakage of plasma proteins into extravascular areas) and a *flare* (due to local axon reflex causing the release of an unknown vasodilator substance).

Gastric acid secretion

Histamine powerfully stimulates gastric acid secretion in all species. This effect is due to activation of H_2-receptors.

Pain

Histamine causes itching when applied to superficial layers of the skin (c.f. itching caused by insect bites; the insect venom releases histamine or may contain histamine). The nociceptive action of histamine is potentiated by ACH and prostaglandins.

Wound healing

Histidine decarboxylase activity (histamine-forming capacity, HFC) is much increased in wound and granulation tissue and subsides after healing. Histamine may aid healing by increasing local blood supply and capillary endothelial permeability.

24.3   5-HYDROXYTRYPTAMINE (5-HT)

5-HT occurs in serum (hence it is also known as serotonin). It is found in the gastrointestinal tract, CNS, blood platelets, and mast cells. 5-HT is formed from the aminoacid tryptophan by a decarboxylase enzyme closely related to dopa decarboxylase and is destroyed by monoamine oxidase (Fig. 24.2). The amount of tryptophan consumed, as for example in fruits such as bananas, plantains and pineapples, can influence the concentration of 5-HT in the brain because ordinarily, the enzyme tryptophan hydroxylase is only half saturated. For reasons which are not altogether obvious, a low protein, high carbohydrate meal, or starvation, exercise or stress, increase the level of 5-HT in the brain; whereas a high protein meal decreases it.

Fig. 24.2. Biosynthesis and catabolism of 5-hydroxytryptamine. The enzymes are: (a) tryptophan 5-hydroxylase; (b) aromatic L-amino acid decarboxylase; (c) monoamine oxidase; (d) aldehyde reductase; (e) aldehyde dehydrogenase.

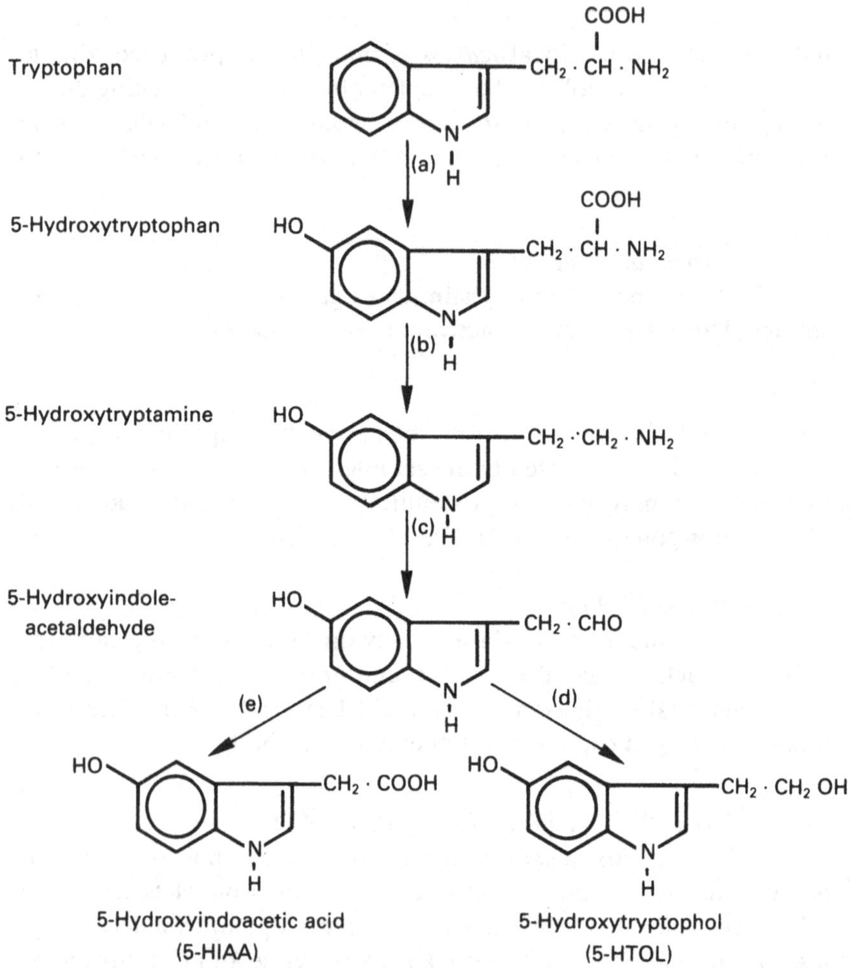

Tryptophan

5-Hydroxytryptophan

5-Hydroxytryptamine

5-Hydroxyindole-acetaldehyde

5-Hydroxyindoacetic acid
(5-HIAA)

5-Hydroxytryptophol
(5-HTOL)

5-HT receptors and pharmacological action

The pharmacological actions of 5-HT are complex which makes it difficult to assign physiological roles to the amine. Since its discovery in 1953, it has been described as a substance in search of a function. The role of 5-HT in some CNS functions is becoming clearer due to the identification of different receptors for different actions of the amine. Gaddum's original classifications of 5-HT receptors as D (smooth muscle stimulant action) and M (present on postganglionic parasympathetic nerves–stimulation causes ACH release) has now been superseded. At least three groups of receptors are now thought to mediate 5-HT effect; these are 5-HT$_1$, 5-HT$_2$, and 5-HT$_3$ receptors. The 5-HT$_1$ type are further subclassified into 5-HT$_{1_A}$, to 5-HT$_{1_D}$.

5-HT plays an important role in the brain in the control of basic functions such as appetite, sexual behaviour, mood, sleep, and temperature regulation. In the hypothalamus the levels of 5-HT fluctuate rhythmically with peaks in the afternoon and troughs at night.

Some receptors are associated with specific functions: 5-HT$_1$ receptors are found in the CNS and in peripheral structures. Their stimulation causes decreased or increased appetite (depends on the subclass of receptor), lowering of body temperature, hypotension and bradycardia. Changes in 5-HT$_1$ receptors are thought to be responsible for the abnormal eating behaviour seen in depression and anxiety. 5-HT$_2$ receptors are found in most parts of the brain (increased motor activity), in smooth muscle (contraction), and in blood platelets (aggregation). Ketanserin (a potent hypotensive) is a selective antagonist at 5-HT$_2$ receptors. 5-HT$_3$ receptors are found in the hypothalamus and in peripheral autonomic and sensory nerves. 5-HT is known to facilitate ganglion transmission and the peristaltic reflexes. In argentaffinoma (cancer of the gut in which large amounts of 5-HT are formed), the patient suffers from intestinal hypermotility and diarrhoea. These effects are presumably mediated by 5-HT$_3$ receptors.

The evidence linking 5-HT with various basic CNS functions is strong.

(1) On *mood*, LSD is a powerful hallucinogen as well as being structurally related to, and a specific antagonist of, 5-HT (see Fig. 20.4). MAO inhibitors prevent the metabolism of 5-HT. Imipramine type drugs inhibit 5-HT uptake into nerve terminals. These two effects increase the concentration of 5-HT at receptor sites and lead to the elevation of mood (see Chapter 20 for details).

(2) On *appetite*, 5-HT may activate different receptors to produce opposing effects. Fenfluramine releases 5-HT and decreases appetite.

Also 5-HT injected into the hypothalamus decreases appetite. Conversely, blocking 5-HT synthesis or 5-HT receptors (e.g. with cyproheptadine and methysergide) increases appetite.

(3) On *temperature regulation*, 5-HT may be involved in the normal hypothalamic control of body temperature. Substances such as reserpine which deplete the brain of 5-HT, lower body temperature; and experimental administration of 5-hydroxytryptophan increases brain 5-HT and causes fever; experimentally 5-HT is one of the most potent fever-producing substances known.

24.4   BRADYKININ

Bradykinin is a peptide consisting of nine aminoacid residues (a nonapeptide) and formed by enzyme action from the precursor bradykininogen present in serum. Another kinin, kallidin, found in saliva, is probably identical with bradykinin. The kinins have transient *in vivo* effects because they are rapidly inactivated by blood kininases. These peptides have been widely studied but their importance in disease and their physiological function remain elusive.

Pharmacological actions

Bradykinin causes vasodilatation and an increase in capillary permeability. It is also a powerful pain-producing substance when applied to blisters. These properties made bradykinin an important candidate for consideration as a mediator of inflammation at one time. Tella and Maegraith have shown that there is an increase in plasma kinin (as shown by a decrease in plasma kininogen) in monkeys infected with malaria. Similar increases in plasma kinin levels were observed by Goodwin in cattle and humans infected with trypanosoma. The role of plasma kinins in the pathophysiology of these parasitic diseases remains to be elucidated.

24.5   ENDOGENOUS PROSTANOIDS AND
LEUCOTRIENES

The essential fatty acid, arachidonic acid, is metabolised into pharmacologically active products through two main pathways, namely; the fatty acid cyclooxygenase, and 5-lipoxygenase pathways The products of the cyclooxygenase pathway include the stable prostaglandins and unstable biologically highly reactive intermediate metabolites such as prostacyclin and thromboxane-A. These are referred to as prostanoids to distinguish them from the products of 5-

lipoxygenase metabolism which are termed leucotrienes because they are released by leucocytes when the latter are activated by a variety of agents. Another fundamental difference between the prostanoids and the leucotrienes is that the latter are nitrogen- and sulphur containing structures, being products of conjugation reactions with glutathione (see Fig. 19.3).

Prostanoids

Prostanoids with interesting pharmacological activities are prostaglandins (e.g. PGE_2, PGF_{2_a}), prostacyclin (PGI_2), and thromboxane-A (TxA_2). The compounds are unsaturated fatty acids. The stable prostaglandins were first detected in seminal fluid and Von Enter so-named them because they were thought to be specific secretions of the prostate gland. Prostaglandins have been found in most animal tissues and even plants. The substances are not stored, but are formed and released in response to a variety of stimuli such as antigen–antibody reactions, irritants, tissue damage, and nerve stimulation. When released prostanoids produce a wide variety of pharmacological effects. Pharmacologically PGE_1 and PGE_2 can modulate NA and ACH release from autonomic nerves, but there is no firm evidence that prostaglandins play such a physiological role in nerve transmission. Their most interesting actions are local and relate to inflammation, body temperature regulation, and pain. These points have already been made in connection with antipyretic, anti-inflammatory and analgesic agents in Chapter 19.

Actions of PGI_2 and TxA_2 on blood coagulation

TxA_2 and PGI_2 are short-lived but have powerful biological activities. TxA_2 stimulates platelet aggregation. Its formation from endoperoxide is the major pathway in platelets; it is probably concerned physiologically in blood clotting. PGI_2 is the most potent anti-aggregatory agent known. It prevents platelets from clumping together and from adhering to the endothelium of blood vessels. It can disperse already aggregated platelets as well as being a powerful vasodilator. The formation of PGI_2 from endoperoxides by prostacyclin synthetase is the major pathway in blood vessels. Stable analogues of this prostanoid are being developed for clinical use in the treatment of thrombosis.

Two other approaches are being made to exploit the system for the prevention of thrombosis: (1) Specific thromboxane synthetase inhibitors, e.g. *dazoxiben*, are being studied which would prevent the formation of TxA_2. Dazoxiben specifically blocks the synthesis of this agent in man and also increases the synthesis of PGI_2. (2) The alternative approach is that platelet cyclooxygenase is more sensitive to blockade by aspirin than the vascular enzyme. A low dose of aspirin (40 mg) selectively inhibits the platelet enzyme to prevent TxA_2 synthesis without affecting PGI_2 production. Possibly, therefore, a small dose regimen of aspirin can be developed as a prophylactic for thrombotic diseases such as heart attack.

Reproduction

The sensitivity of the human uterine smooth muscle to the contractile effects of prostanoids (PGF_{2_a}) increases with advancing gestation. During labour contractions, large quantities of prostanoids are found in amniotic fluid, placenta, and umbilical circulation. These findings suggest that prostanoids are involved in the initiation of parturition. In rats administration of cyclooxygenase inhibitors during gestation delays parturition. Prostanoids have been tested for the induction of labour and in the control of fertility and used in therapeutic abortions with varying degrees of success

Inflammation

Most of the products of arachidonic acid metabolism are implicated in the pathophysiology of inflammation. The evidence is of the following type: (1) Prostanoids, e.g. PGE_1 and PGE_2, can produce the cardinal features of inflammation, that is, they increase capillary permeability, capillary dilation and fluid and protein exudation. PGE_s are also chemotactic, that is, they attract polymorphonuclear cells to a site of inflammation. (2) Prostaglandins occur in high concentrations at inflammatory sites, e.g. the sinovial fluid in rheumatoid arthritis. When the condition is treated with anti-inflammatory drugs which inhibit prostanoid formation, the condition subsides as the concentration of prostanoids at the inflammatory site decreases. (3) There is a positive correlation between the clinical effectiveness of many anti-inflammatory drugs of diverse chemical structure and their ability to inhibit cyclooxygenase. Anti-inflammatory compounds such as chloroquine and corticosteroids that do not inhibit cyclooxygenase also prevent the formation of prostanoids by inhibiting phospholipase A_2.

Pain and fever

Prostanoids are pain-producing substances. Pain in inflamed joints is due to prostaglandins which either stimulate pain receptors or sensitise pain receptors to the action of other pain-producing substances such as histamine, 5-HT or bradykinin. Feldberg has proposed that fever induced by bacterial toxins (pyrogens) is mediated by PGE_1 or PGE_2 whose concentration in the cerebrospinal fluid has been found to rise during fever and to fall when the fever subsides on treatment with cyclooxygenase inhibitors (e.g. aspirin).

Leucotrienes (SRSA)

Slow-reacting substance of anaphylaxis (SRSA) was the name given to smooth muscle stimulating substance(s) released along with histamine during anaphylactic reactions in guinea-pig and human lungs. It was pharmacologically characterised by its slow-developing but powerful sustained contraction of bronchiolar and other smooth muscles and its resistance to histamine H_1-receptor antagonists. Its possible importance in the bronchospasm of asthma which is largely unresponsive to antihistamines has been recognised for four decades. In the last ten years, it has been established that SRSA is formed from arachidonic acid by the action of 5-lipoxygenase and that the activity previously described as such is a mixture of the leucotrienes LTC_4, LTD_4 and LTE_4 (see Fig. 19.3). Allergen challenge of lung tissue from asthmatic patients elicits a bronchial contraction that is correlated with the amount of leucotrienes released.

Pharmacological properties of leucotrienes

The leucotrienes (C_4, D_4, and E_4) constrict guinea-pig and human airways with a potency that is several orders of magnitude higher than that of histamine. They seem to interact with a specific leucotriene receptor; they are active at nanomolar concentrations, and experimentally specific competitive leucotriene antagonists have been described. C_4 and D_4 evoke pulmonary mechanical changes which indicate that these compounds have preferential effects on peripheral rather than central airways in both guinea-pigs and humans. In humans C_4, D_4 and E_4 injected intradermally (1 nmol), produce a local wheal and a flare of prolonged duration. Leucotrienes are active on the microcirculation, but the effect varies between species and in the same species between different parts of the circulation. These properties suggest that the leucotrienes may be involved in both the mechanical and inflammatory mainfestations of the airways in allergic asthma.

24.6   HYPERSENSITIVITY REACTIONS

Hypersensitivity reactions are characteristically interactions between antigen and antibody. The term *allergy* is used to denote different forms of hypersensitivty in man.

Antigens are large molecular weight proteins or polysaccharides which can induce antibody formation; antigens are foreign to the organism. However, under certain pathological states, the organism may produce antibodies, and become sensitised, to its own proteins. This happens when disease changes the character of the tissue proteins, so that they are 'not self' (foreign) to the immunologically competent cells. Examples of such *autosensitisation* are seen with diseased thyroid and testes. Autosensitisation is thought to account for certain forms of *myaesthenia gravis* in which motor end plate ACH receptors are neutralised by antibody.

Drugs are small molecular weight substances and do not usually induce antibody formation, but some drugs do so after becoming complexed to plasma proteins. The antibody induced by the drug–protein complex reacts with the drug when the latter is subsequently administered, giving rise to a drug-induced hypersensitivity reaction. Examples of such drugs are aspirin and penicillin.

Antibodies are γ-globulins produced in response to antigenic stimulation. They are manufactured by immunologically competent cells found in the reticuloendothelial system (spleen, lymph node, bone marrow). The most striking property of an antibody is its specificity: the antibody manufactured in response to one antigen will react only with that particular antigen or, rarely, with a closely related antigen. Antibodies are of different immoglobulin types. Most human allergic reactions are mediated by IgE reaginic antibodies.

Types of hypersensitivity reactions

The location of the antibody is important for the type of reaction provoked when it comes in contact with antigen.

(i) The antibodies may circulate in plasma where, by reacting with antigen (e.g. virus, bacteria, or toxin), they provide immunity against the disease caused by the agent.

(ii) Antibodies may become attached (fixed) to cells and produce anaphylactic sensitisation (see below). There is species specificity in tissue sensitisation, e.g. γ-globulins (antibodies) from horse cannot sensitise guinea-pig tissues. But rabbit and guinea-pig antibodies will cross-sensitise.

(iii) Antibodies may become intimately integrated into lymphocyte membranes. Hypersensitivity evoked by the reaction of antigen with these cells is known as *cell-mediated hypersensitivity*. The prototype of this reaction is the *tuberculin* reaction.

(iv) Antigen–antibody complexes formed when antigen reacts with circulating antibodies may also provoke a hypersensitivity reaction. Examples are *serum sickness* and *Arthus reaction*. The response is provoked by a complement-dependent interaction of antigen–antibody complexes with cells.

Anaphylaxis

In pharmacology, anaphylaxis is the most widely studied hypersensitivity reaction: it is a useful model for research into allergic asthma and anaphylactic shock. The phenomenon can be demonstrated most dramatically in the guinea-pig: if a small dose of antigen, say egg albumen is injected into a guinea-pig, it produces no effect, but if a further dose of the same antigen is given i.v. three weeks later, the animal dies within a few seconds from asphyxia. The reaction can also be demonstrated in isolated strips of smooth muscle and isolated hearts. Ileal and uterine muscles taken from sensitised guinea-pigs contract powerfully when challenged with antigen (the Schultz-Dale response). Isolated hearts respond by increased rate and force of contraction. Desensitisation is characteristic of the anaphylactic reaction. If an animal survives a dose of antigen, it responds less or not at all if the same dose is administered shortly afterwards. Similarly, the same dose repeatedly applied to a sensitised isolated tissue gives successively diminishing responses. This phenomenon may be fundamentally similar to tachyphylaxis seen with indirectly acting sympathomimetic amines (p. 367), if it is assumed that mediators of the anaphylactic response are used up during repeated challenge with antigen; or it may be analogous to desensitisation at the receptor level, that is (i) the antibody is covalently bound to the cell-membrane, and (ii) it becomes temporarily inactivated after combining with antigen. This view is supported by observations made by Dale & Okpako (1969) that in isolated ileum and perfused lungs from guinea-pigs, the desensitised tissue can spontaneously regain its sensitivity after washing out the antigen. It is likely that when the antigen–antibody complex dissociates, the antibody is free to react with antigen again.

Mechanism of anaphylaxis

The anaphylactic response is mediated by pharmacologically active substances (histamine, SRSA) released from sensitised cells, e.g.

mast cells. The events leading to the release are complex but may involve the following well studied facets:

(i) Esterase enzymes are probably activated since release is temperature dependent and can be inhibited by a variety of enzyme inhibitors.

(ii) The release requires calcium. Certain substances known as calcium ionophores (e.g. A23187) which facilitate calcium entry also release mediators. Disodium cromoglycate used to treat asthma prevents the release of mediators apparently by blocking the entry of calcium into sensitised cells following antigen–antibody interaction.

(iii) Catecholamines, e.g. adrenaline, and isoprenaline, by activating the membrane enzyme adenylcyclase to increase intracellular cyclic AMP, can inhibit the release of mediators. This raises the point that beta-adrenoceptor agonists used in the treatment of asthma have at least two modes of action, namely, bronchodilation and blockade of mediator release.

Pharmacologically active substances released in anaphylaxis are histamine, SRSA (leucotrienes), prostanoids, and possibly kinins. The pharmacological properties of these substances have been described. Except for mild allergic asthma, drugs that block the bronchoconstrictor action of histamine (i.e., H_1-receptor antagonists) do not provide relief from asthma. This observation is usually taken to mean that histamine, though released in allergic asthma, is not the major bronchoconstrictor agent. In the past 50 years, much attention has focussed on SRSA (leucotrienes) as the possible mediator of asthmatic bronchospasm because of their powerful smooth muscle stimulant properties; these compounds also have pro-inflammatory actions, and it is now doubtful whether the respiratory distress in bronchial asthma is due entirely to simple bronchoconstriction. Inflammation of the bronchial mucosa may well be an important contributory factor. In that case, actions of the various putative mediators including histamine (dilates pulmonary vessels by an H_2-receptor effect) will have to be evaluated.

24.7   HISTAMINE RECEPTOR ANTAGONISTS

Histamine receptor antagonists were discovered in 1948. Some structures are shown in Fig. 24.3. Many of these compounds have the general structure R—X—C—C—N. The R nucleus may be one or more aromatic or heterocyclic groups. The component X may be (a) nitrogen as in mepyramine and promethazine, (b) oxygen as in diphenhydramine, or (c) carbon as in chlorpheniramine.

These drugs are competitive and specific antagonists of histamine in low doses. They are better referred to as *histamine receptor antagonists*, rather than as antihistamines which may include drugs such as adrenaline that can prevent some actions of histamine by *physiological antagonism*. The drugs antagonise the following actions of histamine:

   (i) Contractions of smooth muscles of bronchioles, intestine, stomach, and uterus.

   (ii) Vasoconstrictor actions of histamine on blood vessels (hypotensive actions are only partially blocked).

   (iii) Increased capillary permeability.

Some other actions of histamine are not antagonised by this group of drugs. These actions are described in (a)–(c) below. (a) Gastric acid

Fig. 24.3. Structures of some histamine H$_1$-receptor antagonists.

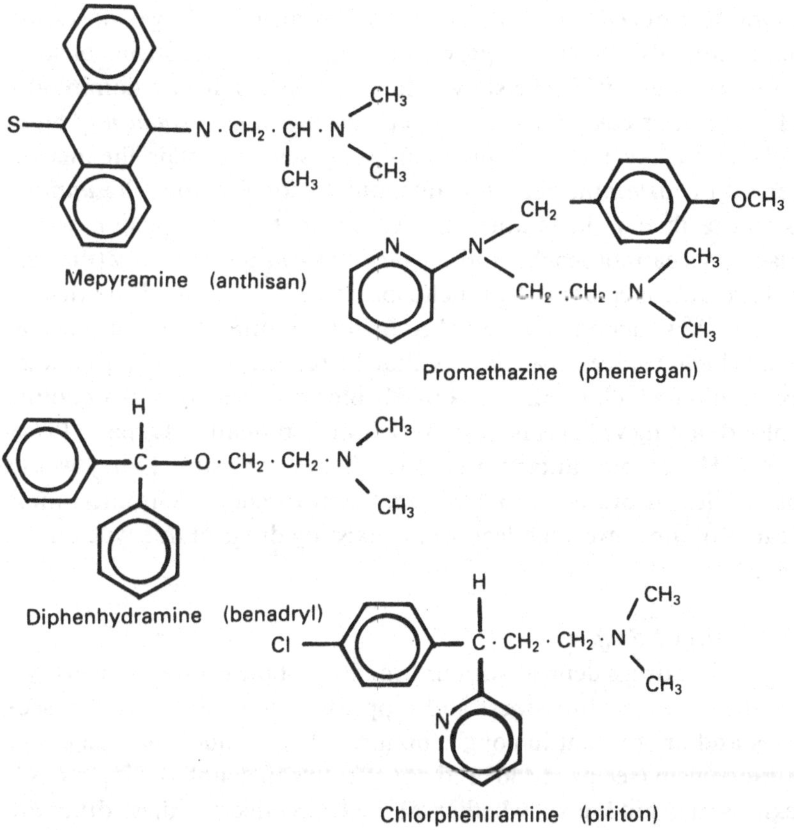

Mepyramine (anthisan)

Promethazine (phenergan)

Diphenhydramine (benadryl)

Chlorpheniramine (piriton)

secretion. This is the basis of the *augmented Kay's test* for achlorhydria in pernicious anaemia. A large dose of histamine is given to test the hydrochloric acid secretory activity of the stomach. Mepyramine is first given to protect the patient from the bronchoconstrictor effect of histamine. (b) Increased rate and force of cardiac contraction. (c) Relaxant effects of histamine on certain smooth muscles, e.g. bronchioles of certain species (sheep), and pulmonary vasculature (guinea-pig and man). Ash and Schild showed in 1966 that the mepyramine-sensitive actions of histamine were mediated via a homogeneous population of receptors (H_1-receptors) different from those which mediated the mepyramine-resistant actions; the latter were subsequently called *H_2-receptors* by Black who first discovered in 1972 that they could be specifically blocked by burimamide (see pp. 105, 106, for references).

Actions of H_1-receptor antagonists
(i) *Anaphylaxis and asthma*
Although low doses of H_1-receptor antagonists can prevent histamine-induced bronchoconstriction, even much larger doses are only minimally effective in preventing anaphylactic bronchoconstriction even though it can be shown that the effect is due predominantly to histamine release. *The drugs are not effective in the treatment of bronchial asthma.* Several mechanisms are suggested to explain the ineffectiveness of histamine receptor antagonists; for example, the *intrinsic* histamine theory (histamine is released at its site of action which antagonists cannot reach), and the *alternative mediator* theory (that the predominant mediator of bronchospasm in asthma is SRSA (leucotrienes) whose action is not blocked by mepyramine). Another mechanism which I have advocated is that histamine-induced pulmonary vasodilation which is enhanced by H_1-blockers may lead to a pooling of blood in lung vessels and so reduce lung compliance (Okpako,1972). Even if H_1-receptor antagonists were effective in asthma, they would not be ideal drugs to use in the treatment of such a chronic illness because of the powerful effects of the existing drugs of this type on the CNS.

(ii) *CNS effects*
The drugs depress various functions of the central nervous system; they produce drowsiness and suppress cough and are used as sedatives and are present in cough mixtures. They reduce the tremors of Parkinsonism (see page 446) and are effective in counteracting motion sickness. It is not known whether all the CNS effects of these drugs are

due to H_1-receptor blockade. Their potencies in producing CNS effects, e.g. drowsiness with diphenhydramine, do not always correlate with their receptor-blocking potencies. Such a comparison may be inappropriate; variation in lipid solubility and hence pharmacokinetic factors can account for variability in CNS action as much as receptor-blocking potencies. Also several H_1 antagonists in use have local anaesthetic, atropine-like and quinidine-like actions.

Uses

(i) *Allergic disorders,*

notably urticaria, atopic dermatitis, allergic rhinitis and hay fever.

(ii) *Cough,*

especially unproductive cough in children, as elixir and syrup. Sedation is probably an important aspect of their action. In productive cough the benefit is offset since under the influence of these drugs, the mucous secreted is viscid and more difficult to expectorate.

(iii) *Motion sickness.*

Cyclizine, promethazine and chlorcyclizine are extensively used. "Antihistamines" are sold for this more than for any other purpose. The mechanism of action is unknown but the action is CNS in origin and involves the vestibular apparatus and chemoreceptor triggerzone.

The major side effects are CNS effects – drowsiness, lassitude, blurred vision, all of which can interfere with the patient's ability to manipulate complicated machinery such as driving a car or motorcycle.

Actions of H_2-receptors antagonists
Gastric acid secretion

Histamine has long been known as a powerful stimulant of gastric acid secretion and because of its presence in the gut lining, histamine is thought to be involved in the physiological control of acid secretion in the stomach. The H_2-receptor antagonists which block histamine-evoked acid secretion are now powerful tools in the study of the role of histamine in gastric acid secretion. Research has now shown that H_2 antagonists can prevent acid secretion induced not only by histamine and histamine analogues but also that induced by gastrin, pentagastrin, insulin, and a protein-containing meal in rat, cat, dog, guinea-pig, and man. Basal acid secretion is also reduced in man by H₂-blockers. The *in vivo* action of the drugs is not an indirect one via the decrease they cause in mucosal blood flow (acid secretion is dependent on mucosal blood flow), but a direct one. Hormone-stimulated acid secretion in isolated mucosal preparations of several species is specifically prevented by H₂-blockers. Acid secretion by vagal stimulation or by carbachol is not affected by H₂ antagonists. These data point to the likelihood that histamine is the final mediator of acid secretion evoked by a variety of hormonal stimuli.

Structure–Activity relationships

The structure of some H₂-blockers are shown in Fig. 24.4. The compounds are derived from the histamine molecule with a substantial increase in the length of the side chain. Burimamide was the first of the H₂-blockers to be studied extensively in animal and human experiments. Its clinical usefulness was limited by poor absorption after oral administration. Metiamide was better absorbed, more potent and more selective as an H₂-blocker than burimamide, but the drug was abandoned because it caused agranulocytosis; this was associated with the thiourea moeity. In cimetidine, the drug now marketed by Smith, Kline & French as targamet, the thiourea group is replaced by cyanoguanidine; no cases of agranulocytosis have been reported with cimetidine. A similar drug is ranitidine.

Uses

The only indication for the clinical use of H₂-blockers is in the treatment of peptic ulcer (both gastric and duodenal). They reduce gastric acid secretion in ulcer patients and induce the healing of the ulcer as effectively as vagotomy. A point to note: histamine by stimulating H₂-receptors increases intracellular cyclic AMP, thereby reducing the release of histamine and other mediators in allergic reactions. Histamine may thus modulate its own release and blockade of H₂-receptors could thus enhance the severity of certain allergic reactions. H₂-blockers have also been shown to enhance histamine contraction of guinea-pig bronchial muscle and anaphylaxis in human lungs. These drugs are thus potentially capable of exacerbating bronchospasm in asthmatics. Watch out!

Drug treatment of bronchial asthma

Bronchial asthma is characterised by an increase in airways resistance due to three main factors: (i) bronchoconstriction, (ii)

Fig. 24.4. Structures of some histamine H₂-receptor antagonists.

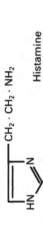

Histamine

CH₂ · CH₂ · NH₂

Cimetidine

CH₂ · S · CH₂ · CH₂ · NH · C · NH · CH₃
‖
NCN

Burimamide

CH₂ · CH₂ · CH₂ · NH · C · NH · CH₃
‖
S

Famotidine

NSONH₂
‖
S · CH₂ · CH₂ · C
                  |
                  NH₂

C = N
/
H₂N
\
H₂N

Ranitidine

CH₂ · S · CH₂ · CH₂ · NH · C
                             ‖
                             CH · NO₂
                             |
                             NH · CH₃

(CH₃)₂N-CH₂

oedema of the bronchial mucosa, and (iii) increase in bronchial secretions. The immediate cause of asthmatic bronchospasm is probably the release of endogenous bronchoconstrictors (histamine and leucotrienes). Specific antagonists for all the endogenous bronchoconstrictors are not available. Therefore the most important drugs used in the treatment of asthma are those which either physiologically antagonise the bronchoconstrictors (bronchodilators) or prevent their release.

Bronchodilators

Many of the bronchodilators used in the treatment of asthma are sympathomimetic beta-adrenoceptor agonists.

Adrenaline

In acute asthmatic attack or anaphylactic bronchoconstriction, adrenaline is given by subcutaneous injection or by inhalation. In anaphylactic shock, adrenaline relieves the respiratory distress, restores the fallen blood pressure, and relieves the congestion in the upper respiratory tract.

Ephedrine

Is an indirectly acting sympathomimetic amine of natural origin with effective bronchodilator action (see page 345).

Isoprenaline

Is a potent bronchodilator; it stimulates both bronchiolar (beta$_2$) and cardiac (beta$_1$) adrenoceptors. Isoprenaline must never be given by intravenous injection because of its powerful action on the heart. It is inactive by mouth because of extensive first-pass metabolism. Sublingual and rectal routes can be used, but the most popular method of administration is aerosol inhalation.

The most serious drawback is isoprenaline toxicity on the heart. Asthmatics tend to inhale excessive amounts of isoprenaline so that sufficient is absorbed into the circulation to cause serious cardiac arrhythmias. Tolerance develops to inhaled isoprenaline because (i) repeated exposure of bronchial muscle to the drug increases its sensitivity to bronchoconstrictor agents, e.g. histamine; and (ii) the COMT metabolite, methoxyisoprenaline has beta-adrenoceptor blocking actions. As a result of this tolerance the patient inhales increasing amounts with consequent toxicity to cardiac muscle.

Orciprenaline
Resembles isoprenaline in structure but because the two phenolic hydroxy groups are *meta* rather than *ortho* to each other, the compound is not a substrate for CMT; it is active after oral administration. Orciprenaline stimulates both beta₁ and beta₂ adrenoceptors.

Selective beta₂ stimulants
There is a large number of these. Examples are isoetharine, salbutamol, terbutaline, and carbuterol. Most of the compounds resist uptake₂ and COMT metabolism. Consequently they have a longer duration of action than isoprenaline and adrenaline and are active orally. The major advantage of these drugs is their relative lack of cardiotoxicity.

Their commonest unwanted effect is muscle tremor, particularly of the hands. Salbutamol produces this effect in up to 35% of patients. The tremor is a beta₂-adrenoceptor effect. One aim of present ongoing research is to develop drugs with high afinity for bronchial, and low affinity for skeletal muscle, beta₂ adrenoceptors.

Nucleotide phosphodiesterase inhibitors
The mediator of bronchodilation caused by the sympathomimetic amines is cyclic 3′5-adenosine monophosphate (cyclic 3′5-AMP or cyclic AMP). Cyclic AMP causes hyperpolarisation and relaxation of bronchial smooth muscle (see Fig. 16.7). This nucleotide is rapidly converted to the inactive 5-AMP by a phosphodiesterase. Inhibitors of this enzyme cause cyclic AMP to accumulate in the cell and cause bronchodilation. Examples are methylxanthines, e.g. caffeine and theophylline.

Aminophylline is a complex of theophylline and ethylene diamine (inert but solubilises theophylline). Aminophylline is given by a slow i.v. injection in the treatment of chronic severe asthma and status asthmaticus. It is effective in patients refractory to sympathomimetic bronchodilators.

Disodium cromoglycate (INTAL)
This drug has a unique mode of action: it is not a bronchodilator, it does not prevent antigen–antibody reaction, nor does it directly block the action of released bronchoconstrictors. The most likely mechanism is that it prevents the release of mediators by preventing calcium entry and utilisation.

Corticosteroids, e.g. hydrocortisone, prednisolone

These are life saving in status asthmaticus or severe chronic asthma that cannot be controlled by other treatment. They are given by i.v. infusions (see Chapter 23 for further details).

New ideas on asthma

Some recent evidence suggests that asthma is not a disease caused simply by the narrowing of the airways. Inflammation and oedema are now thought to be major factors and the mechanism of action of drugs should be viewed from these standpoints.

The mechanism of action of corticosteroids is still largely unknown, but their therapeutic efficacy in asthma is most probably due to an anti-inflammatory activity which involves the inhibition of phospholipase A_2. (Nonsteroidal anti-inflammatory drugs such as aspirin are contraindicated in asthma partly because by blocking fatty acid cyclooxygenase, the substrate, arachidonic acid, is diverted to the 5-lipoxygenase pathway with consequent enhanced formation of bronchoconstrictor leucotrienes).

The beta-2 agonists do more than dilate bronchioles. There is now evidence that salbutamol (a) is antioedematic by promoting fluid reabsorption, (b) blocks mediator release, (c) reduces ciliary movement, (d) loosens sputum and (e) increases surfactant release.

The therapeutic value 'of the xanthines is probably not due to bronchodilation and almost certainly not due to inhibition of nucleotide phosphodiesterase. A new xanthine drug, *enprofylline* is a more effective antiasthmatic with few extrapulmonary side effects (e.g. CNS diuresis, cardiac) than theophylline; it is a weak inhibitor of phosphodiesterase, but it has strong anti-inflammatory activity.

In asthma the airways lose their endothelium leading to increased sensitivity to spasmogens. The loss of endothelium exposes sensory receptors to external stimuli which may activate a local axon reflex. Sodium cromoglycate may inhibit such a reflex thought to be mediated by substance P. The new idea does not attribute the action of cromoglycate to mast cell membrane stabilisation as other more potent membrane stabilisers are not anti-asthmatic.

FURTHER READING

Bradley, P.B., Engel, G., Feniuk, W., Fozard, J.R., Humphrey, P.P.A., Midllemiss, D.N., Myelacharane, E.J., Richardson, B.P. & Saxena, P.R. (1986). Proposals for the classification of and nomenclature of functional receptors for 5-hydroxytryptamine. *Neuropharmacol.*, **25**, 563–576.

Dale, M.M. &Okpako, D.T. (1969). Recovery of anaphylactic sensitivity in the guinea-pic ileum after desensitisation. *Immunology*, 17, 653–663.

Flower, R.J. (1988). Lipocortin and the mechanism of action of the glucocorticoids (XI Gaddam memorial lecture). *Br. J. Pharmacol.* 94, 987–1015.

Okpako, D.T. (1972). A dual action of histamine on guinea-pig lung vessels. *Br. J. Pharmacol.*, 44, 311–321.

Tella, A. & Maegraith, B.G. (1966). Studies on bradykinin and bradykininogen in malaria. *Ann. Trop. Med. Parasitol.*, 60, 304–317.

Index